The Cambridge Medical Ethics Workbook

Second Edition

The Cambridge Medical Ethics Workbook

Second Edition

Donna Dickenson

Richard Huxtable

Michael Parker

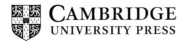

CAMBRIDGE
UNIVERSITY PRESS

CAMBRIDGE UNIVERSITY PRESS
Cambridge, New York, Melbourne, Madrid, Cape Town, Singapore,
São Paulo, Delhi, Dubai, Tokyo, Mexico City

Cambridge University Press
The Edinburgh Building, Cambridge CB2 8RU, UK

Published in the United States of America by Cambridge University Press, New York

www.cambridge.org
Information on this title: www.cambridge.org/9780521734707

First edition © Cambridge University Press 2001
Second edition © D. Dickenson, R. Huxtable and M. Parker 2010

First edition published 2001
Second edition published 2010

Printed in the United Kingdom at the University Press, Cambridge

A catalogue record for this publication is available from the British Library

ISBN 978-0-521-73470-7 Paperback

Contents

Contents

Cases

Papers

All papers are reproduced with permission.

Preface to the second edition

Why call this book a 'workbook'? Isn't it more than that? In length and coverage alone, this is a full-fledged textbook, not what might seem a mere auxiliary teaching item. We are all experienced teachers of medical ethics and law, and this book embodies the pedagogic methods and strategies in which we believe. And while we are committed above all else to helping readers make up their own minds, we also have our own positions on the issues we raise, along with our own 'take' on the theoretical underpinnings of medical ethics. It is fair to say that we are much less utilitarian in our approach than the dominant trend in British bioethics, for example. So aren't we selling ourselves and the book short by trivializing it with the title of 'workbook'?

What might seem a pedantic issue of nomenclature has preoccupied the authors since we began planning for a second edition of the *Cambridge Medical Ethics Workbook* as long ago as 2004. At least one reviewer of the first edition made the point we set out above, which provoked us into some very profitable discussions about our overall purpose, going well beyond the title issue. In the end we chose to retain the original name, on the principle that the book has enjoyed a very favourable reception under that title; but here at the start of the second edition, we want to point out that our ambitions and the book's 'mission' are considerably broader than the title 'workbook' may imply to some readers.

We have tried to provide an innovative method of learning and teaching medical ethics and law from the 'bottom-up', beginning with actual cases and challenging readers to develop their own analysis and recommendations. Medical and nursing educators have praised the first edition because it felt 'real', but as with 'realistic' fiction, it takes some doing to create that effect. We are aware that we have not always succeeded, but we strongly feel that the attempt is worth making. For many years the dominant trend in medical ethics education was 'principlist' or 'top-down', with a number of overarching deductive

principles introduced to the reader and then applied to particular cases. Our approach is 'bottom-up', presenting cases – taken in many instances from real-life clinical examples, with adjustments for confidentiality – and working with the reader to derive from them maxims or principles that can apply more generally. For the philosophically minded, our approach is more inductive and empirical: less like the Cartesian method than like Aristotle's method of *phronesis* or case elucidation. Two of us are in fact philosophers by training, one a lawyer, although we have all taught for many years in medical schools and collaborated with clinicians as research partners. All three of us view our book as no less theoretically weighty than the more dominant strand of principlism, but as an alternative – one which, in the Quaker phrase, 'speaks to the condition' of healthcare professionals.

We do present the major ethical schools of deontology, utilitarianism, feminism, communitarianism and virtue ethics – particularly in the final chapter, where we examine the philosophical and legal basis of the key concept of autonomy, along with challenges to the previous dominance of this concept in Anglo-American bioethics. Here the theoretical depth of the book – its claim to be more than just a 'workbook' – is most apparent, as we elucidate the importance of autonomy in medical ethics but also present alternatives to its dominance from European law and other conceptual models. Michael Parker's article in that chapter, 'A deliberative approach to bioethics', can be read as an example of the way in which the workbook as a whole moves carefully from practical matters to critical analysis of key ethical concepts such as rights and community.

While it was widely praised for being consciously practice-oriented, distinguishing itself from the top-down principlist approach, the previous workbook did embody a theoretical perspective based on respect for everyday ethics, experience, relationships and narratives. We have tried to avoid the use of the clever hypothetical cases beloved of moral philosophers, in favour of common situations that may not even appear at first glance to raise moral issues. Why our 'moral antennae' pick up certain situations as ethical dilemmas and ignore others is itself a question worthy of ethical analysis.

At the same time, 'workbook' still seems an appropriate title: we are committed to challenging readers to 'work through' their own initial responses and thoughts on the profound questions this book raises. The addition of an entirely new component, the CD-ROM of six case studies, demonstrates that process. After watching an initial clip setting out an ethical dilemma from the areas of genetics, reproductive medicine or research, readers are asked what they would have done in the situation. They are then directed down one of two or more branching paths, given further information and asked whether it would make them change their minds, and finally presented with the likely outcome of their decision. At the end they are asked to reconsider or justify their original choice in the light of the further information and consequences. So we also stand by our statement in the introduction to the first edition that 'this is very much a workbook', and we have devised new ways of working for and with the reader in this second edition.

Acknowledgements

The former BBC producer Alison Tucker, who scripted and directed the video sections for the CD-ROM, lived to see the CD-ROM produced as a separate entity but died before it came out as an integrated component of this workbook. She was the most professional colleague and most imaginative collaborator any author could wish for. Professor Heather Widdows and Dr David Lloyd developed the structure of the CD-ROM, the extensive glossary and the teaching strategy associated with it, working along with Donna Dickenson. We owe deep gratitude to all of them.

Nick Dunton, Nisha Doshi and Jane Seakins of Cambridge University Press have seen this project through a number of difficult stages, with calm and encouragement. We hope they are as pleased as we are that it has come to fruition.

Ron Berghmans of the University of Maastricht deserves special thanks not only for expanding his original contributions to Chapter 1 on death and dying, but also for volunteering a personal account of his own serious illness. Our thanks to him for his courage. Other contributors are listed under individual chapter headings. The use of their articles, many written especially for this edition, has allowed us to create a book with many different 'voices', many more sonorous than our own, all in what we hope is close harmony.

Richard Huxtable would like also to thank Genevieve Liveley for her encouragement, plus his colleagues and students for their support for – and input (both explicit and implicit) into – the book, which he dedicates to his Nan, Alma Huxtable.

Donna Dickenson would like to dedicate this book to Elsie Vernon Hart, who is herself a case study in courage, endurance and laughter.

Preface to the first edition

The *Cambridge Medical Ethics Workbook* is a practical, case-based introduction to medical ethics for anyone who is interested in finding out more about and reflecting on the ethical issues raised by modern medicine. It is designed to be flexible; suitable both to be read in its own right and also for use as a set text in group teaching or in open learning. It is aimed at the interested general reader, at practising healthcare professionals and at medical and nursing students studying ethics for the first time.

The workbook is able to be flexible in this way because it is based around the reading of and reflection upon real cases. It uses a variety of structured activities to introduce and to explore the major ethical issues facing medicine today. These activities are clustered around: (a) *cases* (which were provided by healthcare professionals from many countries); (b) *commentaries* on those cases by healthcare professionals, ethicists, lawyers and so on; and (c) *short papers* by experts in the area concerned. This is very much a *workbook*, designed to help readers think about, reflect upon and to work their own way through ethical problems, by deliberating on the issues raised by them either alone or together with others. In this way, the reader is guided through the core themes in medical ethics in a way which is appropriate for them and which is relevant to their own experience.

While a glance at the workbook's contents page shows that it covers most of the major themes in medical ethics, it does not aim to provide in itself a comprehensive survey of every issue. Our aim is rather, through the active and structured exploration of core themes and key cases, to develop skills of independent study and research in ethics. This is an increasingly important requirement of healthcare professionals. For a measure of good practice in medicine today is increasingly coming to be seen to be the extent to which such practice is 'evidence-based'. An understanding of the ethical issues involved and of the way to balance and assess the validity of ethical arguments in relation to particular cases is a core skill in the development of an analytical approach to medicine. Good quality healthcare is ethical healthcare and a consideration of the ethical dimensions of decision-making in healthcare practice must form a cornerstone of good evidence-based practice. This workbook helps practitioners and students to develop these skills and to have confidence in their use, not only in the context of research but also of teamwork within clinical practice.

Medical ethics is increasingly coming to be seen as an essential element of the education of any healthcare professional (GMC, 1993) and this is increasingly reflected in the medical and nursing schools themselves. Recently teachers of medical ethics in UK medical schools published a joint statement on the core themes and topics which ought to form the basis of any ethics curriculum (Consensus statement by teachers of medical ethics and law in UK medical schools, 1998). Similar work is also currently being done by the Association of Teachers of Ethics in Australasian Medical Schools and developments are also proceeding apace in other countries. Whilst recognizing these developments and being to some extent a reflection of them, this workbook does not follow any of these curricula rigidly. (We do however provide a useful grid in appendix two, showing how the UK national core curriculum maps onto the chapters and subtopics of this workbook.)[1] This workbook is intended to be a flexible educational resource which will enable those who teach medical ethics in any of these or any other educational setting to explore the core themes and issues in the ethics of medicine using cases and activities which will resonate with and be engaging for both medical and nursing students and those healthcare professionals who wish to develop their skills in this area. We would encourage teachers of medical ethics to pick and choose cases, activities and themes from the workbook in order to construct courses, workshops or training days appropriate to those they are teaching. The workbook is intended to be both a coherent approach to medical ethics and also a toolkit of resources for teachers and lecturers.

The workbook is divided into three parts.[2] In part one we explore some key ethical themes arising as a result of recent and ongoing technological developments in medicine. The first chapter is on ethical decisions at the end of life and explores ethical issues relating to the withholding and withdrawing of life-prolonging treatment and other ethical issues at the end of life. The chapter's focus is the extent to which the application of modern medicine at the end of life demands a reconsideration of the goals of medicine itself. When healing is no longer possible what ought to be the goals of medicine and of the healthcare professional? The second chapter in part one looks at the ethical issues raised by genetic testing and by the use of genetic information in clinical practice. The third chapter investigates the ethical implications of developments in reproductive technology. The fourth looks at the ethics of medical research itself and investigates the extent to which the research which is driving advances in medicine itself raises ethical issues – for those who organize and fund such research, for those clinicians who enrol their patients in research and for those of us who participate as research subjects.

In part two of the workbook we look more specifically at four themes which permeate medical ethics: vulnerability, truth-telling, competence and confidentiality. We do so by looking at the ethical issues raised by medicine and healthcare with three particularly vulnerable groups of patients. In keeping with the UK national curriculum in medical ethics, we also consider the vulnerabilities of clinicians. In chapter five we investigate the ethical issues that arise in long term and daily care. In chapter six we look at the ethics of mental health and of the treatment of psychiatric patients. And in chapter seven our attention turns to the ethics of work with children and young people. In each case the key issues are competence, vulnerability, truth-telling and confidentiality.

In part three of the workbook we explore some of the generic ethical issues relating to healthcare. In chapter eight, still by means of real cases, we investigate the ethical issues relating to the allocation of healthcare resources, questions of priority setting and just distribution. It hardly needs saying that these issues are increasingly important in all healthcare systems and across all clinical specialties. Finally, in chapter nine we reflect on a theme which emerges at several points throughout the workbook, the extent to which we ought to see autonomy and patient choice as the key measure of whether healthcare provision and treatment are ethical. What exactly are the limits of such patient-centredness? To what extent is an ethical approach based on the concerns of individual patients capable of addressing the role of relationships and the duty of care which appear to be central to ethical healthcare practice?

The existence of the workbook depends a great deal upon the willingness and enthusiasm of those who have provided us with cases, papers and commentaries and so on. We feel that this makes the workbook both up to date and vibrant as a way of learning about medical ethics. But times change and so do the ethical issues in medicine. It is our intention to update the workbook in the future and in order to do that we will need new cases and papers. If you have any comments on the workbook or any suggestions for how it might be improved, or if you have cases which would work well as educational tools we would be very pleased to hear from you. You can contact us on michael.parker@ethox.ox.ac.uk.

We think the case-based approach, supported by activities and guided reading exercises has several advantages over other approaches to medical ethics. Firstly, such an approach cuts across disciplinary and cultural boundaries. Everyone can 'relate' in some sense to an actual case, even if they come from very distinct religious or cultural traditions which dictate different principles of ethical conduct. The cases we have chosen are wherever possible 'everyday' cases. Similarly, different healthcare disciplines have increasingly evolved their own forms of healthcare ethics: nursing ethics, for example, sees its concerns and approach as quite distinct from those of medical ethics proper. But in a case-based approach, the different slants of different disciplines can be explicitly built in. Secondly, such an approach requires little previous knowledge of ethics and reassures students who think of philosophy as abstruse and difficult. It is at the same time an approach which is capable of facilitating the development of the skills necessary for a rigorous and consistent analytical approach to the ethics of healthcare practice. Thirdly, a guided, case-based approach encourages students to think of comparable cases of their own, and thus to generalize what they have learned from one case to another, comparing similarities and differences. Finally, given the approach adopted by this workbook, the case-based approach allows students to learn from practice in other countries.

We hope that you will agree and that these chapters will give you the necessary motivation and support for doing the important tasks of learning about medical ethics, for students/practitioners, and of teaching students and practitioners, for medical and nurse educators.

Acknowledgements

We owe thanks to a great many people for their help and advice with this workbook over the three years it has taken us to write it. The cases and papers used have been gathered from all over the European Union, the United States and Australia. Many of them were collected at a series of workshops held as part of the European Biomedical Ethics Practitioners Education project (EBEPE) which was funded by the European Commission's BIOMED II programme. We would like to acknowledge the European Commission's Directorate General 12 for their support during this period and Hugh Whittal in particular for his support and encouragement. We would also like to acknowledge the role of Imperial College London who supported us through the later stages of the EC project.

Michael Parker would like to thank Julian Savulescu, the University of Melbourne Visiting Scholars Scheme and the Centre for Health and Society at the University of Melbourne for providing him with a Visiting Fellowship in summer 1999 which enabled him to work on this book and to write two additional chapters (and to see the Barrier Reef). Thanks too to Elena Iriarte-Jalle.

We would also like to acknowledge the contribution made by those who participated in the EBEPE workshops without whom this workbook would not have been possible. The success of the project was a result of the teamwork and support of our project partners. They are Ruud ter Meulen; Juhani Pietarinen, Raffaele Bracalenti, Carlo Calzone and Stella Reiter-Theil.

Many of the EBEPE participants and partners provided the commentaries, papers and cases which form the core of the workbook. Those who do not appear in print have influenced the workbook in other ways. Those who contributed papers or commentaries are acknowledged where their work appears in the workbook itself. Those who contributed cases are not acknowledged for reasons of confidentiality but we would like to take this opportunity to thank them for their contributions. The EBEPE participants were: Ines Adriaenssen; Gwen Adshead; Steve Baldwin; Attilio Balestrieri; Loutfib Benhabib; Ron Berghmans; Dieter Birnbacher; Gunilla Bjorn; Stefano Boffelli; Paul van Bortel; Nico Bouwan; Raffaele Bracalenti; Masja van den Burg; Arturo Casoni; Carlo Calzone; Abram Coen; Anne Crenier; Paula Daddino; P. Dalla-Vorgia; Joaquin Delgado; Paolo Deluca; Dolores Dooley; Ralf Dressel; Holger Eich; Dag Elgesem; Bart van den Eynden; Eduard Farthmann; Luis Simoes Ferreira; T Garanis-Papadatos; Chris Gastmans; Wolfgang Gerok; Sandro Gindro; Diane. De Graeve; Marco Griffini; Harald Gruber; Anja Hannuniemi; Jocelyn Hattab; Jean Marc Heller; Eckhard Herych; Christian Hick; Wolfgang Hiddemann; Rachel Hodgkin; Tony Hope; Franz Josef Illhardt; Giuseppe Inneo; Antti Jääskeläinen; Winfried Kahlke; Aristoteles Katsas; John Keown; Valeria Kocsis; Kristiina Kurittu; Raimo Lahti; Veikko Launis; Kristiina Lempinen; Jerome Liss; Salla Lötjönen; Giuseppe Magno; Caroline Malone; Elina Männistö; Glauco Mastrangelo; Simonetta Matone; Anne-Catherine Mattiasson; Susan Mendus; Roland Mertelsmann; Ruud ter Meulen; Michael Mohr; Emilio Mordini; Maurizio Mori; Dimitrios Niakas; Marti Parker; Valdar Parve; Stephen Pattison; John Pearce; Filimon Peonidis; Juhani Pietarinen; Gideon Ratzoni; Marjo Rauhala-Hayes; Dolf de Ridder; Stella Reiter-Theil; Klaus Schaefer; Renate Schepke; Alrun Sensmeyer; Jaana Simula; Sandro Spinsanti; Karl-Gustav Södergård; Randi Talseth; Maxwell Taylor; Mats Thorslund; Ulrich Tröhler; Mauro Valeri; Maritta Välimäki; Kristiane Weber; Sander Welie; Vera Wetzler-Wolff; Hugh Whittal; Guy Widdershoven; Rainer Wolf.

First drafts of all the chapters were sent to critical readers in several countries for critical comment. Their comments and criticisms have been central to the success of the workbook. The critical readers were: Ann Sommerville; Tony Hope; Richard Ashcroft; Carmen Kaminsky; Mark R. Wicclair; Chris Milet; Mairi Levitt; Ruth Chadwick; Chris Barnes; Martin Richards; Julian Savulescu; Ainsley Newson; Udo Schüklenk; Peter Rudd; Judy McKimm; Dieter Birnbacher; Alastair Campbell; Rowan Frew, Don Chalmers, Ajit Shah; Corrado Viafora; Peter Kemp; Robin Downie; Dolores Dooley; Win Tadd; Margareta Broberg; Alan Cribb; John Keown and Richard Lancaster, along with many of the EBEPE participants listed above.

Our thanks also to Richard Barling and Joe Mottershead of Cambridge University Press, who helped us to develop what may have appeared to them a rather unwieldy collection of materials into this present work. And, finally, the authors would like to acknowledge the administrative and other support of Yvonne Brennan and Helen Watson of Imperial College London and Caroline Malone of the Open University – and for always being calm and positive in a crisis.

Michael Parker
Donna Dickenson

Notes

1. In the second edition, we have replaced this with an appendix mapping a common system of keywords against the contents of this book. Readers interested in the UK core curriculum can, however, find a reference for the most recent version in the bibliography (Stirrat *et al.*, on p. 241).
2. The second edition is not similarly divided.

Cases in medical ethics and law: an interactive tutorial

Created by **David Lloyd**, **Heather Widdows** and **Donna Dickenson**
How to use the CD-ROM

1. Insert the CD-ROM into your PC's CD-ROM drive. Depending on the configuration of your PC, the program may start its installation routine automatically (after 5–10 seconds). If the process starts, go to step 5 below. If the process doesn't start automatically, go to step 2.
2. Click on: Start/Run
3. Then either type:

   x:\setup.exe
   in the Run dialog box, substituting the drive letter of your CD-ROM drive for 'x', e.g. if the drive letter of your CD-ROM drive is 'D', you should type d:\setup.exe
   or

use the Browse button on the Run dialog box to navigate to the file 'setup'

4. Click the 'OK' box on the Run dialog box.
5. Follow the on-screen instructions to complete the installation.
6. When installation is complete, you will be able to launch the program from your Windows 'Start' button 'Programs' menu, or by using the 'Medical Ethics' icon on your Windows Desktop.

Published by Cambridge University Press. Manufactured in the United Kingdom. Not for sale separately.
This CD-ROM © Cambridge University Press.

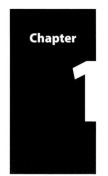

Death and dying: decisions at the end of life

Section 1: Values and goals at the end of life

Rather than reaching a more finely honed consensus about the values and practices that undergird end of life care, conflict has come to dominate the discussion. The consequences are serious for patients, health care providers, family members, and society.

(Dubler, 2005, p. 19)

Death is an unavoidable fact of life. However, the manner in which we each will die is a matter of great concern and conjecture, not least given the considerable advances presented to us by modern medicine. It is nowadays possible for us to delay death and, in many cases, to enable those who would previously have died prematurely to recover and to live full and healthy lives. Such techniques also allow us to exert a greater degree of control over the processes of dying, even when full recovery is not possible. This means that there are people who can now be kept alive by medical interventions but who will never recover sufficiently to live an independent, or in some cases even a conscious, life as a result. There are also patients for whom medical interventions make no (or no appreciable) difference to their suffering – and, sometimes, these patients insist that they would rather die than endure their current existence.

The occurrence of such requests, along with the opportunities and challenges that modern medical techniques simultaneously present, raise a host of important ethical questions. In this chapter we will explore various dilemmas that arise in end-of-life care. In doing so we will consider two fundamental questions:

(1) What is the value of human life?
(2) What are the goals of medicine?

This will prompt us to ask such questions as: does life possess an intrinsic value or is it only valuable for as long as it is a happy life, of a good quality? Or, instead, is the value to be determined by the individual, such that it is for him or her to decide when life is – or is not – worthwhile? And what is medical expertise supposed to achieve, particularly when the patient is nearing the end of his or her life? In other words, if we cannot heal the patient, then what should be the goal of medicine and of the healthcare professional?

These questions undoubtedly have great relevance in the context of end-of-life decision-making – and, we suggest, they also underpin many of the other ethical issues that we will explore throughout this book. As such, your reading of this chapter should give you some of the philosophical tools that will help you to think through the other areas of medical practice you will encounter.

In order to explore these questions we will introduce a range of real clinical cases. Some of these cases have proven so difficult that they have ended up before a court of law. However, even those that have not been passed to a judge can involve intense ethical dilemmas, as our first case poignantly demonstrates. This case was referred to us by the bioethicist Alastair Campbell and, unlike many of the cases we will discuss, the patient, Anna, was happy to be named – indeed, she was keen for the issues to be debated as widely as possible, as Campbell explains (Campbell, 1998, p. 83).

> **The case of Anna**
>
> Six and a half years ago I met a woman called Anna for the last time. Anna asked me to tell her story whenever I could, and I often have since that time. She was a woman in her thirties who was tetraplegic as the result of a road traffic accident some years previously. She also suffered diffuse phantom pain, which required constant administration of high doses of analgesic to make it bearable.

Anna was married and had three young children. She had previously been a very active person – she had loved hiking and was an amateur singer of considerable talent. She also enjoyed amateur dramatics. By profession she was a schoolteacher. Now she felt she no longer had a life to live, that she was no longer the person she had been, and she wished to die.

ACTIVITY: Imagine that you are one of the doctors caring for Anna. How would you respond to her statement? Do you share (or at least sympathize with) the conclusion she has reached about the value of her life? Or do you think that there is still value in Anna's life, perhaps even enough to say that Anna is wrong to feel this way?

As you work through this book, you will be introduced to various articles about the topics under consideration. In the first reading, below, Richard Huxtable describes some of the different views that have been taken on the value of human life, which you may yourself have considered when thinking about Anna's case.

Calculating the value of life?

Richard Huxtable

Modern medicine is capable of securing great victories for a diverse range of patients, whose afflictions may range from the minor to the major, from the transient to the chronic, to the incurable and even to the terminal. Indeed, in much of the developed world at least, experts trained in palliative care have the knowledge and means to offer the dying patient a death that is, so far as possible, free from painful and distressing symptoms. Yet, such victories may be hard fought and incomplete, and they may even be more apparent than real. Some patients will continue to suffer; some will reject the medicines and machines on offer; and some will insist that what they really want is positive help in dying.

Given the differences in outlook and opinion that exist, it is perhaps inevitable – but still regrettable – that conflict is rarely far from the practices and policies adopted at the end of life. Sometimes the conflict is all too real: the judges in England have had occasion to consider a case in which a physical struggle developed between medical staff and the relatives of a seriously unwell boy on a paediatric intensive care ward (Huxtable and Forbes, 2004). The physical struggle emerged from an ethical dispute, involving a fundamental difference in opinion about the ways in which the boy, who the doctors believed was dying, ought to be treated. That was, of course, an extreme case. Nevertheless, the ethical tensions on which it rested are rather more common, since even our everyday practices and policies often require us to take a stand on what it is that makes life valuable – and this is something about which many of us will disagree, and often reasonably so.

So, which (and whose) values should guide us in our actions at the end of life and in shaping the rules that govern those actions? The ethical terrain has been comprehensively mapped over decades, if not centuries, and three themes emerge as particularly dominant: the duty to respect life; the obligation to alleviate suffering; and the need to respect patient autonomy, essential to such concepts as informed consent. It should come as no surprise to learn that each of these options will, in turn, shape death and dying in quite distinctive ways.

The first theme, the duty to respect life, has the longest history, as it has long featured in (for example) Judaeo-Christian teaching. The basic idea here is that life has a special worth, such that it should never intentionally be brought to an end. This is often formulated as the principle of the sanctity of life, but it can also be phrased in less theistic terms as the principle of the inviolability of life, or in terms of the right to life (Keown, 2002). Whichever formulation is preferred, its supporters emphasize that life is a basic good, and that it possesses an intrinsic value.

Adherence to this concept of the value of human life will give rise to a set of policies on terminal care which emphasize our commitment to valuing the patient regardless of any disability or inability. Viewed from this perspective, all of society, including the terminally ill themselves, should see every life as worthy of respect and protection. Proponents emphasize that this does not commit us to doing everything in all circumstances; rather, futile or overly burdensome treatments can still be avoided, and potentially risky symptom relief can also be undertaken – provided that there is never any intention to shorten life.

Opposition to this viewpoint comes from the argument that life is only instrumentally valuable: life essentially derives its value from the uses to which it can be put. A useful or happy life is one that we can describe as having a good quality; conversely, a life of disability, inability and suffering might sometimes be described as a poor quality life. Obviously, proponents of this viewpoint believe that we are morally obliged to tackle suffering, through treatment and ongoing research. But some defenders of this position go further and argue that it is not necessarily wrong for us to think that some patients' lives are of such desperately poor quality that they would be better off dead (e.g. Singer, 1993, pp. 191–2).

An appeal to the instrumental value of life is therefore a key feature of arguments in favour of euthanasia. Yet, it is seldom the only feature; it is more common to encounter such a claim alongside an appeal to self-determination or autonomy, which derives from the Greek *auto* (self) and *nomos* (governance). The duty to respect patient autonomy thus grounds a third perspective on what it is that makes life valuable, which maintains that we should leave the assessment to the patient.

Respect for people's choices has a central place in modern healthcare ethics and, indeed, in modern healthcare. However, it is not just *anyone's* choices that we ought to honour; instead, it is the choices of *autonomous* individuals that deserve the most respect. At a minimum, an autonomous individual is one who is mentally 'competent' (that is, capable of taking the particular decision), appropriately well informed about the choice to be made, and able to make their choice freely. Provided that the patient satisfies the relevant criteria, the value of life is entirely a question for her – indeed, it would be unjustly *paternalistic* of anyone to interfere with her view, such as by imposing treatment on her against her will or denying her the right to commit suicide, even with assistance (e.g. Harris, 2003).

There would appear to be something of value in each of the three perspectives just outlined: we should aim to protect and preserve life; we should also want to eradicate or at least minimize suffering; and we should also strive to heed and respect people's views on how they would like (or not like) to be treated. But, we might have very different views about which of these obligations is to take priority, and this will undoubtedly give rise to dilemmas in practice. Sometimes we can devise practical (and principled) methods for dealing with disputes: one example involves affording recognition to a professional's conscience, and thus protecting their autonomous right to refrain from involvement in a policy with which they personally disagree. On other occasions, however, it will be less easy to discern a way of dealing with the competing injunctions that emerge from these various perspectives on the value of life.

No doubt the values conflict will persist. Nevertheless, some bioethicists are looking for new ways of answering the fundamental questions associated with life and death. There will, as a result, be important creative contributions (for example, recent writing on the meaning and scope of human dignity; Beyleveld and Brownsword, 2001; Biggs, 2001), and there will also be value in seeking consensus wherever possible. There will also be merit in seeking to combine the different insights on offer, along the lines of a compromise approach (Huxtable, 2007). Whichever option is favoured, the quest for values is an important one and it is one in which we all have a stake; as such, the very least we might legitimately expect is an open dialogue on the various issues arising in end-of-life care, so that we may all help to shape the resultant practices and policies.

ACTIVITY: According to Huxtable, there are three prominent views on the value of life, which can be summarized as: life is *intrinsically* valuable; life is *instrumentally* valuable; and life has a *self-determined* value. Which of these do you find most persuasive and how do you think it applies in Anna's case?

As Huxtable explains, our responses to Anna might differ according to which account of the value of life we find most persuasive. An adherent to the intrinsic value of life would most likely seek to remind Anna that her life is something she should continue to value. However, this would not require her to submit to every form of medical treatment that would prolong her life: Anna is entitled to say 'enough is enough' if any such treatment is proving futile or otherwise overly burdensome for her.

Alternatively, a supporter of the instrumental value of life could probably be persuaded that Anna's perspective on the quality of her life is entirely understandable. A quality of life assessment is, in essence, a relative one: the patient is judged to be worse off than he or she had previously been, or worse off than other people who are not so afflicted. As Campbell describes her story, Anna herself seems to judge her present existence, in which she is confined to a hospital bed, as significantly worse than her previously active life.

Anna's judgement on the worth (or worthlessness) of her life is undoubtedly important, and it comes to the fore if we believe that life has a self-determined value. Of course, our first task here would be to ensure that Anna is exercising an autonomous choice to die. This could require us to ask various questions of Anna. Is there anything interfering with her ability to reason? For example, is she depressed and, if so and we treat her depression, will she change her mind? Is there anything or anyone exerting pressure on Anna, such that the decision is not really *hers*? And is she sufficiently informed about how she could best cope (and even thrive) with life in her condition? Meeting other patients in her condition might help her to see the value in such an existence.

However, even if we are tempted to ask these sorts of questions, we might still reach the conclusion that Anna *is* making an autonomous decision about the value of her life. And doesn't that mean that we should therefore leave it to her to determine the timing and manner of her death?

Of course, true respect for autonomy undoubtedly hinges on appropriate *communication* between the patient and the healthcare professional. The healthcare professional will need to ensure that they have informed the patient of their options, so that the patient can truly exercise a choice. The patient, in turn, will need to communicate their decision to the healthcare professional. We think that good communication skills and good ethics tend to go hand-in-hand. Indeed, and here we return to Anna's story, you might have been tempted to think that Anna was asking the doctors to help her to die. In fact, this was not quite the case, as Alastair Campbell explains.

Although she had made it clear that she wished no resuscitation, she had suffered a respiratory arrest while away from her usual carers, had been resuscitated, and was now respirator dependent. After some months of discussion and the seeking of legal and ethical opinion, it had been agreed that her request to disconnect the respirator could be agreed to. A device was fixed up that enabled her to switch off the machine, and three days after our conversation, at a pre-arranged time and with all her family present, she flipped the switch. Drugs were administered to alleviate any respiratory distress and she lapsed into unconsciousness. However, a short time later she woke up and asked angrily, 'Why am I still here?' More medication was given and she relapsed once more into an unconscious state. It was some hours later before eventually her breathing ceased entirely and she died.

(Campbell, 1998, pp. 83–4)

ACTIVITY: What are your reactions to this series of events? Which, if any, aspects do you agree with, and which do you oppose?

The fact that Anna was resuscitated against her wishes is a highly regrettable feature of her story, which raises questions about the effectiveness of the communication between Anna's different carers. Again, then, we see the importance of good communication, not only between patients and carers but also between members of the care team.

For her part, Anna made certain to communicate not only with her professional carers but also with her loved ones: she had clearly made her wishes known to her family, and they were there with her when the respirator was turned off. This suggests that Anna knew that her choice did not exist in a vacuum, in which the only salient concern was what she, as an autonomous person, wanted. Anna knew that her decision would impact upon her family, and she had evidently gained their understanding and perhaps even their support – in other words, she seemed to know that ethics means not only considering our *rights* but also our *duties* to others.

Anna finally got what she wanted all along – but, in the end, did her doctors act ethically? This is another point at which there is sincere and serious disagreement amongst the ethicists, which again rests on competing philosophies of the value of life. Some might say that this was euthanasia, that is, an action intended to end Anna's unwanted life of suffering.

The administration of drugs at this stage seems clearly to be a response to her request to die, through ensuring that her still active respiration was further compromised. At this stage, in my view, the doctor killed the patient at her request, clearly an act of voluntary euthanasia ... and therefore a criminal act, since there was no law to authorize it. No action was taken against the doctor in this case, nor was it likely to be given the circumstances of respiratory and emotional distress in which the sedatives were administered.

(Campbell, 1998, p. 89)

If, like Campbell, you believe that this was a case of euthanasia, then do you think there is anything wrong in this? Here, it is helpful to consider the extent to which a practice like this can be said to fit with the *goals* of medicine, particularly when the patient is nearing the end of his or her life.

ACTIVITY: What do you consider to be the goals of medicine in general (i.e. not simply at the end of life)? What would you consider to constitute an absolute violation of these goals? Which of these goals are no longer appropriate at the end of life? Which goals would you modify or remove, and what new activities and attitudes would you add?

You are likely to have thought that 'healing' will be a vital part of the healthcare endeavour. However, you are also likely to recognize that, for Anna, healing is no longer possible in any meaningful sense. Perhaps, instead, the central goal of medicine ought to be the *alleviation of suffering*. But we might go further and claim that the duty to end suffering means that we should also be prepared to end lives. Of course, not everyone will share this view: some will object that this involves violating goals intrinsic to medicine, such as the duty to protect and preserve life.

ACTIVITY: Now read the following article and, as you do so, consider the extent to which the goals of medicine (in the broadest sense) are in tension with and perhaps even conflict with what we would consider ethical treatment or care at the end of life. Are the ethical dimensions different when questions of life and death are at issue?

Physician-assisted death, violation of the moral integrity of medicine and the slippery slope

Ron Berghmans[1]

Those who take the view that physician-assisted death involves a violation of the moral integrity of medicine argue that doctors must never be a party to intentional killing, because that would go against the very essence of the medical profession (Singer and Siegler, 1990; Pellegrino, 1992; Momeyer, 1995). The essence of medicine from this perspective is considered to be healing and the protection of life. This view is opposed to the possibility of physician-assisted death in all circumstances. Those who defend this view refer to categorical claims such as the inalienability of the right to life, the sanctity of life, the absolute prohibition against killing other human beings, and to healing as the single and ultimate goal of medicine. I want to focus on this last claim.

On this view, the essence of medicine is to be found in the *telos* of benefiting the sick by the action of healing. It is worth asking however just what is the status of this claim. It should be recognized that the practice of medicine and the ends it serves are of human invention, and not 'naturally given' activities deriving from the structure of natural order. The practice of medicine is shaped by human beings in order to serve human purposes. It involves human choice with regard to value systems, and choosing such a

value system requires moral argument and justification, not an appeal to the "nature of things". Whatever the goals of medicine are, or should be, is thus a matter which is open to rational debate, and cannot be decided without reference to value considerations.

But even if, for the sake of argument, we agree that the *telos* of medicine is healing – and not, for instance, the relief of human suffering or the promotion of the benefit of patients – then we still are left with the question of exactly what moral force such an end or goal of medicine has. If we look at the actual practice of medicine, it is clear that healing is more an ideal than an unconditional goal of medical endeavour. Take for instance the case of refusal of treatment by the patient. A well-considered refusal of treatment ought to be respected, even if the physician takes the view that treatment would be beneficial to the patient. The reasons for respecting competent refusals of treatment are twofold. The first reason is that non-consensual intervention where a person has decision-making capacity invades the integrity of the person involved. The second is that competent persons ought to be considered the best judges of their own interests. Only the competent person himself can assess the benefits, burdens and harms of treatment in view of his or her wishes, goals and values. So if a person refuses treatment because he or she does not value treatment in his or her personal life, then such a refusal ought to be respected, even if this might result in an earlier death. Thus, as this example shows, healing as an ideal in medical practice implies that other goals and values can and do operate as constraints upon medical actions serving this ideal.

More directly related to the issue of physician-assisted death is the consideration that the ideal of healing can become illusory, for instance in cases of severe and unbearable suffering in which no prospect of alleviation exists. The goal of relieving the suffering of the patient then becomes the primary goal of the physician, rather than healing.

Part of the moral integrity argument is the claim that if physicians assist in suicide or euthanasia, then the public will begin to distrust the medical profession, and as a result the profession itself will suffer irreparable harm (Pellegrino, 1992; Thomasma, 1996). Against this objection it can be argued that if physician-assisted death is categorically rejected the result may also be a loss of trust in the medical profession. The public may experience this as a lack of compassion and personal engagement on the part of physicians in those cases where no adequate means of relieving the suffering of the patient are available and the patient wants some control over how to die, but is left alone by the doctor.

My conclusion is that in principle as well as in practice euthanasia and physician-assisted suicide do not *necessarily* go against the goal or goals of medicine, or the moral integrity of the medical profession. The Hippocratic vow of 'helping the sick' and of exercising medical skills for the benefit of patients does not prohibit the co-operation of physicians with requests for euthanasia and assisted suicide, so long as they are convinced that this is what is in a patient's best interests and to the degree that the physician is committed to respecting a patient's own values.

The involvement of doctors in the dying of patients is inescapable. In many cases, a decision of a doctor leads to a hastening of death, although that decision may not always be considered the direct cause of the death of the patient (i.e. the decision to respect the treatment refusal of a patient). In euthanasia and assisted suicide, the causal role of the actions of the doctor is more clear-cut, and the practice of physician-assisted death raises a number of issues regarding the proper role of the physician and the self-understanding of the medical profession. Although the primary task of the physician is to preserve the life of the patient, preservation of life is not an absolute goal. This would demand an unconditional obligation to preserve life by all possible means and under all circumstances. If the relief of suffering is also a proper goal of medicine, then in particular circumstances a weighing or balancing of the goal to preserve life and the goal of relieving suffering becomes inescapable.

Euthanasia and assisted suicide do not necessarily violate the moral integrity of medicine.

ACTIVITY: What do you make of Berghmans' arguments about the *telos* or goal of medicine? Can you think of any counter-arguments?

Berghmans proposes that the goal of terminal care ought to be the alleviation of suffering, even if this sometimes goes against our sense that, in general, medicine ought to be concerned with healing. You may wish to continue to reflect on his arguments as you work through the remainder of this chapter. You should also bear in mind the three views that tend to be taken on the value of human life, which Huxtable described. In the remainder of this chapter we shall be going on to explore the ethical implications of these arguments in a variety of different ways. We will start with one of the key issues arising in Anna's story: the ethical dimensions of decisions about whether (or not) to attempt resuscitation.

Section 2: Deciding not to attempt resuscitation

In the previous section, Huxtable and Berghmans demonstrated how deciding whether or not to treat a patient will give rise to important questions about the value of life and the goals of medical treatment, particularly where the patient is suffering greatly. These questions arise again in the following case, known for reasons of confidentiality as the case of 'Mr R' (*Re R* [1996] 2 FLR 99).

The case of Mr R

Mr R was born with a serious malformation of the brain and cerebral palsy. At eight months of age he developed severe epilepsy. At the age of 23 he had spastic diplegia (paralysis) and was incontinent, as well as apparently deaf and blind (with possible vestigial response to a buzzer and to light). He was unable to walk, to sit upright or to chew; so that food had to be syringed to the back of his mouth. His bowels had to be evacuated manually because his limited diet resulted in serious constipation. He suffered from thrush and had ulcers 'all the way through his guts', according to testimony. When cuddled he did indicate pleasure, and he also appeared to respond to pain by grimacing. Although he was not comatose, nor in a persistent vegetative state, his awareness on a scale of 1 to 10 was rated somewhere between 1 and 2 in an assessment by Dr Keith Andrews of the Royal Hospital for Neurodisability at Putney, London, who said:

> It is my opinion that he has very little, if any, real cognitive awareness at a level where he can interpret what is going on in his environment. He reacts at the most basic level by responding to comfort, warmth and a safe environment by being relaxed and producing the occasional smile. He responds to discomfort, pain and threatening situations by becoming distressed and crying. These are very basic level responses and do not imply any thought processes.

Until he was 17 Mr R lived at home, where he was totally dependent on his devoted parents. He then moved to a residential home, but continued to return home at weekends. Now his condition was beginning to deteriorate: his weight had dropped to just over 30 kg, and he was extremely frail, suffering from recurrent chest infections, bleeding from ulceration of the oesophagus, and continued epileptic fits. In 1995 he was admitted to hospital on five occasions, each time for a life-threatening crisis. After the last crisis Dr S, the consultant psychiatrist for learning difficulties who was responsible for his care, wrote:

> To hospitalize Mr R if he had another life-threatening crisis would, in my clinical judgement, be nothing more than striving officiously to keep him alive for no gain to him. In my opinion, this is tantamount to a failing against a basic duty of humanity. Indeed, at the last few admissions to hospital, I have had real concern as to whether it was ethical to treat him actively. That said, I would never withhold treatment against the wishes of his parents. In summary, taking R's best interests into account and whilst taking into account the basic premise of the sanctity of human life, it is in my judgement unquestionably in R's best interests to allow nature to take its course next time he has a life-threatening crisis and to allow him to die with some comfort and dignity. That would relieve him of physical, mental and emotional suffering.

ACTIVITY: Read through Dr S's opinion and make a list of the ethically charged terms and concepts that are being used to construct an argument. After each term, write down the consultant's apparent interpretation of it. Do you agree with this interpretation? If not, write down your own.

It strikes us that there are at least 10 ethically charged terms and concepts contained within Dr S's opinion:

(1) Best interests of the patient
(2) Gain or benefit to the patient
(3) Sanctity of life
(4) Duty of humanity
(5) Death with dignity
(6) Relief of suffering
(7) Wishes of the parents
(8) Withholding treatment
(9) Treating actively
(10) Medical futility.

This is quite a full list for one paragraph, and the exercise illustrates how tightly packed with ethical concepts an apparently clinical judgement can be.

You will be aware from your reading of the papers by Huxtable and Berghmans that there are various ways in which these terms and concepts can be interpreted. You might, for example, think that serving the best interests of the patient involves the eradication of suffering, perhaps even by ending their life; alternatively, you might think that the third point, the sanctity of life, must be central to our thinking about a case like Mr R's, such that we must always recognize the worth of his life, notwithstanding his disabilities.

For her part, Dr S was clearly concerned to avoid 'striving officiously' to keep Mr R alive; as she elsewhere put it, she felt it better 'to allow nature to take its course'. This idea is open to interpretation. Dr S appears to mean that it might be better not to attempt to resuscitate Mr R; in other words, that we should *withhold* treatment from him. A similar issue arose in the case of Anna – but for her the issue then became whether or not treatment should be *withdrawn*. Is there any difference between the two? The General Medical Council (GMC) has noted that:

> Although it may be emotionally more difficult for the health care team, and those close to the patient, to withdraw a treatment from a patient rather than to decide not to provide a treatment in the first place, this should not be used as a reason for failing to initiate a treatment which may be of some benefit to the patient. Where it has been decided that a treatment is not in the best interests of the patient, there is no ethical or legal obligation to provide it and therefore no need to make a distinction between not starting the treatment and withdrawing it.
>
> (GMC, 2002, para. 18)

The GMC is here addressing – and denying – the alleged distinction between withholding and withdrawing treatment; i.e. the GMC believes that there is no difference between the two. The distinction often invites a variety of ethical questions. Does a doctor incur additional obligations to his or her patient (or even to their family) once treatment has been started? Or is there no substantial difference between the two, particularly if their consequences are identical? And does the physical behaviour associated with withdrawing, as opposed to withholding, have any moral relevance? This latter question draws us into another contested distinction, between *acts* and *omissions*. The GMC, for its part, holds that the 'actions' of withholding and withdrawing treatment are actually both to count as 'omissions'.

The distinction between acts and omissions originated in Catholic moral theology and for its supporters intentionally ending life by (negative) omission can be just as wrong as doing so by (positive) action. The wording in the Anglican creed, for example, asks God to pardon believers for two separate matters: that 'we have done those things we ought not to have done' (wrongful acts), and that we have 'left undone those things we ought to have done' (wrongful omissions).

However, it is not the case that *every* omission that might shorten life would be condemned. In the sanctity of life tradition, a doctor is not obliged to give a 'disproportionate' or, some would say, 'extraordinary' treatment – but he or she *is* obliged to provide 'proportionate' (or 'ordinary') treatments. Notice, though, that it is only when treatment is disproportionate that it can be withdrawn or withheld: neither the patient nor the doctor is entitled to omit treatment for some other reason, say, because the patient wants to die or because the doctor thinks that the patient's quality of life is poor. And, the argument continues, the active, intentional ending of life can never be permitted.

Some critics of the principle of the sanctity of human life think that it is wrong to draw these various distinctions, because they simply do not stand up to scrutiny. Indeed, their objections show how some of the conflicts that exist at the level of applied healthcare ethics can rest on deeper conflicts about what it is that makes an action or an omission ethical in the first place.

According to one school of thought we should do that which it is our duty to do. This is a *deontological* position, one which is famously associated with Immanuel Kant. You might detect this sort of thinking in the sanctity of life approach, under which we are duty-bound to protect life and, by extension, to recognize that everyone has a right to life – although we should also recognize that the position also features in the autonomy approach, where a doctor may be duty-bound to respect the patient's autonomous choice, even if the patient has chosen to bring an early end to his life.

Alternatively we might think it more appropriate to do that which has the best consequences. This is a *consequentialist* stance, popularly adopted by *utilitarians*, who ask us to achieve the greatest good for the greatest number. The philosophers who advance these sorts of ideas tend to be persuaded by arguments first outlined by Jeremy Bentham and John Stuart Mill.

Utilitarians will claim that the distinction between acts and omissions makes no moral sense. For one thing, it is difficult to distinguish between them in practice. For example, is turning off a ventilator a positive act, or merely omitting to perform the treatment any longer? More radically, these philosophers argue that there is no significant moral difference between killing and letting die (Rachels, 1986). Jonathan Glover uses the following example to illustrate the objection:

> A man who will inherit a fortune when his father dies, and, with this in mind, omits to give him medicine necessary for keeping him alive, is very culpable. His culpability is such that many people would want to say that this is not a mere omission, but a positive act of withholding the medicine. Supporters of the acts and omissions doctrine who also take this view are faced with the problem of explaining where they draw the line between acts and omissions. Is consciously failing to send money to [charity] also a positive act of withholding?
>
> (Glover, 1977, p. 96)

Supporters of the distinction might first answer Glover's challenge by saying that the point at which to draw the line is the duty to care. It is because the son has a duty to care for the father that failing to give the medicine is wrong. (It might also be wrong to fail to give it to anyone who needed it, if we think we have a generalized 'Good Samaritan' duty to others.) In the context of a doctor's duty to care, both acts and omissions may indeed be wrongful: treating without consent would be a wrongful act, whilst failing to treat someone who had consented and who needed treatment might be a wrongful omission.

This may explain why doctors are sometimes reluctant to rely on the distinction between acts and omissions, why they feel a duty to treat at all costs – sometimes against the wishes of the patient or their relatives. However, some healthcare professionals, like Karen Forbes (a consultant in palliative medicine), are not so wary of the distinction that Glover attacks:

> I do not agree with those authors who argue that it is only the outcome of medical action or inaction that is morally relevant, so that to kill and to allow to die are one and the same thing ... There seems a certain arrogance in the underlying assumption that with medical action, i.e. treatment, people will live, and without treatment people will die, and that therefore to deny medical action is to kill. It is

salutary to remember that usually it is the timing of the outcome, rather than the outcome itself, that is altered by medical action or inaction.

(Forbes, 1998, pp. 100–101)

ACTIVITY: What do you make of the alleged distinction between acts and omissions? Do you think that it makes moral sense? Can you see a role for the distinction in working out what should be done in the case of Mr R?

Now please continue with your reading of the case.

> The immediate question now was whether to resuscitate Mr R in the event of another acute admission resulting in cardiac arrest. He was so frail that it was feared CPR (cardio-pulmonary resuscitation) might crush his ribcage. In addition, there was a risk of further brain damage from resuscitation. A subsidiary question was whether to administer antibiotics if he developed pneumonia. After Mr R's fifth hospital admission, in September 1995, the consultant, Dr S, discussed the position with Mr R's parents. They agreed that Mr R would not be subjected to CPR if he suffered a cardiac arrest in future. Accordingly, Dr S signed a DNR (do not resuscitate) direction, signed by Mr R's mother under the heading 'next of kin'.
>
> This decision was opposed by staff at the day care centre which Mr R had been attending; they felt that he did in fact have some 'quality of life'. In addition they interpreted Dr S's decision as a 'no treatment' policy, which Dr S denied: the only treatment which she was withholding, she argued, was cardio-pulmonary resuscitation. Agreement could not be reached, and a member of the day care centre staff applied for review of the decision by a court, on the basis of information provided by social workers involved in Mr R's day care.
>
> The basis of the application was that the DNR decision was irrational and unlawful in permitting medical treatment to be withheld on the basis of an assessment of the patient's quality of life. The hospital sought a court judgement that, despite Mr R's inability to give a valid refusal of treatment, it would be lawful and in his best interests to withhold cardio-pulmonary resuscitation and the administration of antibiotics. However, a proposed gastrostomy would be performed, underlining that there was no question of a comprehensive refusal to treat Mr R. Likewise, the hospital decided that it would ventilate Mr R and provide artificial nutrition and hydration if applicable, although initially it had indicated it would not. The application made it clear that the hospital intended

> 'to furnish such treatment and nursing care as may from time to time be appropriate to ensure that [R] suffers the least distress and retains the greatest dignity until such time as his life comes to an end.'

In the High Court hearing, where Mr R was represented by the Official Solicitor (who acts on behalf of incompetent patients), discussion centred on guidelines for resuscitation issued by the British Medical Association (BMA) in 1993 in a joint statement with the Royal College of Nursing (RCN). It has been argued that resuscitation, originally devised to be used in a small minority of cases, is sometimes overused (Hilberman *et al.*, 1997). Although the technique can be very successful in the right context, in some US states it has become the default response to cardiac arrest, that is, it is required unless it is explicitly refused or clearly 'futile'. Yet cardiac arrest is part of death. But was Mr R dying?

It is also wrong to think that CPR necessarily will work for every patient. Because it might not do so, we nowadays prefer to talk of 'DNAR' orders; in instructing 'do not *attempt* resuscitation', we make it clearer to patients, their families and even the healthcare professionals that CPR can sometimes be *tried*, but there is no guarantee that it will revive every patient (British Medical Association *et al.*, 2007).

The 1993 BMA/RCN guidelines, as used in relation to Mr R, did not actually say that resuscitation must always be attempted unless the patient is clearly in a terminal condition. Instead, they suggested three types of case in which it is appropriate to consider a DN(A)R decision:

(a) Where the patient's condition indicates that effective cardio-pulmonary resuscitation (CPR) is unlikely to be successful
(b) Where CPR is not in accord with the recorded sustained wishes of the patient who is mentally competent
(c) Where successful CPR is likely to be followed by a length and quality of life which would not be acceptable to the patient.

ACTIVITY: Which, if any, of these conditions might apply to Mr R? Note down the reasons for your answer.

Condition (a) is the most obviously 'clinical' of the three. It seems to focus solely on the medical facts of the matter. Certainly Mr R is gravely ill, but he has come through five acute admissions in the past year, so it is difficult to say that he is definitely unlikely to survive CPR. Condition (b) cannot be met, because Mr R is not mentally competent to record a wish. Finally, we have condition (c), focusing on unacceptable quality of life – but again, the guidance talks of this being acceptable or unacceptable *to the patient*. It is very hard to know whether Mr R gets any enjoyment out of life: he seems to respond to being cuddled, and to react to pain, but that is really all we can say. The BMA guidelines did note that 'If the patient cannot express a view, the opinion of others close to the patient may be sought regarding the patient's best interests.' But, although the situation is nowadays different in England, the 1993 guidelines do not say that opinion has anything more than advisory value as to what the patient would regard as reasonable quality of life. (We will consider the views of his family again in a moment.) The guidelines also appear to envision a different kind of situation – where a previously competent patient, who (unlike Mr R) had expressed definite views about good and bad quality of life, is no longer able to enunciate his or her wishes, but where the family will remember his or her preferences.

So, strictly speaking, it is possible to make a case for arguing that none of these conditions applies to Mr R. But that was not the opinion of the court. Prompted by guidance from Keith Andrews as an expert witness, the court agreed that conditions (b) and (c) were not applicable – ruling out the quality of life arguments both for and against. Only condition (a) was to be considered, that is, the likelihood rather than the desirability of successful CPR. Even in hospital settings only about 13% of patients receiving CPR survive to discharge, Dr Andrews testified; in a residential home such as the one Mr R lived in, the chances would be virtually nil. Accordingly, the case turned on the alleged *futility* of treatment, rather than on the quality of Mr R's life. On the basis of medical futility, the Court accepted the DNAR order, but not a global policy against other interventions by the consultant when and if a potentially life-threatening infection arose.

ACTIVITY: Do you think there are any valid counter-arguments to this view? What might be the pitfalls of using medical futility to decide whether or not to resuscitate?

The British guidelines have been updated since Mr R's case, but they continue to reflect the ethical issues that

his doctors encountered. The latest guidance contains the following statement:

> In some cases, the decision not to attempt CPR is a straightforward clinical decision. If the clinical team believes that CPR will not re-start the heart and maintain breathing, it should not be offered or attempted. CPR (which can cause harm in some situations) should not be attempted if it will not be successful. However, the patient's individual circumstances and the most up-to-date guidance must be considered carefully before such a decision is made.
>
> (British Medical Association *et al.*, 2007, p. 8)

Notice that this statement avoids using the word 'futile'. Indeed, although the concept is one that features prominently in the sanctity of life principle, it is also subject to widespread distrust (e.g. Gillon, 1997). Critics of futility have made the following points:

(1) It is never possible to say that, in any particular case, a treatment will be completely futile; rather, it is a question of what levels of probability are acceptable. What if this particular patient happens to be in the 0.01% of patients who can benefit from a seemingly 'futile' intervention? Surely that means that the intervention is far from futile for *them*?

(2) If we think something is futile then we basically mean that it will not achieve its purpose. In order for us then to say that a *treatment* is futile, we need to have some idea about the very purpose of medicine – and this returns us to familiar questions about the *telos* of medicine (what about offering hope to patients and families?) and the value of life (Halliday, 1997).

(3) Given the background assumptions that must inform the decision to label something 'futile', it is wrong to conclude that this is a purely 'clinical' criterion that can be determined wholly by the doctors. In other words, the label might be used to conceal value judgements, which might themselves be *paternalistic* and unrepresentative of the values of the patient and his or her loved ones.

However, you might think that the label is sometimes appropriate and, indeed, unavoidable. Unless we want to say that treatment should always be provided to a competent patient at their request or to an incompetent patient whatever the circumstances, then someone has to draw the line somewhere. That person is most likely to be the doctor (Brody, 1997). But should it be the doctor alone?

It seems to us that Mr R's case does indeed involve very important questions about the duties that doctors owe, particularly in dealing with a patient's suffering. When do the burdens of treatment outweigh its benefits? And when can we say that the reverse holds true? In order to answer these questions appropriately we need to remember that there can be different ways of understanding the concepts of 'benefit' and 'burden'. Of course, one way of determining the meaning of 'benefit' and 'burden' to an individual patient simply involves asking that patient. We will pick up this theme in the next section.

Section 3: Refusal of treatment, and advance directives

Listening to the patient is crucial in ethical healthcare and we saw earlier how the idea of respect for autonomy underpins one view of the value of life. The idea that we should respect the patient's right to self-determine and so make decisions for him or herself is most obviously captured in the requirement that a patient is entitled to consent to or refuse treatment. Indeed, treating patients without their consent, even in the name of their best interests, means disrespecting their autonomy – it amounts to an unacceptable, paternalistic invasion of personal integrity. Many European jurisdictions recognize that, even at the end of life or at the risk of death, a competent adult patient has an absolute right to refuse treatment (e.g. Nys, 1999).

In the first section, Ron Berghmans argued that a 'well-considered refusal of treatment ought to be respected' because competent patients will be 'the best judges of their own interests'. But what does Berghmans mean by 'a well-considered refusal of treatment'? Might one argue that refusing treatment which is medically advisable is automatically ill-considered? That this kind of reasoning can occur in practice has been extensively documented (e.g. Roth *et al.*, 1977; Culver and Gert, 1982; Faulder, 1985) and, as we shall see in a later chapter, in the case of young people under 18 it has actually been upheld in law. The argument here is that refusal should carry a heavier 'tariff' than consent to treatment, because it goes against medical opinion. But that is different from saying that a refusal can *never* be 'well-considered', even if it flies in the face of medical

opinion. As one English judge has put it, 'the patient is entitled to reject [medical] advice for reasons which are rational, or irrational, or for no reason' (*Sidaway* v *Bethlem RHG* [1985] 1 All ER 643).

It may appear respectful of autonomy to allow patients to refuse treatment even on seemingly irrational grounds, but true respect for autonomy will obviously hinge on the person being autonomous in the first place. A key component of autonomy is *competence* (or capacity): the patient must be capable of taking the particular decision. This issue famously came before the English courts in the case of Mr C (*Re C (Adult: Refusal of Treatment)* [1994] 1 All ER 819 (FD)), a case we will re-visit when we examine mental health.

The case of Mr C

Mr C, aged 68, had paranoid schizophrenia and had been detained in a secure mental hospital for 30 years. His delusions included the belief that his doctors were torturers, whilst he himself was a world-famous specialist in the treatment of diseased limbs. When his own foot became infected, he therefore hid his condition from medical personnel until it had actually become gangrenous. His doctors believed that unless his foot was amputated, he stood an 80% to 85% chance of dying.

Mr C, however, refused to consent to the amputation, saying that he would rather die intact than survive with only one foot. He sought reassurances from the hospital that his foot would not be amputated without his consent if he slipped into a coma. The health authority in charge of the hospital refused to give an undertaking not to amputate his foot without his consent. Mr C then sought a High Court order to prevent amputation if he became unconscious.

ACTIVITY: Do you think Mr C was competent to refuse consent to treatment? Note the principal reasons why, or why not.

As Mr C's solicitor, Lucy Scott-Montcrieff, explained:

The issue at the heart of all of this was whether or not Mr C had the capacity to refuse the treatment that was being offered to him. Mental illness doesn't of itself mean that a person doesn't have capacity; you could have capacity for some things and not other things. We had to establish whether Mr C could understand and retain the information about the advantages and disadvantages of amputation and the advantages and disadvantages of not having amputation. The surgeon who'd been treating Mr C gave evidence; what he said was that he believed that Mr C did have capacity, because Mr C's views about capacity fitted in a very normal sort of way with the views of other elderly people with vascular disease who got gangrene more or less at the end of their lives. They didn't want to spend their last few years either coping with an amputation or possibly coping with repeated amputation as the vascular system fails all round the body. So the order was made that the hospital trust shouldn't amputate his foot without his permission.

(BBC, 1995)

In the event, Mr C survived, and his case made UK legal history for two reasons, the first being that the ruling in his case established clear criteria for competence:

(1) Capacity to *comprehend and retain information* about the proposed treatment. Mr C was found to have this capacity, in part because it was shown that in other aspects of everyday prudence, such as budgeting, he was able to take 'sensible' decisions. Further, it was held that what mattered was the narrowly construed ability to comprehend and retain information about this particular decision, on a functional basis, not capacity in some general sense. Given the general presumption of competence in adults, the doctors had to establish that Mr C did not possess this capacity; the court held that this had not been proved.
(2) *Belief* in the validity of the information. It might be thought questionable whether Mr C really believed what the doctors told him; after all, he thought they were torturers. Perhaps he also believed, in his delusions about his own medical 'stardom', that he knew better than the hospital physicians. Nevertheless, the court held that Mr C also met this criterion.
(3) *Ability to weigh up* the information so as to arrive at a choice. Mr C had balanced the risks and benefits differently from the doctors, but that did not invalidate his decision, particularly because an expert witness had testified that many other elderly people came to the same conclusion.

The legal criteria for assessing competence in England and Wales have since changed (with the Mental Capacity Act 2005), but both the ruling in Mr C's case and the new law make the same essential point: competence is decision-specific and a functional matter.

In other words, competence concerns the individual patient's ability to process and use information in making a particular decision – it does not hinge on the patient's more general mental functioning or status. As such, a mentally disordered patient might well be capable of taking particular decisions, and he or she will have the right to have such decisions respected.

Indeed, the second notable feature of Mr C's case was that the judge went so far as to confirm that this right to have one's decisions respected applied even when the patient had become incompetent. This would be the case in a situation where the patient, while competent, had made a clear anticipatory decision about which treatment they would not accept. Thus, although Mr C was found to have fluctuating competence, he had made a clear and competent choice to refuse to submit to amputation – and this decision had to be respected by his doctors. This sort of decision is known as an 'advance directive' or 'living will', and it too has legal backing in many jurisdictions. For example, in England and Wales there is now legislation (the Mental Capacity Act 2005) which sets down when doctors must comply with particular types of advance decisions to refuse treatment. However, even before this law was enforced, it was clear that respect for autonomy entailed respect for advance decisions.

Despite support for advance directives in principle, they still give rise to complicated ethical and practical dilemmas. An advance directive can, as we might expect, take a variety of forms: it may be found in a written document or even in an oral statement, as it was in Mr C's case. The medical journals also reveal that some patients have taken to getting tattoos which indicate their views, an example being the patient who had 'do not resuscitate' etched on her chest (Polack, 2001). Is that a valid, and therefore binding, form of directive?

To answer this question we need to consider the types of conditions that are usually placed on respecting advance decisions:

(1) The directive must have been issued when the patient was *competent.*
(2) The patient must have been sufficiently *informed* before making the directive.
(3) The patient must have made the directive *voluntarily*; that is, they must not have been forced into making the decision.
(4) The directive must *apply* to the situation that has now arisen, and this includes the requirement that

the patient must not have changed their mind since making the directive.

ACTIVITY: Can you think of any problems with these various conditions, either in principle or in how they might work in practice?

Some philosophers think that there is a fundamental conceptual problem with honouring an advance directive, since the doctor seems to be dealing with two different patients: the competent one who made the directive, and the incompetent one they find before them now. This prompts complex philosophical questions about the nature of personal identity – is the doctor dealing with the same patient, such that they should honour the directive? One answer might be to adopt the idea of 'precedent autonomy', and insist that this *is* the same patient, and so their previously stated views offer us the best guide to what we should do (or not do) now that they are incompetent (Davis, 2002).

At a more practical level, doctors and other professionals can find it difficult to decide whether they are really bound by an apparent advance directive. Consider again the tattoo example: can the doctor be sure that this was voluntarily chosen by the patient when they were capable and informed about what the statement might entail? Can he or she be certain that it was not merely decorative in nature? Consider also the seemingly throwaway verbal remarks that we all occasionally make: are these necessarily sufficient as a guide to our long-term wishes? Even written directives need not be as helpful as they first appear: there might always remain genuine doubt as to whether or not they apply in practice, since even the most detailed statement might neglect to cover the one situation (or treatment option) that has now arisen. Indeed, studies show that there will also be sincere disagreements between healthcare professionals as to how a directive should be interpreted and applied in practice (Thompson *et al.*, 2003).

Despite these problems, there will often be occasions when it *is* obvious what a directive should mean, and the doctor's duty to respect autonomy seems to require compliance with it. There should be nothing controversial, in principle, with the authority that an advance directive carries: a patient receiving surgery whilst under general anaesthetic will have given consent in advance of the operation (at least, provided they were competent to do so before receiving the anaesthetic), and it is this enduring consent that gives the surgeon the right to proceed. However, there seems to be a distinction drawn between *authorisation* and *compulsion*; in other words, the patient cannot expect a directive to *compel* the doctors actively to do something, as the English case of Mr Leslie Burke demonstrates (*R* (*on the application of Burke*) v *General Medical Council* [2005] 3 WLR 1132).

The case of Leslie Burke

Mr Burke was suffering from cerebellar ataxia, which meant that his physical condition was deteriorating, but not his mental competence. It seemed that he would at some point need – and he wanted – to receive artificial nutrition and hydration. Guidance had been formulated by the General Medical Council (GMC) in the UK about when life-supporting treatment might, and might not, be offered to patients like Mr Burke, and he feared that the guidance indicated that he would not be eligible to receive artificial food and fluids. He was most concerned that, if he lost his mental competence, the doctors would be entitled to stop (or not start) this treatment, with the effect that his life would come to an end.

Mr Burke approached the court, arguing that the guidance violated his human rights under the European Convention on Human Rights, which had been incorporated directly into English law by the Human Rights Act 1998. Mr Burke specifically objected to the infringement of his right to life, his right to be free from inhuman and degrading treatment, his right to determine what treatment he should receive and his right to equal respect before the law irrespective of any physical or mental disability.

ACTIVITY: Imagine you are the judge hearing Mr Burke's case. Do you agree that his rights are being infringed? Give reasons for and against your decision.

The first judge to hear his case, Mr Justice Munby, ruled that the GMC's guidance was incompatible with the duty to respect Mr Burke's human rights, particularly his autonomous right to decide what treatment he should get and his right not to be treated in an inhuman and degrading manner. This decision seemed to signal that patients had the right to demand – and get – treatment. The GMC appealed against the ruling, and their case was heard in the Court of Appeal, one of the superior courts in the UK.

The judges in the Court of Appeal this time sided with the GMC. These judges did not think there was anything in the guidance to suggest that Mr Burke would be denied artificial nutrition and hydration should he need it, and they ruled that the GMC guidance was entirely lawful. They felt that the arguments presented by Mr Burke and the decision reached by the first judge both went too far, but they did recognize that the rights of patients like Mr Burke demanded respect. The appeal judges therefore confirmed that it would be unlawful (indeed, it would be murder) to withdraw life-support against a competent patient's wishes and that people with disabilities enjoyed the same human rights as non-disabled persons.

This court's decision suggests that there are some limits to respect for autonomy: we can decide, now or for the future, what treatment we will not accept, but we cannot dictate what treatment we will get. This distinction mirrors the one to which we referred earlier: it rests on an apparent difference between omissions (we can insist on what doctors should not do) and positive actions (we cannot insist on what doctors should do). Resource limitations will also determine what an advance directive can specify. Someone dying of kidney failure cannot obtain dialysis or a kidney transplant merely by taking out an advance directive demanding it. The dilemmas associated with resource allocation will be considered again, in detail, in Chapter 8. For now, we will continue to explore the distinction between acts and omissions, as we move, in the next section, to consider more of the issues that arise when a patient lacks autonomy.

Section 4: Withdrawing treatment from incompetent patients

Leslie Burke resisted the idea that he might be denied treatment at a time when he would not be able to communicate his views. Despite the court's reassurance in his case, it is clear that decisions are sometimes made to limit the treatment that could be provided to patients who are incompetent due to age or affliction. Modern medicine's potential for prolonging life can give rise to intense dilemmas about whether it is right to use the new treatments and techniques that have become available. So what should be the goal of medicine in these sorts of cases, and which version of the value of life should guide our thinking? Furthermore, who should get to make the final decision? We might

think, following on from the last section, that the patient's opinions should carry most weight, but in the cases we are now considering the patient is not (or no longer) competent – and they might well not have issued an advance directive. Do we then ask their family members or other loved ones to decide, as was contemplated in Mr R's case? If so, do we only heed the views of someone who has been granted an enduring power of attorney (in other words, made a healthcare proxy, and thereby empowered to decide on the patient's behalf)? What if no such document has been executed? And, in any case, what happens if the family members cannot agree?

These are difficult questions, which have required the attention of judges across the globe. In some of these legal cases, the doctors and the patient's family were in complete agreement about what should happen, as occurred in the famous British case of Anthony Bland. On that occasion, the court decided that it would be lawful for artificially provided nutrition and hydration to be withdrawn from Mr Bland, who was in a persistent vegetative state (PVS) (*Airedale NHS Trust* v *Bland* [1993] 2 WLR 816). The judges felt that continued treatment was no longer in Mr Bland's best interests – indeed, some of them thought that Mr Bland no longer had any interests, given that he appeared no longer to have the ability to feel or experience life in any meaningful sense. This is a controversial idea, not least because recent neuroscientific evidence casts doubt on the idea that patients in a PVS are completely unconscious and insensate (Panksepp *et al.*, 2007). However, as one might expect, the ethical dilemmas become even more acute when the various individuals involved in the care of a seriously unwell patient cannot agree on what should happen. These sorts of dilemmas have unfortunately played out not only in the courts but also in the media (e.g. English *et al.*, 2009). A particularly divisive American case that attracted international attention involved Terri Schiavo, as we describe below.

The Terri Schiavo case

Terri Schiavo was only 26 when she collapsed at home and experienced severe oxygen deprivation (anoxia) for several minutes. She was hospitalized and underwent placement of a percutaneous endoscopic gastrostomy tube (PEG) because she could not swallow. Four months later, with no amelioration of her condition, she was judged to be in a persistent vegetative state.

Under the laws of Flordia, where the Schiavos lived, Terri's husband Michael was appointed her legal guardian, since she was judged incompetent to decide on her own care and had not executed an advance directive. Alongside Terri's parents, Robert and Mary Schindler, Michael worked with the clinicians to try to overcome Terri's condition by means of all available therapies, but after several years there was still no improvement.

At this point Michael Schiavo and the Schindlers began to disagree over what should be done. Michael believed that Terri's condition was irreversible and that she would not have wanted to be kept alive in a persistent vegetative state. Her parents, in contrast, wanted to maintain her artificial hydration and nutrition. The matter was taken to the courts when Michael Schindler petitioned for 'an independent determination of Mrs Schiavo's terminal condition', including 'the decision to continue or discontinue life-prolonging procedures' (cited in Perry *et al.*, 2005, p. 745).

But how firm was the diagnosis of persistent vegetative state? Since the case of Tony Bland, a series of much-publicized examples had appeared to indicate that some minimal degree of function might still be retained by certain patients diagnosed as being in PVS (Andrews *et al.*, 1996; Bauby, 1997). In reply to a subsequent critic who claimed that Terri Schiavo was actually in a 'locked in' state rather than true PVS, however, the bioethicist Art Caplan thundered:

> I would like to have him find three neurologists who agree with that claim. Terri Schiavo suffered anoxia to her brain – twice! Her brain damage was confirmed while she was alive by CAT scan and then at autopsy. She was *blind* despite the alleged tapes that were made showing her tracking objects. Her cortex had shriveled to half its normal mass.
>
> (Caplan, 2009)

In January 2000 a trial was held to settle the issue of Mrs Schiavo's future, with both sides presenting witnesses. The question, presiding Judge Greer said, was whether she would choose to have her artificial feeding and hydration continued if she were competent. Clear evidence of Mrs Schiavo's previously expressed wishes was admissible under Florida law, even if only made orally.

It was held that the diagnosis of PVS in Mrs Schiavo was indeed valid: 'the court found that she met the statutory definition of the persistent vegetative state and that there was no hope of her regaining consciousness or the ability to communicate' (Perry *et al.*, 2005, p. 746). Given that finding, the next issue was how Mrs Schiavo's autonomy rights could be exercised and what her true wishes would have been if she were competent. The trial judge ruled in favour of Mr Schiavo, who had produced three witnesses to affirm that his wife had previously declared 'she would not want to live like that'. The feeding tube was ordered to be removed.

Refusing to accept this outcome, the Schindlers took the case to appeal. By this point their daughter had been diagnosed as being in PVS for 10 years. The appellate court upheld the ruling of the lower court on both clinical and legal grounds, likewise ordering that the feeding tube should be removed.

Before the order could be put into effect, however, the Schindlers presented evidence before a second trial judge from other expert witnesses (none of whom had actually examined Terri) and succeeded in obtaining a further evidentiary hearing. They also claimed that new and better medical treatments for brain damage had become available since the initial trial. The case was referred back to Judge Greer, but he again ruled that Mr Schiavo's experts were more likely to be correct and that the supposed new remedies were not accepted by the mainstream neurological community as having a firm evidence base. On a second appeal in 2002, Judge Greer's decision was scrutinized and upheld as 'a cautious legal standard designed to promote the value of life' (cited in Perry *et al.*, 2005, p. 746). This was the sequel:

> With Terri Schiavo's "personalized decision" determined at the 2000 trial and her medical condition conclusively confirmed at the 2002 hearing, artificial hydration and nutrition were stopped for the second time, on 15 October 2003, pursuant to court order. This order was superseded 6 days later when the Florida legislature passed and Governor Jeb Bush signed Terri's Law, which provided the governor unfettered discretion to order resumption of Mrs. Schiavo's medical treatment.
>
> Eleven months later, the Florida Supreme Court held Terri's Law unconstitutional as a violation of separation of powers, and a third date was set for removal of the PEG tube. On 18 March 2005, the tube was removed for the final time, and despite the intervention of Congress and President George W. Bush, Terri Schiavo's saga ended with her death on 31 March 2005.
>
> (Perry *et al.*, 2005, p. 748)

There are many ethical dimensions to Mrs Schiavo's case and, indeed, much that remains controversial. Consider, for example, the fact that Mrs Schiavo was being fed by a tube – how, if at all, does this differ from gaining hydration and nutrition from spoons and cups? This issue generated much discussion in the wake of the Anthony Bland case. The judges would probably say that the two are quite different – Mrs Schiavo was receiving artificially administered nutrition and hydration, which can be described as a form of medical treatment, and they were only contemplating its withdrawal. This, in turn, recalls the problematic distinction between (positive) actions and (negative) omissions. That distinction seems central to a case like this because few (if any) doctors or judges would be willing to contemplate doing anything beyond stopping Mrs Schiavo's treatment and thereby allowing her to die.

Running throughout the case is also the dilemma over the value of life. The judges essentially defended their decision on the basis that it was respectful of Mrs Schiavo's autonomy. We want to explore further the belief that autonomy provides the best guide in a case like Mrs Schiavo's.

One option for ensuring that the incompetent patient's autonomy endures beyond the point at which they have become incompetent is to provide for the appointment of a healthcare proxy, that is, a surrogate decision-maker. Such was the role that Mr Schiavo took over after his wife's incapacity, but this person can be appointed by the patient when they are competent, and empowered to make decisions for that patient if or when they become incapable of doing so for themselves. This option is available in many American and European states (for example, the Mental Capacity Act 2005 introduced a system of enduring power of attorney into English law for the first time).

However, allowing for the appointment of a healthcare proxy cannot be the end of the matter: as we saw in Mrs Schiavo's case there will still be differences of opinion to deal with, and the proxy will also need some guiding principles for the decisions they will be expected to make. Here, two options are usually discussed: the *best interests* standard and the *substituted judgement* standard. The first of these will involve taking account of the patient's interests, which will necessarily include reference to the salient medical evidence, but might also encompass the patient's wider spiritual, cultural and other personal interests. It may also (but need not) include some reference to what the patient either currently wants (despite their incompetence) or to what they might be likely to have wanted, given the way they conducted their lives prior to becoming incompetent. Once such features are brought into the best interests equation, then it starts to resemble the substituted judgement approach: here, the proxy explicitly tries to decide *as if* they were the patient. In other words, the proxy puts themselves in the patient's shoes.

There are various strengths and weaknesses to the best interests standard and to the substituted judgement standard. As Susan Bailey explains:

> Adherence to the substituted judgement principle protects the self-determination of an incompetent individual in the health care setting by allowing a proxy decision maker to express the patient's preferences as he or she would have done had he or she been able. However, many contingencies impact on this principle that serve to undermine its value in the clinical setting. At times, the substituted judgement principle is open to abuse because it is possible that decisions based on what somebody else views as the patient's best interests will be made covertly under the guise of a substituted judgement.
>
> (Bailey, 2002, p. 491)

Certainly, making a substituted judgement or taking a wide account of a patient's best interests can help to minimize some of the problems of medical bias (and even paternalism) that we mentioned in the earlier discussion of futility. This is not to say that healthcare professionals are necessarily ill-motivated or must necessarily be constrained. In fact, the presence of a proxy can help the doctor to navigate a way through difficult decisions about the burdens and benefits of treatment, and so to set appropriate goals. However, with the proxy come new difficulties and, at worst, new biases, as the proxy can never truly occupy the position of the patient. This will be particularly true if the individual has never been capable of expressing their wishes, such as, for example, when the patient is a young child.

Of course, if the patient is a child, then there is another proxy we can approach – their parent or parents. Once more, however, we must remain alert to the possibility of disagreement and even outright conflict between the family and the healthcare team (e.g. Huxtable and Forbes, 2004). Some professional groups have developed guidance aimed at tackling the specific dilemmas that can arise. One prominent example, first issued in 1997 and updated in 2004, comes from an Ethics Advisory Committee of the Royal College of Paediatrics and Child Health (in England), the summary of which states (RCPCH, 2004):

> There are five situations where it may be ethical and legal to consider withholding or withdrawal of life sustaining medical treatment
>
> (1) The "brain dead" Child: In the older child where criteria of brain-stem death are agreed by two practitioners in the usual way it may still be technically feasible to provide basic cardio-respiratory support by means of ventilation and intensive care. It is agreed within the profession that treatment in such circumstances is futile and the withdrawal of current medical treatment is appropriate.
>
> (2) The "permanent vegetative" state: The child who develops a permanent vegetative state following insults, such as trauma or hypoxia, is reliant on others for all care and does not react or relate with the outside world. It may be appropriate to withdraw or withhold life-sustaining treatment.
>
> (3) The "no chance" situation: The child has such severe disease that life-sustaining treatment simply delays death without significant alleviation of suffering. Treatment to sustain life is inappropriate.
>
> (4) The "no purpose" situation: Although the patient may be able to survive with treatment, the degree of physical or mental impairment will be so great that it is unreasonable to expect them to bear it.
>
> (5) The "unbearable" situation: The child and/or family feel that in the face of progressive and irreversible illness further treatment is more than can be borne. They wish to have a particular treatment withdrawn or to refuse further treatment irrespective of the medical opinion that it may be of some benefit.

In situations that do not fit with these five categories, or where there is uncertainty about the degree of future impairment or disagreement, the child's life should always be safeguarded in the best way possible by all in the Health Care Team, until these issues are resolved.

ACTIVITY: Think back to the three approaches to the value of life we considered in the first section. Where, if at all, do these approaches appear in the guidance from the Royal College of Paediatrics and Child Health? Do you think that the guidance takes the right approach to decision-making in this area?

The principle that underpins this guidance on treating children and young people is actually the same one that often governs the treatment and non-treatment of incompetent adults: that is, the *best interests* of the patient. However, as with adults, it is rarely clear or uncontroversial which approach to the child's best interests will or should be taken. Indeed, the Royal College alludes to the value of life problem that we have been discussing when it recognizes that the duty to act in a child's best interests 'includes sustaining life, and restoring health to an acceptable standard. However there are circumstances in which treatments that merely sustain "life" neither restore health nor confer other benefit and hence are no longer in the child's best interests'.

Hence, the conflict between the intrinsic and the instrumental value of life is rarely that far away from the dilemmas that can arise in this context, as in many others at the end of life. What, though, of respect for autonomy and the role of the proxy? We noticed that this framework seemed to be rather doctor-orientated, with little role for the child, their parents or their family (except under point 5). We should be alert to the distinction that is sometimes assumed to exist between children and adults, which is that children are incompetent, whilst adults are competent. As we will see in Chapter 7 on children and young people, this alleged difference is sometimes reflected in law, but it is a distinction which is open to question and has been challenged by many theorists of childhood. Nevertheless, the physician's concern about the competence of the patient and about the possibility that the relatives' decisions might not be in the patient's best interests is particularly sharply defined in relation to children.

In our view, the least we can do is to ensure that there are mechanisms available for airing and, wherever possible, resolving any disagreements that might arise in caring for the young person, incompetent adult or indeed any patient. This seems to us to be particularly important, given the conflicting views of the value of life and the goals of medicine that we have canvassed throughout this chapter. However, we don't want to imply that it will always be best to refer difficult cases to the courts – but we do think that recourse to mediators, clinical ethics committees and the like can help to ensure that every perspective is taken into account and that a way forward is found (Huxtable and Forbes, 2004). Effective communication is obviously essential to working through ethical dilemmas. Unfortunately, there is always the risk of misunderstanding and miscommunication – as we will see again in the next section.

Section 5: Relief of symptoms at the end of life

As we saw in the previous section, a decision whether or not to treat a seriously ill patient will often depend on an assessment of their best interests. But how are we to judge the best interests of the patient for whom there is, seemingly, little that can be done? In particular, which values and principles should be our guide when the patient is dying? The Royal College of Paediatrics and Child Health, whose guidance we consulted in the previous section, makes the following point:

> The decision to withhold or withdraw life sustaining therapy should always be associated with consideration of the child's overall palliative or terminal care needs. These include symptom alleviation and care, which maintains human dignity and comfort.
>
> (RCPCH, 2004)

Palliative care is a specialty that aims at providing holistic care to patients with advanced, usually terminal, progressive illnesses. Doctors and nurses working in this field may use a range of powerful drugs, including sedatives and also opioids like morphine and diamorphine, to manage symptoms at the end of life. Yet, a question which sometimes arises is, in which circumstances should such drugs be used, given that the drugs themselves can potentially pose risks to the patient's health? Consider the following case.

The case of Jeanette

Jeanette is a 50-year-old woman with widespread disease, including bony metastases [cancer whch has spread to the bones] from a renal [kidney] tumour. Having so far been treated for cancer as an outpatient, she is admitted to hospital when her condition deteriorates. She is in constant pain, even when resting or performing only minimal movements. Radiotherapy has given her some relief from her symptoms, but this was short-lived; she is now receiving high doses of opioid drugs.

Jeanette explains to her doctor, Dr Hearn, that nothing anyone has ever done has made any appreciable difference to her increasing pain. However, she continues to ask for opioids to be provided. Dr Hearn discusses this request with Jeanette and he learns that she is taking the drugs because, although they do not adequately tackle her pain, they do help her to go to sleep.

After consultation with his colleagues on the ward and on the oncology team, Dr Hearn concludes that Jeanette has very few treatment options remaining. She is now very frail and seriously unwell, and Dr Hearn believes that she has only days left to live. He approaches an anaesthetist at the hospital in the hope that she might be able to administer spinal analgesics, which could provide Jeanette with pain relief through a line inserted at the base of her spine. The anaesthetist, Dr Robertson, is unwilling to perform the procedure, since she is concerned about the bed sores that Jeanette has at the base of her back – inserting the line could expose Jeanette to the risk of serious infection.

Dr Hearn is disappointed with the anaesthetist's decision, since he feels that, even if there is a risk of infection, it is more harmful to leave her suffering and in pain throughout her final days. He explains to Jeanette that the only remaining option is to try increasing her analgesics again, which she agrees to. Unfortunately, as is sometimes the case, the opioids cause her to suffer from distressing hallucinations and confusion, while her pain is unrelieved. Dr Hearn decreases the opioids back to the previous level.

Jeanette now says that her situation is so intolerable that she would rather be asleep than awake and in pain. She fully understands that her prognosis is short, and she asks Dr Hearn to sedate her until her death.

ACTIVITY: Do you think Dr Robertson, the anaesthetist, was right to refuse to give Jeanette an epidural? And what do you think Dr Hearn should do now? Imagine that you are in Dr Hearn's position. What would you say to Jeanette? Would you accede to her request? You may find it helpful to write a list of arguments for and against sedating Jeanette.

You are likely to have detected many overlapping, and perhaps even conflicting, ethical dimensions to Jeanette's case. Some of these features will be familiar, such as the extent to which we ought to heed Jeanette's (autonomous?) request and how best we can honour our obligation to treat her in her best interests. You might think, for example, that Dr Robertson, the anaesthetist, was wrong to refuse to give Jeanette a spinal line, if this had the potential to offer the patient some comfort in her final days. Alternatively, you might sympathize with the doctor's decision; after all, wouldn't it be worse to risk causing Jeanette further harm when there was no guarantee that this would provide her with any benefit (and, indeed, when there might be better ways of tackling her symptoms)?

Balancing benefits against harms is an exercise familiar to many healthcare professionals, especially those working in palliative and terminal care. Furthermore, the idea has a long history in Judaeo-Christian thought, particularly in Catholic moral theology, since it features prominently in the doctrine of 'double effect'. The doctrine requires four conditions to be satisfied if a good action with a bad side-effect is to be allowed:

(1) The action, considered by itself and independently of its effects, must not be morally wrong.
(2) The bad effect must not be the means of producing the good effect.
(3) The bad effect must be sincerely unintended, and merely tolerated.
(4) There must be a proportionate reason for performing the action in spite of its bad potential consequences.

(Veatch, 1989)

It seems to us that the anaesthetist could have applied the principle of double effect and concluded that it was acceptable to administer the epidural. There is nothing morally wrong with administering pain relief, in itself; indeed, it is morally good to relieve others' suffering. Any infection that might result, whilst obviously 'bad', is clearly not the means by which Jeanette would be relieved of her pain. The anaesthetist – particularly one so initially reluctant to risk causing an infection – would seem to be genuinely aiming at relieving Jeanette's symptoms. Finally, using this form of pain relief looks eminently proportionate: no other analgesics had worked for Jeanette, and her very short

prognosis might suggest that it is worth running the risk of infection if it means her final days are as pain-free as possible.

Of course, this anaesthetist, in good conscience, was unwilling to risk harming the patient. This left Jeanette feeling that the only option for her was sedation until her death. It is actually in this sort of situation – where dealing with the patient's symptoms might mean shortening their life – that the doctrine of double effect tends to be applied:

> According to the principle of 'double effect' it is sometimes perfectly proper if one's conduct *unintentionally* has the effect of shortening, or of not lengthening, life. For example, the doctor who, with the intention of easing pain, administers morphine to a terminally ill cancer patient may foresee that this will shorten the patient's life. But the shortening of life is merely an *unintended side-effect* of the doctor's intention to alleviate pain, and there is a very good reason (namely the alleviation of pain) for allowing that bad side-effect to happen. He is not attacking the patient's life but the patient's pain.
>
> Similarly, a doctor may sometimes properly withhold or withdraw treatment even though the doctor foresees that the patient's life will be shorter than it would be with the treatment. [In this view] a doctor is under no duty to administer (and patients are fully entitled to refuse) disproportionate treatments, that is, treatments which would either offer no reasonable hope of benefit or would involve excessive burdens on the patient. Even if the doctor foresees that the patient's life will not be as long without the treatment as it would have been with it, the patient's earlier death is merely an *unintended side-effect* of the doctor's intention to withhold or withdraw a disproportionate treatment.

(Keown, 1997)

ACTIVITY: What do you consider to be the strengths and weaknesses of this argument? Think back to the case of Mr R. Do you think the principle can have any relevance there?

Some bioethicists have difficulty accepting the principle of double effect and particularly its use in terminal care. For one thing, the principle requires us to draw some pretty fine lines between what we consider to be 'intended effects', as opposed to 'unintended side-effects'. It is, of course, impossible to climb inside someone else's mind in order to find out what they are really thinking. The problem, say some critics, is that the principle places too much trust in the doctor because it asks us to take his or her word that the 'bad' side-effect was merely foreseen and not intended. And, in any case, why should it be an agent's intention, and this alone, which determines the morality of their action – surely we should not be so willing to ignore 'bad' effects when we attribute moral responsibility?

Critics also note how the principle needs prior definitions of what is to count as a 'good' and a 'bad' effect before it can be put to work. Proponents of the principle will say, in line with the idea that life is intrinsically valuable, that life is a good. But why should we accept the view that death is necessarily a 'bad' outcome? If such a view can only really be defended on theological grounds, then it seems that someone who does not hold the relevant beliefs might have just cause for rejecting the principle. It is better, say the critics, to acknowledge what the principle really involves: they think that it really rests on the idea that death can, sometimes, be a beneficial outcome (Singer, 1993).

ACTIVITY: What do you make of these criticisms of the principle? Can you think of any persuasive counter-arguments?

Defenders of the principle of double effect hold to the idea that death can be a 'bad' outcome. They argue that the intrinsic value of life is not only or simply a theological construct – on rational reflection we should all be able to see that life is valuable in this way, but that there are also limits on what we can and should do to preserve life. As such, the principle of double effect helps to clarify the scope, and limits, of our duty to preserve life. This is essentially a deontological position, being most concerned with duties and rights, and it is worth noting that many critics of double effect are more inclined towards consequentialist thinking, in which outcomes matter most. However, defenders of the principle are also mindful of consequences – and particularly the potentially disastrous consequences of doing away with the principle, because they fear that this will leave patients to die in suffering and distress.

These defenders also think that there are many occasions when it *is* possible to identify a person's true intention and to distinguish this from what they merely foresee but do not intend. If a doctor injected a major dose of a drug that has no therapeutic properties but can only end life, then it would be relatively easy to

establish what his intention was – he intended to kill. If the drug in question *does* have the relevant therapeutic properties, then we can still seek to infer the doctor's intention by looking at the magnitude and timing of the doses given.

An alternative way of establishing the true intention involves considering how the doctor would feel if the patient survived the administration of a pain-relieving drug. If the doctor is not disappointed when the unintended side-effect (death) fails to occur, it really is unintended. That is, if the patient's pain is relieved, and the patient does *not* die, the doctor genuinely abiding by the principle of double effect should be pleased rather than disappointed. He or she has truly intended the good effect and merely tolerated the possibility of the bad one. All the doctor needs to do before administering the drug is ask themselves: will I feel that I have failed to do what I have set out to do if the patient does not die after receiving this drug?

You might therefore think that there are good arguments for and against the doctrine of double effect. Of course, its success or failure can also be judged according to its ability to deal with moral problems in practice. Here, it is notable that many healthcare professionals consider the principle of double effect to be essential to the practice of good medicine. Indeed, a survey of UK nurses in 2000 revealed that 94% of respondents agreed that 'sometimes it is appropriate to give pain medication to relieve suffering, even if it may hasten a patient's death' (Dickenson, 2000).

This is not to say that the doctrine is universally supported by healthcare professionals. Other nurses have expressed serious concerns about the ways in which the principle operates in practice, implying that it might in reality be used to conceal euthanasia (House of Lords Select Committee, 1994). That there is split opinion amongst healthcare professionals undoubtedly reflects the conflicting views that bioethicists have about the validity of the principle. However, these disagreements might also arise from confusion about how the principle really applies in practice.

The scientific literature tells us that there are many myths surrounding opioids that are not substantiated by clinical evidence and experience. It is true that drugs like morphine carry potentially serious side-effects, including nausea, vomiting and respiratory depression. It is precisely because morphine has the potential to stop a person's breathing – and therefore end their life – that the principle of double effect has been applied. However, the risk tends to be over-stated: as two experts in palliative care explain, 'pain is the physiological antagonist of the respiratory effects of opioid analgesics' (Hanks and Twycross, 1984). As such, this risk is very unlikely to materialize in patients with pain, since the pain will cancel out the danger of slowing (or stopping) the patient's breathing. Other studies show that, when they are used appropriately, opioids will have no effect on a patient's life expectancy (Sykes and Thorns, 2003).

ACTIVITY: Given these arguments, do you see any role for the principle of double effect in palliative medicine? Consider when the principle might, and might not, be useful in practice. How, for example, might it apply to Jeanette's request for sedation?

Although the risks have been overstated, studies do confirm that there is still a role for the principle of double effect to play in defending the practices undertaken in palliative medicine. Two examples tend to be given. In the first example, the patient requiring pain relief is already enduring breathing difficulties. In this case, it is clear that morphine must be used cautiously since the drug could further interfere with the patient's ability to breathe – here, then, there is a role for the principle of double effect.

In the second example, the focus shifts from opioids to sedative drugs, and so to Jeanette's case. In this case, it is clear that the clinicians would have to proceed cautiously, and aim to use a dose of sedation that would not obviously shorten life – otherwise we might well doubt what their intentions really were. But even if they do this, it is not always certain whether a particular dose might shorten an already short prognosis. For this reason the principle of double effect can offer moral support; indeed some doctors argue it is vital in order to provide symptom control with the aim of lessening suffering in complex end-of-life situations.

But we also need to recognize that the principle will only really be called into service if the 'bad' effect (death) materializes and it looks like the doctor's actions were the cause of this. In cases like Jeanette's there is often no reason to think that the drug, and not the disease, was the cause of death. Say that Jeanette was sedated and that she died 3 days later. In such circumstances it seems most likely that her death was 'natural' – the sedative drugs did not appear to affect her prognosis. As such, Dr Hearn and colleagues would need to remember the principle of double effect

when they decide to embark on sedation but, in hindsight, they should be reassured that the double effect did not even materialize.

This does not mean we can say that the principle will *never* be needed in cases of so-called 'terminal sedation'. It seems to acquire most relevance when the patient is not only sedated but also has food and fluids withheld. In a case like Jeanette's it appears implausible to claim that the removal of these (apparent) essentials for life would affect her life expectancy: put bluntly, she would not starve to death within 3 days or so. But if she had had a much longer prognosis, say a matter of months, one must query whether it would be appropriate to sedate her and refrain from giving her nutrition and hydration (Jansen and Sulmasy, 2002).

The principle of double effect *might* be called into service in this latter case, particularly if the patient dies sooner than was otherwise expected and it looks like the lack of food and fluid was the true cause of their demise (Huxtable, 2008). However, this is a murky area for the principle, where we should be mindful of the critics' complaint that the principle relies too heavily on how the particular action is described (and by whom). Consider, then, what the doctor's intention would be in such a situation – is it to relieve symptoms (if so, is sedation for weeks or months a necessary or proportionate response to suffering?) or, is it really designed to bring about an earlier death for the patient?

Doctors who (directly) aim at bringing about an earlier death for their patient are obviously operating outside the terms of the principle of double effect. In some jurisdictions, they might bring about an earlier death through euthanasia, which is our next topic.

Section 6: Euthanasia and physician-assisted suicide

According to supporters of the principle of double effect, there is a vast difference between a doctor acting to relieve symptoms, even if he or she foresees that this will shorten life, and a doctor acting with the intention to end their patient's life. In the latter case, the doctor's action might be described as 'euthanasia' if they perform the final, fatal act or 'assisted suicide' if they supply the patient with the means or the information they need to perform that final action themselves.

The ethical, and practical, arguments surrounding these practices are amongst the most difficult that arise in relation to care at the end of life. Do they represent an affront to, or the ultimate expression of, the value of human life? Can they ever be considered a rightful part of the goals of medicine? Or do they violate the moral integrity of medicine (Singer and Siegler, 1990; Pellegrino, 1992; Momeyer, 1995)? Can the best interests of the patient extend to ceasing to exist, or is that logically impossible? Is trust in the medical profession so radically undermined if doctors are allowed to kill that we ought to rule euthanasia and physician-assisted suicide out altogether? Or does the possibility of euthanasia and of assisted suicide where suffering is intractable actually meet what patients want?

Throughout the world, these questions are constantly being debated by bioethicists, healthcare professionals and patients, and, in some jurisdictions, the case for allowing euthanasia and physician-assisted suicide has been accepted. Jurisdictions including Oregon, Belgium and (for a short time) the Northern Territories of Australia have all allowed doctors to engage in practices designed to shorten life, but – as we shall see – it is in the Netherlands that these practices are most well-established – and most fiercely debated.

Elsewhere in the world it is generally the case that neither a doctor nor anyone else is lawfully entitled to put an early end to a patient's suffering. Indeed, the prohibition has led to so-called 'assisted suicide tourism', in which patients have travelled from their prohibitive home states to Switzerland, in order to take up the option of assistance in suicide made available there by the organization 'Dignitas' (Huxtable, 2009). However, for many patients, travelling will neither be a practical nor a desirable option, and some of these patients have chosen to challenge the prohibition that operates in their home territory. This famously occurred in England in the case of Diane Pretty (No 2346/02 *Pretty* v *UK* [2002] 35 EHRR 1).

The case of Diane Pretty

Diane Pretty had motor neurone disease, a condition that progressively attacks the sufferer's muscles, leaving them increasingly dependent on others to perform even the most basic tasks. Although she had, in her own words, 'fought this disease each step of the way', Mrs Pretty felt that her prognosis was bleak and she was especially concerned at the possibility that she might suffocate in the final stages of her life (Dyer, 2002).

Rather than succumb to increasing dependency and a possibly distressing demise, Diane Pretty wished to obtain assistance in committing suicide, which her husband Brian was willing to provide. However, the law in England clearly condemns any such assistance: whilst suicide itself is lawful, assisting suicide is a crime that (according to the Suicide Act 1961) carries a maximum penalty of 14 years' imprisonment. Rather than risk her husband being convicted and incarcerated, Mrs Pretty wanted confirmation from a legal official that no action would be taken against him. The official in question, the Director of Public Prosecutions, declined to make any such statement and so Mrs Pretty approached the courts in an attempt to demonstrate that the legal prohibition on assisted suicide violated her human rights.

Mrs Pretty insisted that her rights were being infringed in five ways. First, she claimed that her right to life granted her the right to determine when her life could come to an end – that is, the right to life was a right that she could waive. Secondly, she argued that the state prohibition on assisted suicide meant that she was being forced to endure an inhuman and degrading existence. Thirdly, the right to personal autonomy or privacy entailed that her autonomous decision to die be respected. Fourthly, Mrs Pretty argued that she had a right to freedom of thought and that, as such, her right to believe in the justifiability of assisted suicide should translate into her (and her husband) being free to act in accordance with this belief. Finally, Mrs Pretty pointed to the right to be free from unjust discrimination; since able-bodied persons were freely entitled to commit suicide, Mrs Pretty argued that she – as a disabled person – was being treated unfairly by the law.

ACTIVITY: What would you decide if you were the judge in Mrs Pretty's case? Think of reasons for and against your decision.

Mrs Pretty's case reached the (then) highest court in England, the House of Lords. The five Law Lords decided, unanimously, that the prohibition on assisted suicide did not infringe Mrs Pretty's rights (or indeed anyone else's).

The right to life, they explained, did not encompass a 'right to die'; indeed, this would be contrary to the very purpose of the right, which was to uphold the sanctity of human life. Moreover, the Law Lords were not convinced that it was the legal policy (and therefore the UK government) which was the cause of Mrs Pretty's suffering - the true cause of this was her disease, and the only obligation owed by the state was a duty to ensure that her suffering was adequately alleviated (which fell short of enabling her to have her life ended).

The judges were even less persuaded by Mrs Pretty's arguments about freedom of thought. Just because Mrs Pretty believed that assisted suicide was morally justified did not mean that the state had to recognize her right to engage in this. The Law Lords further rejected the idea that Mrs Pretty was being unjustly dealt with by the law, not least since they found no (legal) support for the idea that the decriminalization of suicide amounted to a legal 'right' to commit suicide.

The House of Lords also resisted Mrs Pretty's seemingly central claim that her decision ought to be respected since it was autonomously reached. Respect for autonomy, they reasoned, only entitled an individual to be free in the way they lived their life – and the right did not extend to seeking its ending. The judges added that, even if they were wrong about this, there were important social interests at stake (like the preservation of the sanctity of life) that justified placing limits on what an autonomous individual could do.

Mrs Pretty was neither impressed with the Law Lords' decision nor deterred from advancing her cause. Using the same human rights arguments, she approached the European Court of Human Rights in Strasbourg. Once again, and for the final time, Mrs Pretty's case failed. However, the European court differed from the English court in one respect: it was willing to concede that Mrs Pretty *did* have a right to respect for her autonomous decisions, even a decision to die. It nevertheless concluded that it was for the UK government to decide whether there were more important social interests at stake that prevented the right from prevailing.

Mrs Pretty succumbed to her disease less than two weeks after she had lost her case in Strasbourg. Unfortunately, she appears to have endured the very breathing difficulties that she had fought to avoid (Dyer, 2002).

Mrs Pretty's case attracted a wealth of commentary, both in the international media and in the specialist journals. Her case was slightly unusual in that she was seeking to ensure that her husband would be free to help her commit suicide. Bioethicists and lawmakers worldwide are more familiar with considering when, if ever, it is permissible for a *doctor* to help a patient to die.

But what do we mean by 'help a patient to die'? (Huxtable, 2007, pp. 4–9; see also Garrard and Wilkinson, 2005; Doyal, 2006) At its (Greek) root, the word 'euthanasia' roughly translates as 'good death' – yet, we might rightly feel that this encompasses much more than bringing a deliberate end to a life of suffering, which is what the word nowadays usually suggests. Despite this, it tends to be cases like Mrs Pretty's that generate most discussion. In particular, it is common to find attention focused on one of two practices:

(1) Assisted suicide and (unlike Mrs Pretty's case) particularly physician-assisted suicide. Here, the doctor provides the means of committing suicide (for example, a prescription for a lethal dose of medicine), or otherwise provides guidance and counselling on doses and methods. Although the physician may be present at the end, he or she does not perform the final act: the patient does.

(2) Voluntary euthanasia. Here, we tend to think of a doctor administering a lethal drug injection or other agent, at the (autonomous) patient's request. As such, it is the doctor who performs the final act that results in a patient's death.

Both of these practices find a place in Dutch policies, dating back to the 1970s. Having been developed in medical guidelines and court decisions, the Dutch law was placed on a statutory footing in 2001. André Janssen outlines the main components of the current law (Janssen, 2002, p. 263):

[T]he patient:
- holds the conviction that there was no other reasonable solution for the situation he was in;

and the doctor:
- holds the conviction that the request by the patient was voluntary and well-considered
- holds the conviction that the patient's suffering was lasting and unbearable
- has informed the patient about the situation he was in and about his prospects
- has consulted at least one other, independent, doctor who has seen the patient and has given his written opinion on the requirements of due care
- has terminated a life or assisted in a suicide with due care.

The 'due care' criteria to which Janssen refers are (Janssen, 2002, p. 261):

- The patient's request must be voluntary, well-considered and durable.
- According to informed medical opinion, the patient must be in an unbearable state of suffering for which there is no foreseeable cure.
- The doctor involved must consult at least one other independent doctor.
- The ending of life must be performed with all due medical care.

ACTIVITY: Which ethical principles do you think underlie this law? Do you see any difficulties in applying the Dutch legal requirements?

Jurriaan de Haan has convincingly argued that the Dutch justification of euthanasia rests on either of two views:

> On the one view, The Pure Autonomy View (TPAV), the justification of euthanasia rests solely on the principle of respect for autonomy. That is, the reason for performing and permitting euthanasia is the patient's voluntary, well-considered and sustained, in one word: autonomous, request for euthanasia. On the alternative view, The Joint View (TJV), the principle of respect for autonomy and the principle of beneficence morally justify euthanasia together. That is, euthanasia is ethical if and partly because, since the patient is suffering unbearably and hopelessly, euthanasia is in his interest.
>
> (de Haan, 2002, p. 154)

As to how easy it is to translate the principles into practice, we believe that the requirement to consult with an independent doctor will be the least problematic, and the easiest to prove or disprove in practice (although we will shortly consider a case in which this presented a stumbling block for the doctor performing euthanasia). The other criteria all seemed problematic to us for different reasons:

(1) Full information is almost never available: no one can say for certain how long the patient will have to suffer. It is largely in B-grade films that doctors give a definite estimate such as 'You only have six months to live'.

(2) The same caveat applies to 'unbearable' suffering and to the absence of 'reasonable' solutions. The palliative care movement would probably say that there is more that can be done to tackle the patient's suffering, both physical and mental.

(3) The absence of 'reasonable' solutions also begs the question, insofar as the existence of euthanasia itself contaminates this decision. If it weren't available, the patient couldn't rule out other alternatives. Indeed, we might ask whether the patient should be expected to receive palliative care if they do not want this – is that 'unreasonable'?

(4) How do we judge whether the doctor's influence lessens the voluntariness of the action? And what about patients who are unable to give a voluntary consent, because they are in a coma? Should they be candidates for euthanasia (Manninen, 2006)? According to the Dutch law, euthanasia is by definition *voluntary*. This suggests that it will be hard to talk of any other form of euthanasia occurring in the Dutch context. Yet, the data that are available suggest that other forms of euthanasia *are* occurring. Research suggests that euthanasia is more common than physician-assisted suicide: about 2.4% of deaths have resulted from euthanasia, against 0.3% from physician-assisted suicide. This is not necessarily problematic in itself, since both seem to rest on the voluntary request or consent of the patient. However, in 0.7% of cases, life was ended *without* the explicit, concurrent request of the patient (Van der Maas *et al.*, 1996). In many of these cases the patient was comatose or otherwise incapable of making a request. The Dutch Remmelink Commission of 1992 estimated that up to 1000 instances of euthanasia every year were unasked for, and that some of these included competent patients. This is a frightening statistic, and, if accurate, a powerful argument against euthanasia.

Even if we restrict our analysis to deaths that *are* voluntarily sought by the patients, then we might still find our thinking severely tested by the ways in which the Dutch law has developed. In the following paper, Ron Berghmans, whose work we introduced in the first section, outlines one of the most controversial cases by first explaining how the Dutch policy was originally applied.

Physician-assisted suicide in the case of mental suffering

Ron Berghmans[2]

These ['due care'] requirements were developed in the context of persons suffering from a terminal, or at least fatal or incurable, disease, such as patients with advanced cancer (Gevers, 1995). In the 1980s and 1990s, through a series of court decisions, reports and opinions from bodies such as the Dutch Society of Psychiatrists, the Royal Dutch Society of Medicine, the Inspectorate for Mental Health, and the Dutch Association for Voluntary Euthanasia, attention was extended to the issue of physician-assisted suicide for psychiatric patients. Lower courts took the view that in exceptional circumstances, assisting a mentally ill person to commit suicide might be acceptable practice.

The case of Dr Chabot

A landmark in this respect has been the so-called Chabot case (Griffiths, 1995). The defendant was a psychiatrist named Boudewyn Chabot, who in September 1991 supplied to Mrs Boomsma, at her request, lethal drugs which she consumed in the presence of the defendant, her GP, and a friend. She died half an hour later.

Mrs Boomsma was 50 years old; she had married at 22, but from the beginning the marriage was unhappy. In 1986 her eldest son committed suicide. From that time on her marital problems grew worse and her husband more violent; her wish to die began to take shape, but she said that she remained alive only to care for her younger son. In 1988 she left her husband, taking her younger son with her. In 1990 her son was admitted to hospital in connection with a traffic accident, and was found to be suffering from cancer, from which he died in May 1991. That same evening Mrs Boomsma attempted suicide with drugs she had put by, but did not die. She then approached the Dutch Association for Voluntary Euthanasia, which put her in touch with Dr Chabot.

Mrs Boomsma was diagnosed as suffering from an adjustment disorder, consisting of a depressed mood, without psychotic signs, in the context of a complicated bereavement process. Although her condition was in principle treatable, treatment would probably have been protracted and the chance of success small. But she rejected therapy, despite Dr Chabot's best efforts to persuade her. He became convinced that she was experiencing intense, long-term psychic suffering which was unbearable for her, and which held out no prospect of improvement. Her request for assistance with suicide in his opinion was well-considered. In letters and discussion with him, she presented the reasons for her decision clearly and consistently, showing that she understood her situation and the consequences of her decision. In his judgement, her rejection of therapy was also well-considered. Chabot consulted seven experts. None of them believed that there was any realistic chance of success, given Mrs Boomsma's clear refusal of treatment.

In its ruling of 21 June 1994, the Dutch Supreme Court used the Chabot case to clarify a number of important issues in the euthanasia debate. First, it held that assistance with suicide was justified in the case of a patient whose suffering is not somatic, and who is not in the terminal phase of an illness – but only if the physician has acted 'with the utmost carefulness'. The court took the view that what matters is the seriousness of the patient's suffering, not its source.

Secondly, the court stated that it was incorrect, as a general legal proposition, to claim that a psychiatric patient's request for assistance with suicide cannot be voluntary. A person's wish to die can be based on an autonomous judgement, even in the presence of mental illness.

ACTIVITY: How does this judgement compare with the case of Mr C we considered in the third section of this chapter?

The basic proposition appears similar on the surface: both courts agree that mental illness does not in itself bar a patient from making a valid medical decision. If you believe that killing is different from letting die, however, the Chabot case is more serious: Dr Chabot was being asked not to refrain from doing everything which could be done, but to actively assist Mrs Boomsma in her suicide – an act rather than an omission. There is also considerable doubt about whether Mrs Boomsma actually was mentally ill, or simply grief-stricken – whereas there is no doubt that Mr C was the victim of gross psychotic delusions. Finally, in English mental health law a patient is allowed to refuse treatment for a physical disorder, but not treatment for mental disorder. The C case is consistent with that principle. Mrs Boomsma, however, had rejected treatment designed to mitigate her depression, that is, treatment concerning her mental health. It is certainly arguable that if she was adjudged mentally ill, she should have been forcibly treated by antidepressant medication. If she was not mentally ill, but rather deeply bereaved and yet sane, there were no medical grounds for assisting her suicide. Berghmans resumes the story.

The Supreme Court also took the view that a patient's condition cannot be considered hopeless if he or she freely rejects a meaningful treatment option. In such a case, assisted suicide is not justified. The difficult question is what counts as a meaningful option. The court followed the viewpoint of a committee of the Dutch Royal College of Medicine, which laid down the following three conditions:

- the patient's condition can be alleviated if proper treatment is given, on current medical opinion
- alleviation is possible within a reasonable time period
- the relationship of benefits to burdens of treatment should be proportionate.

Finally, the Supreme Court took the view that an independent expert must be consulted on all relevant aspects of the case, and must himself examine the patient before assistance with suicide can be given. This was the respect in which Chabot was adjudged to have failed. The seven experts whom he consulted had not themselves examined the patient. Therefore Chabot was convicted by the Court, although he was given a suspended sentence. After the Supreme Court decision, Chabot was also cautioned by the Dutch Medical Council, which took the view that he should have considered treating his patient with antidepressants, even if she refused consent.

The implication of the Dutch Medical Council ruling is that most psychiatrists would have treated Mrs Boomsma with antidepressants, and that Dr Chabot's decision was aberrant practice. Indeed, the available data have implied that requests for physician-assisted suicide are rarely granted in psychiatric practice (Groenewoud et al., 1997). As Berghmans notes:

After the Supreme Court's ruling in the Chabot case, the Dutch Society of Psychiatrists established a committee to advise on guidelines for dealing with requests for assisted suicide by patients who suffer from mental illness. The committee began from the following premise:
- A request for assistance in suicide in someone with mental illness ought to be assumed to be a request for help. The presumption should be that suicidal wishes are a sign of psychopathology, in the first instance, requiring suicide prevention, not suicide assistance.

ACTIVITY: Compare this premise with the argument made below by two medically trained practising psychoanalysts from Italy, Raffaele Bracalenti and Emilio Mordini (Bracalenti and Mordini, 1997).

A request for suicide assistance from a terminally ill patient should always be considered a reflection of bad practice. There is something wrong with the diagnostic or therapeutic process which has led to such a strong refusal to carry on with life.

Bracalenti and Mordini do not confine their statement to patients with mental illness: that is a key difference from the Dutch guidelines. However, in both cases clinicians are advised to make a prima facie assumption against honouring a request for suicide. But the Dutch psychiatrists' association goes on to state that

- Suicidality should not a priori be considered as a psychopathological phenomenon. Although many death wishes in mentally ill people have a temporary, transitory character, in exceptional cases a request for suicide assistance may be the result of a careful weighing process, and may be enduring.
- In exceptional cases, physician-assisted suicide may be responsible practice, but it can never be a general duty. Individual psychiatrists have no moral or legal obligation to practise assisted suicide, although they do have a duty to deal responsibly and carefully with every request for suicide assistance.

ACTIVITY: What does this imply about the goals of medicine? Think back to one of the original premises with which this chapter began, that the principal goal of medical care at the end of life is the relief of suffering.

Throughout this section we have been testing that premise to the utmost, by asking whether there is a duty in cases of hopeless and unbearable suffering to relieve that suffering by assisting the patient to die. On this alternative view, relieving suffering by assisting suicide is not part of the *telos* of medicine; rather, the proper goal is to deal carefully and responsibly with any request for suicide, and thereby to take the patient and her suffering seriously.

The problem that arises here is that it can be very difficult to define 'suffering', particularly the degree of 'suffering' that we might think legitimates performing euthanasia. This issue came to the fore again in a later case from the Netherlands, involving Dr Sutorius and Mr Brongersma. Richard Huxtable and Maaike Möller outline the main features of the case:

In April 1998, Dr Philip Sutorius assisted 86-year-old Edward Brongersma to commit suicide. Brongersma was motivated by 'life fatigue' or 'existential suffering', and had no somatic or psychiatric medical condition. Sutorius was prosecuted for failing to observe one of the 'due care criteria' on which the Dutch policy was based, namely that he should, on reasonable grounds, 'be satisfied that the suffering is unbearable and that there is no prospect of improvement'.

(Huxtable and Möller, 2007, p. 118)

This case went all the way to the Dutch Supreme Court, where the general practitioner's conviction was upheld: the court felt that being 'tired of life' was insufficient reason to perform euthanasia within the Dutch law (Sheldon, 2003). However, Huxtable and Möller think that this sort of euthanasia *cannot* convincingly be ruled out *in principle*:

> Once voluntary euthanasia as performed by a doctor is allowed, then it may be difficult to draw a principled line restricting this to (seemingly) straightforward cases of 'medical' suffering. This is because the key ethical principles at stake, autonomy and beneficence, at least as understood in the Netherlands, do not preclude a situation in which one 'merely' 'tired of life' is assisted to die. Those opposed to voluntary euthanasia may draw upon the inviolability of life; those sympathetic to that practice but otherwise resistant to the *Brongersma* end-point may only avail themselves of so-called 'practical' or empirical objections. Although these latter arguments have often been discredited in the literature, *Brongersma* surely gives us reason to pause.

(Huxtable and Möller, 2007, p. 126)

This particular debate is far from over in the Netherlands: following a three-year inquiry, the Royal Dutch Medical Association concluded that doctors *can* help patients who seek assistance in dying because they are 'suffering through living' (Sheldon, 2005).

The cases of Mrs Boomsma and Mr Brongersma surely require us to think twice about the rights (and wrongs) of allowing euthanasia. Indeed, they seem to illustrate the 'slippery slope' problem about euthanasia and physician-assisted suicide, which is one of the 'practical' or 'empirical' problems to which Huxtable and Möller referred. This is because it seems unlikely that either sort of case was envisioned when the current guidelines were first established (Keown, 2002). Have the Dutch gone too far? Within the Netherlands, the Chabot case occasioned widespread doubts to that effect. Outside the country, some commentators even surmised the Chabot case demonstrated that euthanasia and physician-assisted suicide risk becoming a kind of social control and medical abuse (Bracalenti and Mordini, 1997). The same might be said following the

Sutorius case. If neither 'patient' had a 'medical' problem, this argument runs, it becomes clear that the doctors' actions instantiate social rather than medical judgements.

Terminal illness, however, had never been a requirement in the Dutch system, and it can certainly be argued that mental suffering is no less unendurable than physical pain. Although mental illness may undermine autonomy and competence – thereby casting the request for euthanasia from a mentally ill person into doubts about validity – it does not automatically make the decision to refuse treatment invalid, as we saw in the case of Mr C.

On the other hand, by focusing on the doctor's duties rather than the patient's competence, it becomes irrelevant as to whether Mrs Boomsma's illness was mental or physical. As one of his critics pointed out at the Dutch Medical Association hearing, if Mrs Boomsma was mentally well enough to make a valid request for physician-assisted suicide, Dr Chabot, as a psychiatrist, should not have been acting in the first place. (Although he also viewed himself as her friend, he would have had no access to the lethal drugs if he were acting merely in his private capacity.) If Mrs Boomsma was mentally ill, Dr Chabot's duty was to cure her mental illness rather than assist her suicide. In fact Dr Chabot recognized that Mrs Boomsma was not mentally ill; the 'illness' from which she suffered was intractable grief. But that takes us back to the question of whether euthanasia was intended as a 'remedy' for human tragedy – a question that we squarely confront in the context of Mr Brongersma, not least given the supportive conclusion reached by the Dutch Medical Association on his sort of case. Surely this was not the intention behind the law – and, if not, then both cases show that the Dutch have indeed slid too far down the slope.

A different sort of argument against euthanasia and physician-assisted suicide draws attention to the regrettable practical consequences of focusing on its legalization, rather than pressing for improvements in palliative care. This view, typical of the hospice movement, asserts that proponents of euthanasia and assisted suicide encourage the widespread public misapprehension that nothing can be done about suffering at the end of life except to end it by death. This is pernicious, they argue, and indeed ethically wrong. Others, drawing on the deontological perspective, will resist the very way that the argument for permitting euthanasia is constructed. They will say that the duty to relieve suffering in no way implies a duty to kill. The American bioethicist Daniel Callahan gives a striking summary of this protest: 'Your right to die doesn't imply my duty to kill'.

Section 7: The values and goals of medicine revisited

Throughout this chapter we have encountered a range of ethical dilemmas, which might arise at the end of life and, indeed, in other areas of healthcare. Very often these dilemmas have required us to find ways of navigating through competing opinions on the value of life and about the proper goals of medicine. As we have seen, sometimes it will be possible to reach clarity and consensus on the conceptual and ethical issues; at other times it will not. During the course of this chapter we have examined the refusal of treatment by competent patients, the withdrawal of treatment from incompetent patients, the use of powerful drugs in relieving symptoms, and the practices known as euthanasia and assisted suicide. In examining these topics we hope to have provided a wide-ranging investigation into the *telos* of medicine at the end of life and the ethical implications of such decisions and situations.

We would like you to conclude your reading of this chapter with a personal account by Ron Berghmans, written from a very different point of view from his two other articles in this chapter: that of his own experience of serious illness. Berghmans courageously and sensitively considers what his own case taught him about the values of medicine and the value of life.

Illness, pain, suffering and the value of life

Ron Berghmans

Introduction

Ethical issues related to end-of-life care concern philosophical questions about the goal(s) of medicine, and the place of pain, suffering and the value and meaning of life of the patient. The story of my illness experience and recovery as a cancer patient, on which the following is based, contains three parts: the first encompasses the period from complaint to final diagnosis (October 2003–July 2004); the second the period of treatment, recovery, relapse, and repeated and more intensive treatment and recovery (July 2004–April 2006). The third is the one from 'definite' recovery until the present time. In that period I suffered a stroke from which I recovered quickly and with only slight residual effects.

My personal story of illness, pain and suffering and the corresponding experience of life's meaning and value started in the autumn of 2003. At that time the chronic back pain which I experienced in the lower parts of my back was increasing. As this was different from normal – I had been used to chronic back pain for a great part of my life – late in October I turned to my general practitioner. She diagnosed the back pain as 'functional' and 'non-specific' and prescribed pain-killers. Her advice was not to work too hard ...

As the pain kept increasing, after a few weeks I returned to the general practitioner. Now she prescribed different pain killers which had as little effect as the previous ones. As my condition worsened, I had a third consultation during which I expressed my wish to have X-rays of my back. Only very reluctantly and after much pressure did my GP agree to refer me to a radiologist in the academic hospital. X-rays of my lower back showed no real and serious anomalies, although there was some minor pathology at the vertebrae. It appeared that my GP was content to see these particularities as the possible (probable) causes of my pain. Nevertheless, my situation kept worsening as there was no therapy available to better my condition.

After consultations with different other medical professionals, finally – it was July 2004, so more than half a year after the first consultation with the GP – an assistant neurosurgeon decided to scan the whole of my back with MRI. On the basis of this scan it appeared that there was a process to be seen halfway down my spinal cord. After taking a biopsy it was concluded that I suffered from malignant B-cell non-Hodgkin lymphoma and that it was localized in the abdomen and the bone marrow. This last detail explained the seriousness of the pain I suffered.

The shock of a fatal diagnosis   It is often said that a cancer diagnosis is experienced as a 'death sentence' by the people involved. The patient's life is at stake, and although therapeutic prospects in many cancers have improved – particularly in the case of non-Hodgkin lymphoma – for most people the prospect of premature death will be the first thought when a cancer diagnosis is communicated. The knowledge of a cancer diagnosis implies that the patient and his family and friends need to relate to this new and mostly unexpected fact. One cannot escape the need to give a place to the illness and the future prospects regarding treatment (if applicable) and premature death.

Becoming aware of the real significance and potential impact of the diagnosis of non-Hodgkin lymphoma certainly was not something which happened immediately after it became clear that there was something seriously wrong in my body. Additional diagnostic procedures were in some way a distraction from what really was the case, as if as such these procedures already improved my future prospects. So the 'shock' of a fatal diagnosis was not really a shock, but something which evolved in the diagnostic process and during treatment. In my opinion this phenomenon affects bioethical and legal notions of informed consent and refusal of treatment, as these notions are tightly connected to communicative aspects during the illness course, as well as psychological, social and cultural factors which relate to defence mechanisms, distortion of information, and cultural habits and values.

Hope   Some claim that hope is the crucial factor in the care for patients with cancer. Hope involves the prospect that in the future there will be a cure, or at least a prospect of a life with an acceptable quality for the patient. During the different treatments I have undergone – chemotherapy, radiation therapy and autologous stem-cell transplantation – I have experienced a lot of support from the idea that at the end of the tunnel there would be the light of a successful treatment, even though I was aware that this chance was real, but definitely not a guarantee. Above that I granted myself the outlook that I would have the luck to belong to the statistical group of patients who would survive the lymphoma (about 50% of all sufferers). This promoted fighting spirit and gave strength during difficult times.

Isolation   In a case of severe illness (together with burdensome medical treatments like chemotherapy and radiation) the patient becomes more and more involved with and focused on the illness and the treatments. In my case, the experience of intense and enduring pain isolates the person from his surroundings. The physical environment has little or no meaning and personal contact becomes difficult, as the person is almost exclusively involved with and focused on the pain he experiences. This introversion increases the vulnerability of the patient who has difficulty in expressing his or her needs and wishes; this implies a need for carers to be sensitive to the unexpressed needs the patient may have. An illustration in my experience was the pressure sores on my back, which went undetected for some time.

Contemplating wishes in advance   As it became clear that my illness might progress in such a way that my

life would end during or after treatment, I decided that it would be helpful to draft an advance directive stating my medical wishes in case I became unconscious or otherwise incompetent. When drafting the advance directive together with my wife, we discovered that it was not easy to formulate in an exact and unambiguous way my wishes regarding end-of-life treatment and care. It was particularly hard to delineate care which would be acceptable, and care which would not be acceptable. In drafting an advance directive, one first needs to be conscious of the values which lie at the basis of your concerns about care at the end of life. On the basis of these values it becomes possible to give practical guidance to carers and relatives. In any case, I learned that debating my wishes with my wife gave me the confidence that in case I became incompetent and decisions ought to be made, then my wife would be in a good position to act as my representative on the basis of my personal values and wishes. It seems to me that the involvement of a person who is close to the patient can provide much better and more valuable input into the process of medical (and ethical) decision-making at the end of life than any formal advance document. At the same time I am aware that this is the ideal case in which there is a formal advance directive together with a person who has knowledge of the concerns and wishes of the patient.

Hopelessness   My experience with severe pain is largely connected to the pre-diagnosis period (October 2003–July 2004). Central in this period was the continuous back pain which 'coloured' my existence and that of my family and friends.

As the pain became unbearable, the rehabilitation physician who was in charge of my physical condition would give an injection with corticosteroids. The effects were really miraculous. The first time, within two hours the pain was completely gone and kept away for six weeks. This gave me and my family the opportunity to spend ten happy days in Tuscany. However, each subsequent injection had less effect, and after 4 or 5 injections the pain only stayed away for less than 24 hours. The rehabilitation physician discussed the issue and explained that he thought it was useless to continue the use of corticosteroids. I could not do other than agree, there was no choice.

Less than a week later – as my condition kept growing worse – the situation became unbearable. The pain was continuously intense and I saw no prospect of relief whatsoever. As there was no use in administering corticosteroids, I contemplated suicide as an escape from this terrible lot. After a sleepless night – I remember it was early on a Saturday morning – I called the rehabilitation physician. In my mind, I had made the decision that if he was not willing to inject me once more with corticosteroids, I would jump from the local bridge into the river.

Confusion and broken communication Next to the pain during the pre-diagnosis period, there was the pain which accompanied the medical procedures – particularly the intensive chemotherapy which was followed by autologous stem-cell transplantation – I received morphine by injection. This pain-killer was continuously infused by a syringe driver, and briefly after the start of this I became seriously confused. This confusion encompassed different experiences.

The first experience was one of hallucinations: partly visual, and partly what I would call experiential. The visual experience involved distortions of visual perception: when I looked out of the hospital window, I saw dancing construction cranes.

The second experience involved what may be called 'broken communication'. This was very frightening. As I had difficulty expressing myself, I was unable to clarify my wishes, but particularly my concerns to others. An example was my conviction that time had been fixed.

The third experience involved unclearness about place and time. Particularly at night I was disturbed about my environment. I didn't exactly know where I was, and why I was where I was staying. Besides that, I didn't know the time or date, let's say the coordinates of my existence in time. As already mentioned, there was a period in which I experienced time as being fixed, which was particularly troublesome as I thought that this eternal fixation of time would imply that I would have to stay in the hospital without end. This was extremely frightening as I was eager to leave hospital as quickly as possible.

In particular, the experience of broken communication was frightening because I could not get my worries and fears across to the people who were caring for me: nurses and doctors. Only my wife was sensitive enough and able to see that my mental condition was worrisome. Her intervention led to a reduction of the morphine dose, which resulted in a passing of the side effects.

Unbearable suffering The notion of 'unbearable suffering' is difficult to assess. In a recent publication, motivations of patients with a request for euthanasia or physician-assisted suicide were explored on the basis of 10 patient-centred, qualitative studies (Dees et al., 2009). This exploration 'showed that patients express their unbearable and unrelieved suffering in terms of pain, weakness, functional impairment, dependency, being a burden, hopelessness, indignity, intellectual deterioration, perception of loss of oneself, loss of autonomy, and being tired of life.'

The authors of this article conclude that 'the point where suffering becomes unbearable is a very individual perception that is closely related to the personality, the life history, social factors, and existential motivations. Irreversible disintegration and humiliation of the person appeared to be the start of openly exploring the phenomenology of death. The circumstances of their illness brought all the patients to the point where they would rather die than continue to live under the conditions imposed by their illness.'

The unbearableness of suffering can be explored from two positions: the viewpoint and experience of the suffering person, and the viewpoint of 'bystanders', including physicians and other healthcare workers. From the patient's subjective point of view, when pain and/or suffering is or becomes unbearable is less difficult to assess than from the viewpoint and perspective of the bystander. This simply is the case because the former experiences her suffering directly – as the subject of experiences – while the latter can only indirectly try to 'get a picture' of the suffering. As he or she does not directly experience the other person's suffering, essentially he or she has limited access to the experience of suffering of the other person.

On the basis of my personal experience, I very much agree with the abovementioned authors in regard to the 'very individual perception' of the unbearableness of suffering. In the end in my case it was the total disintegration of myself which took place during the period that the cancer process was attacking my spinal cord, which so long went unrecognized by the medical community and led to much unnecessary suffering for myself and distress for those around me.

Value and meaning of life The value of life is connected to the individual experience of the person and to the meaning he or she can attach to objects, living creatures (including animals), and activities in the world. Increasing isolation diminishes the value and experience of life's meaning. The loss of meaning in connection with extreme pain and suffering led in my case to suicidal ideation. In case of loss of hope this was the only 'exit' out of an unbearable situation.

Giving value and meaning to life depends on the possibility of having experiences and attaching meaning to these experiences. Painful experiences are not necessarily meaningless or valueless. This at least partly depends on the broader context of spiritual and (non-) religious world views which people may adhere to. However, serious suffering without reasonable hope of relief deserves compassionate attention and in exceptional cases the moral obligation to relieve this suffering may lead to a decision to actively terminate the life of the sufferer.

In conclusion: suffering and the goal(s) of medicine   I have experienced suffering which I then and now consider(ed) unbearable. Leaving aside the fact that the medical assistance was far from optimal (to say the least), the experience of pain and suffering has taught me a lot about the goals as well as the limits of medicine (and healthcare more broadly). As far as the limits are concerned I am convinced that not all pain and suffering can be controlled in ways which are acceptable to the individual patient concerned. I think my experience with the morphine syringe driver has taught me that pain control can have a high price by way of serious side effects. When suffering becomes unbearable there is a great need for comfort and compassion. Feelings of isolation, of not being recognized as a person and of not being heard by healthcare workers may lead to feelings of despair and abandonment.

As regards the goals of medicine, when cure or relief of pain are unattainable goals of medical practice, then the relief of suffering becomes the primary goal of medical assistance. Ultimately, compassion ought to be the guiding moral compass in cases of extreme, unbearable and hopeless suffering. The sufferer may find consolation in the recognition of the suffering by others, including professional healthcare workers. Compassion in interminable and unremediable suffering may demand an active intervention of the physician.

The most important aspect I learned from my illness experience with a fatal medical condition is how crucial attentiveness and open and careful communication with the patient are. Being seen and heard and being recognized as an individual who is in serious need are far more important than being informed about statistics regarding prognosis and chances of survival. Authentic presence, and the expression of one's own humanity, insecurity, doubt and fear by professional carers acknowledge at the same time that life is precarious and vulnerable, and that hope and fear go together hand in hand.

This personal account by Ron Berghmans shows how even professional medical ethicists find it difficult

to formulate their wishes concerning end-of-life care and to come to decisions on matters of life and death. To us it suggests the value of what the poet John Keats called 'negative capability': the ability to remain open to conflicting feelings and painful experiences without losing one's moral agency and humanity. Similarly, we have not taken an opinion on every issue that has arisen in this chapter, but we have sought – wherever possible and appropriate – to indicate which arguments we think work, and which we think need more work. This we see as an important part of bioethical reasoning: the ability to test arguments, along with the openness to have our own arguments and convictions tested. Such openness requires what one American philosopher calls a 'democratic spirit', and he has argued that we are obliged to recognize the plurality of moral positions that can sincerely exist (Benjamin, 2001). If, like Martin Benjamin, we approach moral dilemmas in this open way then we might be able to resolve some disagreements either in principle or, if that is not possible, then (at least) in practice.

Indeed, some scholars are even beginning to suggest that it is time to look for pluralistic 'middle way' or compromise solutions to such thorny disputes as whether or not to allow euthanasia (Huxtable, 2007; Lewis, 2007). Whatever the merits of these theoretical arguments, we certainly think it necessary – in the real (moral) world – to look for practical solutions to ethical dilemmas. There are various models for achieving this, some of which we have mentioned already, such as mediation and recourse to clinical ethics committees. Whichever method is chosen, we think it essential that the ethical arguments are presented as persuasively and transparently as possible, so that the debates can be conducted and, ideally, resolved in the most effective fashion.

We are not saying there is necessarily a 'one-size-fits-all' principled solution to the various problems we have looked at in the realm of terminal care. However, we *do* think that by using the bioethical tools appropriately we can seek to clarify the issues and work towards an answer that can apply in the clinical setting. After all, it is in the clinic that bioethical theorizing must often be tested. Indeed, Karen Forbes, the consultant in palliative medicine whose work we mentioned in the first section, has objected to the abstract thinking that tends to surround euthanasia, and her comment seems no less applicable to the other topics we have looked at:

[M]uch of the discussion about euthanasia lacks the reality and therefore the immediacy and gravity of clinical experience. 'Individual cases' are what my colleagues and myself as clinicians are faced with, and upon which we must form our opinions.

(Forbes, 1998, p. 98)

What we hope to have achieved through our frequent descriptions of real clinical cases is an approach to ethical theory that is as close to the experiences of health professionals and patients as it can be. In doing so we have drawn attention to potentially abstract notions like autonomy and quality of life – yet we hope also to have touched upon the very real psychological (and physical) components of the decisions at stake. Some decisions will obviously have major consequences for the patient and his or her family. But what about the psychological consequences for the hospital and other staff who are confronted with and must deal with ethical dilemmas on a regular basis?

Thinking of the experience of moral dilemmas as bereavement seems justified ... When [health care professionals] experience moral dilemmas, they lose the self that they thought of as caring, the self that does the right thing for patients, the self who will not do wrong to others, their whole self. They lose their integrity. With each moral dilemma that is thrust upon [health care professionals], a bit of them dies: to themselves, to the world and to their patients.

(Fairbairn and Mead, 1990, p. 23)

Clearly, as Fairbairn and Mead suggest, the experience of confronting the ethical dilemmas which arise at the end of life can sometimes be very difficult for healthcare professionals. However, it seems to us, that by the use of the kinds of analytic and ethical tools which we have started developing in this chapter, it is possible for healthcare professionals to work towards the practical resolution of some of the most difficult of these dilemmas in ways which are challenging without being threatening.

Notes

1. Reproduced with permission from Ron Berghmans, 'Physician-assisted death, violation of the moral integrity of medicine and the slippery slope'. Paper presented at the Seventh European Biomedical Ethics Practitioner Education workshop, Maastricht, 21–22 March.

2. Reproduced with permission from Ron Berghmans, 'Physician-assisted suicide in the case of mental suffering'.

2

Reproduction: decisions at the start of life

Introduction

Of all the issues in medical ethics, probably none is more frequently in the news than reproductive ethics – construed broadly to include such controversial issues as: abortion and selective termination of pregnancy; sale and donation of gametes (sperm and eggs); surrogacy or contract motherhood; 'therapeutic' and reproductive cloning; non-consensual use of gametes and embryos; rights for children born as a result of sperm or egg donation to trace their genetic parents; sterilization of young people with learning disability or physical handicaps; enforced caesarean sections; 'designer babies' (the use of preimplantation genetic diagnosis for social rather than therapeutic purposes, such as sex selection for which there is no clinical need, (e.g. not involving a sex-related genetic condition); egg freezing and other uses of in vitro fertilization (IVF) to allow women to have children after the normal age of child-bearing; the commercial market in private banking of umbilical cord blood for the child's later use; 'reproductive tourism', in which people travel to other countries to obtain reproductive tests or services unavailable in their own nations.

In writing a chapter about reproductive ethics, we have thus faced a dilemma about which of the vast range of issues to include, using our criterion of direct clinical relevance to everyday practice. This chapter therefore omits some issues, such as cloning and surrogacy, which at the time of writing were unlikely to be encountered in the course of ordinary practice. By contrast, we deal with some issues, such as judgements about 'compliance' and 'non-compliance' in pregnant women, which have become quite routine in clinical practice without having undergone serious ethical debate. Other issues, such as abortion, are commonly encountered, but suffer from exposure fatigue: the arguments for and against have been very well rehearsed over the past 30 years. We agree that the case for and against abortion remains tremendously important, but

we have chosen to view it primarily through a filter which grounds it in practice and downplays polemic: the issue of selective fetal reduction. Throughout, our focus is on asking what creates an ethical dilemma – just as in other chapters, one of our first concerns was to ask, 'Is this an ethical problem in the first place?'

Section 1: New reproductive technologies: benefit or burden?

We will start by looking at ethical issues before the inception of pregnancy: for example, fertility-assisted treatments such as IVF and gamete intrafallopian transfer (GIFT). Please begin with the following activity.

ACTIVITY: Make a list of all the new reproductive technologies you can think of. You might like to begin with the list at the start of this section, but no doubt others will occur to you. Then rank them along a spectrum of ethical acceptability and of how controversial they are. For example, you may believe that artificial insemination by husband (AIH) is ethically unproblematic, artificial insemination by donor (AID) slightly more so. If so, why? What extra ethical issues does it raise? Perhaps the question is whether children born as a result should be entitled to know the identity of the donor. The aim of this exercise is not so much to state your own views for and against each practice as to think 'laterally' about how wide a range of ethical issues each raises. Think about the practice from the viewpoint of different religions or different ethnic communities as well. Now look at the sorts of ethical arguments you have identified. Ask yourself, 'For whom is this a problem?' For example, we suggested above that identification of gamete donors is a problem for children born as a result. But it is also an issue for the donors themselves, of course (Daniels *et al.*, 1998) – and, perhaps less commonly noticed, for the recipients, the mothers, in the case of sperm donation. Arguably it is also an issue for the government, although there are also issues about privacy and confidentiality. This responsibility has in fact now been recognized by a recent change in UK statute law to allow young people conceived through gamete donation to trace their genetic parents when they reach the age of 18 – assuming, of course, that their 'social' parents have told them they were conceived by using donor gametes.

In the guided reading which forms the bulk of the rest of Section 1, the question of 'Benefits and burdens for whom?' is considered in greater depth. We will now ask you to begin this by reading selections from a chapter in a reader on ethical issues in maternal–fetal medicine by Professor Christine Overall of the Department of Philosophy, Queen's University, Kingston, Canada. Our aim in assigning this reading is to give you an example of the very comprehensive and balanced way in which a professional philosopher 'problematizes' the new reproductive technologies, which are commonly regarded as a technological marvel. This is not to say that they are necessarily a technological nightmare instead: rather, that they raise profound ethical and legal dilemmas which must be evaluated in terms other than those of the technology's success or failure alone.

New reproductive technologies and practices: benefits or liabilities for children?

Christine Overall[1]

In the recent ethical and social scientific literature on new reproductive technologies (NRTs) and practices, there is not much discussion about their impact on children (e.g. Birke *et al.*, 1990; Iglesias, 1990; Marrs, 1993; Robertson, 1994; Hartouni, 1997; Steinberg, 1997). As the final report of the Canadian Royal Commission on New Reproductive Technologies puts it,

> There is a dearth of information about, for instance, the direct outcomes of being conceived through assisted reproduction. Physical outcomes are important to monitor, but there may also be emotional and psychological outcomes to being born through the use of assisted methods of conception. For instance, we know very little about the effect on a child's sense of identity and belonging of being born through assisted insemination using donor sperm or following in vitro fertilization using donated eggs
>
> (Royal Commission on New Reproductive Technologies, 1993, p. 42).

Books and anthologies written from a feminist perspective mostly emphasize the effects of NRTs on women (e.g. Spallone, 1989; Rowland, 1992). Nonetheless, there is a connection, in reproductive issues, between the status of women and the status of children. This connection is explicitly recognized within the United Nations Declaration of the Rights of the Child, which calls for 'special care and protection' both for children and for their mothers, 'including adequate prenatal and postnatal care' (Principle 4). Hence, it can plausibly be argued that if NRTs either benefit or harm women, then their children may be comparably affected.[1]

In this paper I evaluate, from a feminist perspective, a number of arguments about the direct benefits and harms of reproductive technologies and practices with respect to children. As a moral touchstone for their assessment, I employ the United Nations Declaration of the Rights of the Child, which sets forth, in a reasonably clear and uncontroversial fashion, some basic and essential moral entitlements for children everywhere, entitlements that are widely acknowledged, even if they are not always acted upon. I shall confine my discussion to the western world, since that is the context in which most of the arguments on both sides have been advanced.

Alleged benefits of NRTs and practices

Three main benefits are repeatedly cited: existence itself; loving, motivated, prosperous parents; and the avoidance of disabilities.

One prominent argument is that technologies such as IVF are a benefit to offspring since without the technologies, some children would not exist – even if their existence includes physical or psychological health problems and/or disabilities. Existence itself is a benefit conferred by NRTs upon some lucky children. Thus, John Robertson, a prominent defender of the use of NRTs, argues that, however difficult the problems may be arising from a life created through reproductive technology, that life is unlikely ever to be so bad as to be not worth living. He states, 'Whatever psychological or social problems arise, they hardly rise to the level of severe handicap or disability that would make the child's very existence a net burden, and hence a wrongful life' (Robertson, 1994, p. 122).

How should we assess this argument? Thomas H. Murray points out that, if it is accepted without analysis, then virtually no 'novel method of bringing children into the world' could be morally condemned (Murray, 1996, p. 37). The argument implies that criticizing a reproductive technology requires showing that the children thus created would have been better off never having been born. Of course, it seems true that being alive is usually good; I have little doubt that most children created through NRTs and practices are glad to be alive. Still, this argument should not be allowed to trump all other evidence about possible harms generated by reproductive technologies.

For it would be a moral and conceptual mistake to assume that there are children who would have missed out on a benefit, life, if not for NRTs. It is not as if children exist in a limbo, waiting to be given the opportunity to live via NRTs. Never having existed would not make some hypothetical child worse off; there is no child to harm (Parfit, 1984, p. 487). So, even if coming into existence is a type of benefit, failing to come into existence is not a harm.

Having life is the precondition that makes all other benefits – and harms – possible. If a child suffers illness or disabilities because of the circumstances of his/her conception or prenatal existence, then we seem to have harmed him/her, in the process of benefiting him/her by causing his/her existence. It is arguable that every person has an interest in possessing a healthy, non-disabled body. If the damages incurred at conception are sufficiently great, there seems to be virtually no benefit to the child at all.

I conclude that, from a perspective before conception of a child, life is not a benefit, since there is no one to benefit; only from the perspective after conception has occurred is life arguably a benefit – and then, only if the life is not heavily damaged through the process of conception itself. Causing someone to exist is not a benefit, since there is no one to benefit; but once the person exists, he or she has life, which is usually a good thing.

ACTIVITY: Stop for a moment and try to restate this insightful argument in other terms. Think also about other contexts in which similar confusion arises.

We can think of two examples from other areas of medical ethics. One is the common argument made against IVF for postmenopausal women. It is often argued that it is better for children to be born to mothers who are young enough to 'roll with the punches' of childrearing. But the choice is actually between this child, born to this postmenopausal mother, and no child at all (Hope *et al.*, 1995). We are not making some hypothetical child worse off by allowing it to be born to a postmenopausal mother rather than to a younger mother.

A similar confusion, one might argue, arose in the Bland decision (1992), which is also mentioned in the previous chapter. There the House of Lords' decision sometimes appeared to be arguing that there could be an interest in ceasing to exist, by taking the view that it might be in Tony Bland's best interests to allow artificial nutrition and hydration to be withdrawn. For example, Lord Browne-Wilkinson declared that doctors were only obliged to sustain life when it was in the patient's best interest to remain alive. But in whose interest? We cannot appeal to the interests of someone who will not exist as a justification for ending their existence. To put this criticism another way, the question of remaining alive is prior and necessary to the question of having a best interest. It cannot be determined in the reverse fashion, as Lord Browne-Wilkinson's statement seems to do. A better formulation was that eventually used by other judges, posing the issue in terms of whether continued life on these terms was in Tony Bland's best interests, rather than whether it could be in his best interests not to exist.

Now continue with your reading of Overall.

A second alleged benefit claimed for NRTs is based on the ostensible characteristics of the parents. Prospective parents who use NRTs are often prosperous, seem to really want children, are in some instances supposedly assessed for stability, and are ready to have children. More simply, the claim is that NRTs benefit (potential) parents, who want children (Snowden and Mitchell, 1983, p. 76; Macklin, 1994, p. 56) and are pleased to have them; hence they indirectly benefit the resulting child. This argument usually takes its most explicit form in the context of debates about so-called surrogate motherhood, or what I prefer to call contract pregnancy, where the claim is made that the children resulting from the contract receive all the benefits of life within middle class or wealthy families, which are equipped to provide the material, social, and intellectual privileges seldom attained in working class families. Thus, the American Fertility Society claims,

> Even if there are psychological risks, most infertile couples who go through with a reproduction arrangement that involves a third party do so as a last resort. In some cases, their willingness to make sacrifices to have a child may testify to their worthiness as loving parents. A child conceived through surrogate

motherhood may be born into a much healthier climate than a child whose birth was unplanned.

(American Fertility Society, 1990, p. 312)

However, this argument is not persuasive. Its classist bias is immediately obvious: the assumption is that life in a middle or upper class family is inevitably a greater benefit to a child than life in a working class family. This assumption worked to the disadvantage of Mary Beth Whitehead, a working class woman, when she [unsuccessfully] sought custody of her biological daughter, so-called 'Baby M', whom she contracted to create for William Stern, a well-off professional.

More significantly, perhaps, the argument assumes that would-be parents who resort to NRTs and practices are especially motivated and beneficent toward their subsequent children. However, as I shall suggest later, there are also reasons to be concerned about the motives and goals of these people. And, at the very least, there is no empirical evidence that I know of to suggest that they make better parents than those who do not use technology in reproduction.

The third main benefit claimed for some NRTs and practices is that they can help to reduce or eliminate disabilities in children (Tauer, 1990, p. 75). For example, Deborah Kaplan lists several possible benefits to children of prenatal diagnosis (PND) and treatment.

First: Prevention or amelioration of the disability using methods such as treatment through dietary changes or supplements for the mother or infant; prenatal treatment of the fetus through pharmaceutical or surgical interventions; other forms of treatment or therapy for the infant that occur after prenatal diagnosis.

Second: Prevention of family disruption through prenatal preparation by family members. This can entail obtaining information about the diagnosed condition and its consequences through reading or through talking to families who have children with similar disabilities or to adults who live with the disability themselves. It may also include such means as finding out about available public or private resources or forms of assistance, purchasing equipment, or making home modifications (Kaplan, 1994, p. 50).

So, the suggestion is that the technologies of prenatal diagnosis benefit children directly through the prevention and amelioration of disabilities, and indirectly, by assisting parents. These claims seem justified.

However, it would be a mistake to accept the related claim, made by some, that NRTs produce better, or even perfect, babies (Snowden and Mitchell, 1983, p. 77; Spallone, 1989, pp. 113, 117); that, for example,

babies generated by IVF or donor insemination (DI) using sperm from gifted fathers are smarter or prettier (Scutt, 1990, p. 285). There is no clear evidence to support these claims. And there are reasons to be cautious about them since … they betray a eugenicist agenda.

ACTIVITY: Is there a duty to produce 'as good children as we can'? Before going on to Section 2, stop now and think about whether there is a moral duty to produce the best offspring possible. What would be the consequences of such a duty? What would be its origins? What might it include? For example, genetic enhancement technologies, if perfected. This possibility has occasioned fierce debate in recent bioethics (e.g. Glover, 2005; Savulescu, 2007; Parker, 2007b).

You will note that Overall has raised a large number of specific issues under the umbrella of whether NRTs produce benefits or liabilities for children. She has touched on preimplantation genetic diagnosis to prevent disability or to create 'designer babies', surrogate or contract motherhood, and, indirectly, whether there is such a thing as the 'right to life'. Several of these issues will recur throughout this chapter, explored in case studies – of which the first will be the subject of an exercise using the CD-ROM included with this workbook. If you have not yet done so, please install the CD-ROM on your computer now, following the instructions included with it.

Section 2: The rights of the parents and the welfare of the child: the example of freezing reproductive tissue

One aspect of NRTs that continues to cause controversy is the welfare of any child born as a result of treatment. We have used the Overall article to introduce you to this question, under the broader rubric of whether NRTs in general produce benefits or liabilities for children. One particularly prolonged debate has centred on the question of whether IVF should only be provided to partners in 'traditional' relationships, usually a married couple. When the Human Fertilisation and Embryology Act 1990 was first passed in the UK, a last-minute Parliamentary challenge resulted in the insertion of a requirement (in section 13.5) that IVF clinics had to take into account the welfare of the child born as a result of treatment, 'including the need of that child for a father'. Arguably, this provision now violates the European Convention on Human Rights (Article 12) by denying everyone an equal right to found a family (Lee and Morgan, 2001, p. 159). Amid complaints from clinics that assessing that need was impractical, from lesbian couples that the requirement discriminated against them, and from people on all sides of the political spectrum that this provision interfered with personal reproductive choice, the requirement was finally scrapped in 2007. But it continues to be the case in other countries, such as France, that only heterosexual couples can receive IVF treatment, and that unmarried heterosexual couples must prove their seriousness about the '*projet parental*' by demonstrating that they have lived together for a certain number of years.

The welfare of the child versus the rights of the parents also seemed to be at issue in another highly dramatic sort of case, which you will now explore. Please open Scenario 5 on your CD-ROM, 'Freezing reproductive tissue', and follow the instructions given. You will see that you are periodically asked to select a response to a question about the video clip, to justify your response in a short written response and to compare your response with that of ethical and legal experts, clinicians and other practitioners. At the end of the scenario, you can also compare your responses with a chart of the key ethical, legal and professional issues illustrated by this case. Please complete the entire scenario (which takes about half an hour) before reading any further.

This scenario, although based on one case, has covered a very wide range of ethical issues, including the interests of the future child versus those of the parents (if such a conflict exists) and the interests of the two parents considered separately. In the extreme form of taking gametes from a dead partner, it can't be assumed that the two future parents' interests necessarily coincide. Because informed consent to treatment is a cardinal principle in our law, and because taking gametes without prior consent contravenes that principle, the bulk of expert and clinical opinion in the scenario rejected the surviving partner's right to create a baby using the dead spouse's gametes, even if that might well have been the unexpressed wish of the lost partner.

Similar issues have arisen when a man has withdrawn consent to the use of embryos created using his sperm and the eggs of a woman who is no longer his partner. In the Natalie Evans case of 2006, courts in the UK and Europe ruled that stored embryos would have to be destroyed when Evans's previous partner Howard Johnston opposed her desire to use them to become pregnant, even though she had no other hope of pregnancy following removal of her ovaries after cancer. Johnston argued that 'The key thing for me was just to be able to decide when, and if, I would start a family'. The provisions of the Human Fertilisation and Embryology Act 1990, the courts said, made it clear that both partners had to consent to use of the embryos. Natalie Evans's human right to a family life could not override Howard Johnston's refusal, it was held, and the embryos had no independent legal right to life.

ACTIVITY: Please read the following commentary on the Natalie Evans case by Anna Smajdor (Smajdor, 2007), then researcher in medical ethics at Imperial College London and now lecturer in medical ethics at the University of East Anglia. As you read, ask yourself two questions: (1) What does 'reproductive autonomy' mean in the Natalie Evans case? How did each partner conceive of their own autonomous consent to parenthood? (2) What would the demands of justice to both parties have entailed in this situation?

Is there a right not to be a parent?

Anna Smajdor[2]

On 10 April 2007, Natalie Evans lost the final stage of a four-year legal battle for the right to implant embryos created with her eggs and the sperm of her former partner. Ms Evans had been diagnosed with cancer, and treatment necessitated the removal of her ovaries, leaving her sterile. Creating and storing embryos would, it was hoped, keep the possibility of motherhood open to her.

However, Ms Evans' hopes were shattered when her relationship broke down and her partner, Howard Johnston, withdrew his consent for the embryos to be used. Since the consent of both parties is required for fertility treatment or even for ongoing storage of embryos, it seemed that Ms Evans would have to forego her dream of parenthood. But she was unwilling to submit to the loss of her embryos without a fight; hence the protracted legal struggle which culminated in the European Court of Human Rights' rejection of Ms Evans' case.

Many people, while sympathetic to Ms Evans' plight, felt that the court had come to the right conclusion. After all, the consent protocols are clear and were accepted by both parties at the time the embryos were created. But while in the eyes of the law the correct decision may have been reached, the case raises some interesting questions.

The implication was that people should not be forced to become parents, all other things being equal. Is this an acceptable conclusion? And is it consistent with other legal and social assumptions?

To answer this question, we need firstly to examine the concept of parenthood. I suggest that parenthood is best understood not as inhering solely in genetic ties. Rather, it is a bundle of concepts which may include some or all of the following: being part of a causal chain that brings about the creation of a child; having the intention to procreate; undergoing gestation and childbirth; acquiring legal rights and responsibilities; sharing genetic links; nurturing and rearing.

We may be justified in believing that some of these types of parenthood should not be forced on unwilling people. Forcing people to undergo gestation and birth against their will seems clearly unacceptable. But perhaps the 'right' not to be a parent in the genetic sense has been mistakenly extrapolated from the idea that enforced gestational parenthood is a moral wrong.

The presumed right to abortion is sometimes construed as stemming from a right not to be a parent. But to whom does this right apply? Men are not allowed to force women to undergo abortions, so does this mean that the right applies only to women? Margaret Brazier has suggested that fundamental human rights 'must be gender-neutral' [1]. If this were true, then surely a right not to be a parent ought to apply to both sexes.

However, abortion *cannot* simply be described as an exercise of the right not to be a parent in the genetic sense. If a woman has been impregnated with an embryo that has no genetic link with her, does this mean she has no choice whether or not to continue with the pregnancy? Surely the important fact is that the embryo is inside her body, not that it does or does not share her genes.

This is a vital fact to remember, since what we are protecting here is people's autonomy over their bodies. It is perfectly coherent for respect for autonomy to be afforded to men and women alike. On the other hand, the right not to be a genetic parent, when it conflicts with physical concerns, seems either to come with so many constraints as to be almost worthless, or to lead to unpalatable conclusions (e.g. that a pregnant woman can be coerced by those who are the genetic parents of the embryos she is carrying).

Maintaining autonomy over one's body is of the utmost importance. Women have fought long and hard for the right to do so. We must not conflate this with the altogether separate – and lesser – issue of enforced genetic parenthood.

The harms involved in physical coercion and enforced parenthood are very evident. However, the harms involved in enforced genetic parenthood are far less clear. In fact, men undergo enforced genetic parenthood all the time, and society scarcely registers the fact. A man whose partner is pregnant cannot demand she has an abortion. But we could feasibly allow men to sign a waiver stating that they do not consent to the birth of the child, and that they wish to play no part in the child's life or upkeep [2].

It seems highly discriminatory that the partners of fertile women have no rights whatsoever in this respect. A man whose partner has become pregnant without his desire or knowledge has the legal and financial obligations of parenthood thrust upon him, whereas men whose partners are *in*fertile are accorded the right to veto the entire reproductive enterprise.

This being the case, perhaps we should be more sympathetic to men whose partners are pregnant without their consent. Mr Johnston is simply one of many, many men in the UK who go partway toward parenthood and then get cold feet. There is a degree of moral opprobrium associated with reluctant fathers. We are encouraged to see them as being selfish, feckless and irresponsible. But taking the risk of unprotected sex and then deciding one doesn't want to be a father is arguably no more culpable than creating embryos and then changing one's mind. The latter is perhaps worse, as it involves reneging on an agreement and causing grief to one's partner.

The asymmetry of the law with respect to fathers and mothers, whether fertile or not, needs to be straightened out. Even after the ties of gestation and birth are over, mothers are not forced to accept the further legal and financial obligations of parenthood. They can choose to give their children up for adoption. Men do not have this right. They are utterly at the whim of their partners' choices. In this environment, men's rights are very much constrained compared with those of women. And this constraint extends far beyond what is justified by the mother's physical connection with the child.

It is my contention that this injustice should be remedied. Not by respecting men's or women's 'right' not to be parents, but by affording men and women the same rights in terms of choosing not to assume legal, social or financial responsibility for the child.

In the context of this far greater injustice to men in the UK, I have limited sympathy with Mr Johnston. He, along with other men and women, should have the opportunity to state his refusal to fulfil the function of a social parent, and this should be recognizable in law. If this were possible (and we allow it in the case of gamete donors), it would be hard to see what further harm could come to Mr Johnston purely from the knowledge that a child might be born with some of his genes. Certainly any such harm is far harder to identify or quantify than the harms of enforced physical, legal or financial parenthood.

References

1. Margaret Brazier, 'Reproductive rights: feminism or patriarchy?'. In *The Future of Human Reproduction*, ed. J. Harris and S. Holm. Oxford University Press, 1998.

2. This view is forcibly argued by Elizabeth Brake in her paper 'Fatherhood and child support: do men have a right to choose?' *Journal of Applied Philosophy*, **22**(1), 2005.

'What does reproductive autonomy mean where one person's exercise of it denies it to someone else?' (Chadwick, 2009). The Evans case demonstrates the limitations of the conventional, individualistic approach to autonomy in medical ethics. In the 'normal' situation, one patient's autonomy doesn't conflict with anyone else's – more frequently, it conflicts with the doctor's evaluation of the patient's best interests. That sort of case arose frequently in Chapter 1, for example, in the area of death and dying, although even there the desires of the dying person's family might come into conflict with those of their next of kin. But in reproductive ethics, which is almost by definition typically about relationships, we face decisions about how to balance the reproductive wishes and rights of two parties. Where a relationship is intact, there may be no conflict, but in the Evans case the relationship between the two partners had broken down irretrievably.

That leads into the second question, about how to render justice to both parties when only one can 'win'. Smajdor admits she has little sympathy with Howard Johnston, although, rather unexpectedly, she has considerable sympathy for men in non-IVF couples who are 'forced' to become fathers against their will. Justice

to both parties doesn't necessarily mean treating them both the same, but it does entail compassion with both men and women who reproduce 'normally'. The Greek philosopher Aristotle wrote that the essence of justice lay in treating equals equally. Whereas the courts in the Evans case perhaps took it for granted that both parties had equal rights to decide whether to become parents, Smajdor reminds us that they would only be equal in genetic input, but that we do not consider genetic input to be the essence of parenting. Other commentators have likewise remarked that women put more 'sweat equity' into the laborious and painful processes of IVF than men do, and that losing the embryos thus created represents a much greater loss for them (Donchin, 2009). This was particularly true for Evans, who was now infertile after cancer treatment. On the other hand, Smajdor effectively argues that considering equals equally also means remembering the position of men who become reluctant fathers after normal intercourse, where the law does not intervene to protect their autonomy or decision not to parent.

A parallel case arose in Texas in 2005, when Randy and Augusta Roman contested the 'custody' of their embryos after their divorce. (Since the embryo or fetus is not a legal person in the common law of the UK and USA, 'custody' is really a misnomer.) Although Augusta initially won the right to have the embryos implanted, a higher court ruled that the couple had made a contractual, binding agreement to destroy the embryos if they divorced (Hamm, 2007). The case was potentially far-reaching: if the embryos had been found to have any sort of 'right' to be implanted, that would also have implied that 'right to life' groups opposing abortion had legal backing for their position.

In another instance concerning reproductive autonomy, the Diane Blood case discussed on the CD-ROM, there was also a fear that allowing gametes and other tissue to be taken for this purpose, however laudable, might be the first stage of another sort of slippery slope, rolling down towards other non-consensual taking of tissue. Those fears must also be located in the context of the 2001 Alder Hey scandal in the UK, in which a pathologist kept dead children's tissue without the consent of their parents, and of the growing evidence that some US IVF clinics, for example the University of California at Irvine, are implicated in taking ova without the consent of women undergoing IVF (Yoshino, 2006; Dickenson, 2008). There were also possible conflicts of interest with a third party in the parenting triangle, the birth mother, if a so-called 'surrogate' mother was to be used. Finally, the scenario raised a range of issues about the proper limits of the doctor–patient relationship and the duties of a doctor: for example, whether Dr Ford was obliged to carry out the wishes of the bereaved husband at the cost of overriding the principle of informed consent.

You might have found yourself asking why so many of the commentators on the scenario treated informed consent as the 'gold standard' of medical treatment. Consent also recurs over and over throughout this book, in questions about its proper roles and limits in research trials, for example, or in the treatment of young children or people with severe psychiatric difficulties. But why is informed consent emphasized so heavily in medical ethics and law?

It is easier to answer the second half of the question, why consent is so important in medical *law*. In legal terms, obtaining the patient's informed consent protects the clinician against a possible civil action for battery (unauthorized touching of the patient) or even a criminal action for assault. Adults are generally presumed to be competent to consent to treatment unless proven otherwise. (*Re C* [1994]) But is consent just a legal shibboleth? Is it also *ethically* imperative?

In fact there are contending philosophical approaches possible here, not all of which emphasize consent to the extent that the scenario experts did. (We will revisit these conflicting models later in the book, and explore them in much greater depth in the final chapter.) Philosophical utilitarians, broadly speaking, would not emphasize informed consent as much as rights theorists or deontologists, who emphasize duty. (For present purposes, we will consider the latter two as if they were one, although they disagree on the direction of causality: does my right generate your duty, or does my duty generate your right?)

To a utilitarian, the guide to decision-making in a case like that in the scenario would be maximizing overall welfare of all the parties involved. If we take Steve's desire to have a child by his dead wife at face value – although some of the counsellors in the scenario doubted whether it would really be the best thing for him – then we would want to see his welfare maximized, in this instance, by allowing the ovarian tissue to be stored and later used in IVF treatment of a surrogate, combined with his sperm. A utilitarian might argue that Celia, Steve's dead wife, can no longer have interests or welfare that count in the equation. Therefore no harm would have been done to her if her ovarian tissue was extracted, even without her consent, and no harm can be done if it is later used to create the child her husband wants so dearly. Added to that calculation, some utilitarians argue that having more children increases the amount of overall wellbeing (Harris, 1999a, 1999b).

Other utilitarians have claimed that 'presumed' organ and tissue donation from the dead would increase the supply and benefit both research and therapy, whether or not prior consent has been obtained (van Dienst and Savulescu, 2002). We do not actually agree with this position: even on its own utilitarian terms, it seems counter-productive. If people lose trust in the system of organ and tissue donation, which they may well do if they feel they are just being 'harvested', then voluntary donations of blood and organs may well diminish, offsetting any increase from 'presumed' donation.

However, a more sophisticated form of utilitarianism, centring perhaps on overall rules for society rather than the calculus in each individual case, might note that it promotes general welfare if the wishes of the dead are respected. That would mean respecting informed consent, or its absence, and refraining from taking gametes or organs unless the dead person had given prior authorization. We could also argue that overall societal welfare is enhanced if patients trust their doctors not to carry out procedures on them without their consent.

That sort of 'rule-utilitarian' general principle – as opposed to the 'act-utilitarian' method, which concentrates on the narrower calculus of gains and losses likely in a particular case – would actually coincide with an emphasis on the rights of the patient, or the duties of a doctor, as prior and determinative. In such ethical models, informed consent forms a bulwark protecting the patient's autonomy and limiting the doctor's duty to what the patient authorizes. Even if the doctor is entirely well-intentioned, he or she is not allowed to override absence of informed consent in a competent adult patient – whether or not it would produce a better outcome for either the patient or society. That prohibition may be seen as extending into the patient's right to determine what may or may not be done with her body as she lies dying or even dead, as in this scenario. Although an absolutist notion of concept is probably untenable (Dickenson, 2003, p. 75), we should err on the side of caution in overriding the absence of consent, in this view, even from someone no longer able to claim their rights.

Doing otherwise might be a slippery slope of another kind, towards overriding patients' rights in other contexts, even where patients are indeed competent to claim them – towards medical paternalism, in other words.

Section 3: Preimplantation diagnosis and selective termination: the example of 'reproductive tourism'

In the Diane Blood case, examined in the CD-ROM scenario on 'Freezing reproductive tissue', the High Court upheld the Human Fertilisation and Embryology Authority's decision to withhold permission for Stephen Blood's stored sperm to be used in this country. But Diane Blood eventually succeeded in exporting the sperm to Belgium and obtained treatment there, not once but twice – resulting in the birth of two healthy and apparently much-loved sons. The Blood case was one of the first, and most highly publicized, examples of what has come to be called 'reproductive tourism'. This rather pejorative term, which makes light of the serious motives and dilemmas behind the issue, covers an increasingly wide range of examples. For example, burgeoning private fertility clinics in Spain now number among their customers couples from Germany, France and the UK. The UK couples are frequently driven by the desire to avoid the now-mandatory right of children born as a result of a sperm or egg donor's contribution to know the identity of their genetic parent, while the Germans may be seeking to evade very strict restrictions on IVF and preimplantation genetic diagnosis (PGD) in their own law.

> **Preimplantation genetic diagnosis** is a procedure by which one or two cells are removed from an embryo created through IVF and tested for a genetic disorder. Only the embryos not affected will be replaced in the uterus.

Although these questions may seem highly sensationalistic, they do illustrate the problem of conflicting legal rules in different European jurisdictions, and the conflicting ethical views that lie beneath them. Hovering in the background is also the issue of abortion, to which PGD is a preferable alternative in some views, although others might regard it as equally objectionable insofar as it involves the selection of 'healthy' embryos and the loss of the others. We would now like you to view a second scenario from the CD-ROM to explore these further ethical and legal issues.

> **ACTIVITY:** Please open scenario 6 on your CD-ROM and work through the scenario, including the summary of issues raised and the three additional legal points at the end. This will take you about 15–20 minutes.

What did you decide Karin and Peter should do? We ourselves feel that they should be entitled to travel abroad to obtain preimplantation genetic diagnosis (PGD), even if German law forbids it. Oddly, although the German law is aimed at protecting the embryo, in this case it would result in another abortion – if the next fetus Karin conceives carries the same genetic syndrome (Werdning–Hoffman syndrome) which resulted in the death of the couple's son. That abortion would have to take place at a later stage of pregnancy, at greater risk to the woman, and when the fetus is nearer viability. So it does seem that pragmatically, both opponents of abortion and proponents of a woman's right to choose might actually unite behind the couple's desire to use PGD. True, PGD entails the destruction of the embryos carrying the genetic condition; only embryos which are not affected will be implanted in the woman's womb. But in the case of a genetic condition which inevitably results in the death of the baby once it is born, the child that the embryo would become is going to die anyway.

In this example, utilitarians and rights theorists – who are just as unlikely bedfellows as pro-choice and anti-abortion advocates – would probably agree that PGD should be offered. A utilitarian, with a consequentialist emphasis on outcomes, might well accept the argument that the affected embryo will die in any case, adding that the couple's welfare will obviously be enhanced if they don't have to undergo the painful process of another abortion. A rights theorist – assuming she or he focuses on the rights of the woman rather than the right of the embryo – would come to the same conclusion. Dr Frederick came to a similar view from a duty-based perspective. She felt that it was part of her duty as a doctor to take a compassionate attitude towards Karin and to recommend her for PGD abroad, regardless of what the law in their home country had to say. On the other hand, it would also be possible for a deontologist – someone who focuses on moral duties – to claim that it is no part of the duties of a doctor to condone killing, if they believed that not implanting the defective embryos was indeed a form of killing.

Before we conclude unreservedly that patients should be entitled to disregard the laws of their own country and to travel abroad for whatever reproductive treatments they think best, however, a note of caution is required. That attitude ignores the way in which a global industry is developing around reproductive therapies in countries with more liberal regulatory regimes. In her book *Body Shopping: The Economy Fuelled by Flesh and Blood*, Donna Dickenson argues that we are witnessing an international phenomenon of commercialization of the human body. If individuals like Karin and Peter are allowed or even encouraged by their doctors to evade the laws of their own country, is that the start of a slippery slope towards international 'body shopping' in reproductive tissue and treatments?

Of course parents like Karin and Peter would not see themselves as contributing to global commodification of the human body: only trying to get round their own tragic situation. That, in a way, is exactly what feeds the phenomenon of 'body shopping', and what makes them open to potential exploitation. 'In these cases, and thousands like them', as the American commentator Debora Spar writes, 'the parents aren't motivated by commercial instincts, and they hardly see themselves as "shopping" for their offspring. Yet they are still intimately involved with both a market operation and a political calculation' (Spar, 2006, p. xii).

Because of a loophole in US legislation exempting eggs from the general prohibition on payment for organs, a large and lucrative industry has grown up there: Americans paid well over $37 million for so-called 'donor' eggs in 2002, but that figure was dwarfed by the earnings of IVF clinics, over $1 billion (Dickenson, 2008, p. 2). Advertisements regularly circulate in US college newspapers, offering egg 'donors' amounts up to $50 000, from an average of about $4500. 'Desirability' of genetic traits primarily determines the price: 'blonde, tall, athletic and musical donors command the higher rates, at considerable risk to themselves' (Dickenson, 2008, p. 2).

This phenomenon is not limited to highly commercialized economies like the USA. Spain alone numbers a total of 165 private fertility clinics – more than any other European country. Although EC law prevents these clinics from paying outright for eggs, as US clinics can do, they are allowed to offer up to 1200 euros in 'expenses'. Many of their customers come from other countries with stricter regulatory regimes, including Germany, Italy and France. Similarly, many of the sellers are not from Spain: with Communist-era travel restrictions removed, Eastern Europeans are now 'free' to sell their eggs in clinics in Spain, Cyprus and other locations which have been documented as taking part in the international egg trade (Barnett and Smith, 2006). And if this is happening in Spain, traditionally a profoundly Catholic country, it suggests that human reproductive tissue is evolving into a global commodity.

But what would be wrong with such widespread 'body shopping'? After all, many people would argue, we live in a consumer society, where money is the measure of all things. Bodies and parts of bodies are no different, you might think. You might even feel that any attempt to regulate markets for tissue will subvert the progress of science and medicine. If selling eggs or other forms of tissue improves the fertility of women who have to undergo IVF, and also provides the sellers with an income, some – utilitarian commentators in particular – might say that has to be a good thing for both parties, particularly if it solves the chronic shortage of organs (Radcliffe Richards, 1998; Harris and Erin, 2002; Savulescu, 2003).

Dickenson, along with other critics of commercialization (Andrews and Nelkin, 2001; Waldby and Mitchell, 2006), argues that this is a very naive view which ignores economic disparities, justice and issues of exploitation – apart from the medical risks of ovarian hyperstimulation and other known side effects for donors. Either way, it is clear that a dilemma like the one faced by Karin and Peter extends beyond the personal circumstances of any individual couple, involving profound philosophical, legal and social questions.

Section 4: Fetal reduction and abortion

The previous section, on prenatal genetic diagnosis and reproductive tourism, touched on the question of abortion, but only indirectly. What was at issue there was an *omission* – not implanting embryos who carried a fatal genetic condition – rather than an *act* – choosing to actively abort an embryo or fetus. Particularly in the case from the CD-ROM, where the affected embryo would develop into a baby who would die of the condition in any case, it might also be thought that it was the condition itself that was fatal to the embryo.

You may wonder when we are going to consider the question of abortion more directly. There is certainly no denying that abortion has been a major issue in reproductive ethics for many years, and will continue to be so – perhaps *the* big issue in many more conventional textbooks. But precisely because abortion has been so extensively covered elsewhere, and has led to such unproductively polarized views, we do not propose to let it dominate this chapter. Our view is that you may learn more about the issues raised by abortion by thinking about how it impacts on other issues in practice, helping you to reach a more nuanced position on an issue where black-and-white, ideological stances frequently prevail. But if you do want to read some classic pro- and anti-abortion views, you will find some suggestions in the bibliography at the end of this book.

What we will now do is to view the abortion issue from another clinical perspective related to the new reproductive technologies. Where multiple embryos are implanted, and none is actually defective, is it ever right to 'selectively reduce' or abort any of the fetuses? If so, on what basis? What counts as 'defective'? Controversy has recently erupted over requests by hearing-impaired parents undergoing IVF that clinicians should only implant their hearing-impaired embryos, partly on the grounds that these children will be more readily integrated into the Deaf community. Although the UK Human Fertilisation and Embryology Act 2008 prohibits transferring 'abnormal' embryos by preference over 'healthy' ones, activists and parents from the Deaf community had attacked this provision as a form of discrimination, even a type of eugenics. They might also argue that there is only a fuzzy distinction between defining a characteristic as abnormal when it does not actually impair survival and allowing 'designer babies' or 'genetic enhancement' technologies to flourish unimpeded. (It is unlikely and undesirable, however that IVF will ever become the normal way of reproducing the human species, as genetic enhancement technologies would require. That would require women to routinely undergo the risks and rigours of IVF, which can include potentially fatal ovarian hyperstimulation.)

If, as Christine Overall claims, it is not a benefit to the child to be born, then neither is there an obligation to maximize the number of births. Producing the best children we can might be one thing; producing as many children as we can is another. Of course, this view would not be accepted by some religions, and even outside of organized religion, we have already seen that some philosophical utilitarians (e.g. Harris, 1999a, 1999b) also hold that we can maximize the total amount of happiness in the world by maximizing the total number of people. More narrowly, Bennett and Harris claim that we have an obligation to minimize the number of people born to suffer such a miserable life that it outweighs any pleasure gained by living (Bennett and Harris, 2002). Harris also thinks that there is an obligation on potential parents to use genetic enhancement technologies in order to produce children who have the most favourable genetic endowment possible (Harris, 2007).

Let us assume, for argument's sake, that most people would accept there is no necessary obligation to produce as many children as we can, and no duty to produce the most genetically 'enhanced' children that we can, but that we ought to 'do our best' by those children we do produce. What would 'doing our best' entail, in terms of pregnancy and childbirth? You have already considered this issue in the activity at the start of this chapter. Perhaps you identified some of the following:

- Ensuring that both parents are in maximal reproductive health at the time of conception. This sounds like common sense, but would it mean that 'older' parents should be actively discouraged from conceiving? The risk of fetal abnormality increases radically with maternal age (and, to a lesser degree, with paternal age).
- Ensuring that the fetus develops in the best possible environment. This also sounds unexceptionable, but it might legitimize legal interventions against pregnant cocaine addicts, refusal to serve pregnant women alcohol in bars, and all sorts of ramifications which are far from uncontroversial (Daniels, 1993).
- Ensuring that the fetus has the best possible chance of a safe delivery. This, too, sounds like something everyone would want, but in practice it legitimizes enforced Caesarean sections, which are not presently legal in either the USA or the UK – after a long struggle in both countries against legal decisions which were perceived as flawed in law, and discriminatory against pregnant women as the only class of patients on whom non-consensual procedures could be performed (In *Re A.C.*, D.C. App. No. 87–609 [April 26, 1990], reversed on

appeal in 573 A.2d 1235 [D.C. App. 1990]; *Re S* [1992] 4 All ER 671, and the 1997 case of *MS*, which reversed the holding in *Re S* and firmly disallowed imposed Caesarean sections).

Once again, it seems we cannot get away from ethical controversy in maternal–fetal medicine, even without tackling the 'biggest' issue directly – abortion. The apparently uncontroversial statement that we should do the best we can by the children we do have – a position which we adopted in order to avoid the even more controversial one that says we should have as many children as possible – turns out to have all sorts of ramifications. One such consequence has not yet been identified, however, and at first it does appear to be more of a technical than an ethical matter. This is the issue of selective reduction of multiple fetuses in IVF. Although in recent years many countries have restricted the number of embryos that can be implanted in IVF to two or even one, others permit the practice of multiple embryo implantation, which some clinics and patients actively prefer because it is widely, if erroneously, thought to increase the chance of a successful pregnancy (Ledger, 2006). But if the health, or indeed the life, of one fetus in multiple pregnancy requires destruction of others, how can we decide what to do? Are we obliged to do anything at all? If not, do we impose unacceptably high risks on both the pregnant woman and the fetuses, including the risk that all of the latter will die? How do we choose which, if any, fetuses to abort when it is really a matter of 'the fewer the better'?

We will now guide you through a reading by Mary Mahowald, Professor Emerita of Medical Ethics at the University of Chicago, which explores whether or not that is true. You will see that the issue of abortion does in fact surface very early. Nonetheless, we have chosen Mahowald's article because it has a more practical, less theoretical feel to it than many of the classic texts on abortion; it is not about hypothetical cases, but again about real clinical practice. As you read, try to relate the sample cases Mahowald offers to your own experience.

The fewer the better? Ethical issues in multiple gestation

Mary B. Mahowald[3]

Until the last part of the twentieth century, Hellin's Law governed the predictability of multiple births: the natural occurrence of twins in the general population is 1/100, and the frequency of each higher multiple is determinable by multiplying the denominator by 100, so that the frequency of triplets is 1/10 000, the frequency of quadruplets is 1/1 000 000, and so on. Since the advent of fertility drugs in the 1960s and in vitro fertilization in the 1970s, the incidence of multiple gestations has increased markedly. By the late 1980s, the rate of multiple births had more than tripled; it appears to be rising still (Hammon, 1998).

With each higher order of multiples, risks to both fetus and pregnant woman escalate. For women, the risks include anemia, preterm labor, hypertension, thrombophlebitis, preterm delivery and hemorrhage. Tocolytic therapy to avoid preterm delivery introduces further risks. For fetuses or potential children, the risks include intrauterine growth retardation, malpresentation, cord accidents, and the usual sequelae of preterm delivery, such as respiratory distress, intracranial hemorrhage and cerebral palsy (Hammon, 1998, p. 339).

Obviously, prevention of multiple gestation is desirable and can probably be accomplished in most cases. As already acknowledged, however, the possibility of high multiples occurs in nature, albeit rarely, and the mortality and morbidity of these gestations for women and some of their fetuses can only effectively be reduced by terminating other fetuses. In other words, the criterion on which to base the medical prognosis for women and their potential children in multiple gestations is 'the fewer the better'. How, then, does one reduce many gestating fetuses or embryos to fewer?

The language used to name procedures to reduce the number of developing fetuses in an established gestation is controversial in its own right. Among the terms utilized are selective birth, selective abortion, selective reduction, fetal reduction and multifetal pregnancy reduction.[2] Others that could be utilized are partial abortion or partial feticide. The term 'selective birth' has been used for cases of multiple gestation in which a specific fetus had been identified as anomalous and targeted for termination. (Targeting could occur for other reasons, such as sex selection.)

Prenatal detection of the anomaly is not possible until weeks, sometimes months, after detection of the number of gestating fetuses. Ultrasound-guided cardiac injection of the targeted fetus is then the means through which termination is accomplished. Obviously and perhaps misleadingly, the term 'selective birth' focuses on the fetuses that are not targeted. 'Selective abortion' would more accurately describe the procedure, but only if abortion is defined as termination of the fetus rather than termination of pregnancy.

'Selective reduction' is accurate if specific fetuses are targeted and if the pregnancy itself is not thought to be 'reduced'. But women, after all, are neither more nor less pregnant, regardless of the number of fetuses they are carrying. What is reduced, therefore, is the number of gestating fetuses. In situations in which selective reduction of fetuses occurs, the actual procedure is direct termination of the targeted fetus or fetuses. In these cases, 'selective termination' would be a more accurate representation of what is intended and done. If abortion is defined as termination of the fetus rather than termination of a nonviable pregnancy, 'selective abortion' would be accurate when specific fetuses are targeted and 'partial abortion' would be accurate in other cases as well.[3] If abortion is defined as termination of a (nonviable) pregnancy, terminating one fetus while maintaining the pregnancy through other(s) is not equivalent to abortion.

Years ago I used the term 'fetal reduction' to describe interventions to reduce the number of developing fetuses in multiple gestations.[4] I now consider the term 'reduction' misleading or ambiguous. It is misleading because it obscures the fact that the procedure in most cases entails direct killing of at least one fetus, and in other cases makes it impossible for some fetuses to survive, which to many is morally equivalent to killing. It is ambiguous because 'reduction' is not equivalent to 'termination'. Although 'termination' is the more honest description, a fair and adequate definition of the procedure needs to include the aim of maintaining the pregnancy by preserving some fetuses.

'Multifetal pregnancy reduction' is the term most commonly used by those who perform the procedure.[5] This terminology raises some of the same problems cited above: pregnancy is not reducible, and even if it were, the term 'reduction' mischaracterizes the intervention. To be adequate, a definition of the procedure would indicate that it involves terminating fetuses while preserving pregnancy. Awkward but accurate definitions could therefore be any of the following: fetal termination with pregnancy preservation; fetal termination and preservation in multiple gestation; reducing the number of fetuses in multiple gestation; abortion with pregnancy preservation; and partial abortion. As already suggested, the last two definitions are only accurate if abortion is defined as termination of the fetus rather than termination of pregnancy. Hereafter, I will use the first definition, which I consider simplest, clear, and accurate: fetal termination with pregnancy preservation, which I will shorten to FTPP.

ACTIVITY: Why is it important to get the terminology right, according to Mahowald? Is she just splitting hairs? In our view, what she is doing is clarifying the assumptions which often remain hidden, and exposing uncomfortable truths. 'Reduction' does camouflage what is really going on: for any single fetus, the issue is not being 'reduced' but being 'terminated'. Regardless of whether one favours or opposes the right to abortion, it is important to see that abortion is involved. Feminist bioethicists, of whom Mahowald is one, have been particularly perceptive about the ways in which language is used to decide the debate before it even starts. For example, the term 'surrogate mother' implies that the birth mother is not the 'real' mother, with the corollary that if she refuses to hand over the baby to the contracting couple, their rights rather than hers will be respected (e.g. the case of Mary Beth Whitehead, mentioned earlier by Christine Overall). Feminist bioethicists have urged instead the terms 'contract mother', or 'gestational/genetic mother', depending on whether the woman's contribution includes her own ova.

Now continue with your reading of Mahowald, moving into the section of her article which asks you to consider what differences are ethically relevant in cases with similar clinical facts.

Although fetuses are not legally persons, and their personhood is morally debatable, they are in fact living, human and genetically distinct from the women in whom they develop. Many human fetuses have the capability of becoming persons both legally and morally. In high-order multiple gestations, however, that capability is so greatly and unalterably reduced (without intervention) that the scenario is morally different from, say, a twin gestation, where the capability of both fetuses becoming legal and moral persons is high. The following cases illustrate this morally relevant difference along with other variables that influence the capabilities of individuals. Consideration of these variables is crucial to ethical decisions about whether FTPP should be requested or performed. Case 2a is one in which I was personally involved; case 3a is the well-publicized case of the McCaughey septuplets. Although the other cases are fictitious, all of the features enumerated have occurred in real cases.

Case 1a Normal twins During her second prenatal visit, a 36-year-old mother of five, ages 2 to 12 years, is told that she has a twin gestation. She tells her doctor that she thinks she can handle a single newborn but not two at once. 'I simply don't have time for twins,' she says. Having heard about FTPP, she asks whether this is an option for her. The alternative of adoption is suggested but rejected.

Case 1b: Same case as Case 1a except that one fetus has trisomy 21 (Down's syndrome).

Case 1c: Same case as Case 1a except that one fetus has trisomy 13 [editor's note: trisomy 13 may produce cleft palate, atrial septal defect, inguinal hernia and lower limb abnormalities. For children with full trisomy 13, survival beyond the first year is uncommon; however, it is rare for fetuses with this condition to go to term, so it occurs in only one of every 6000 live births.]

Case 1d: Same case as 1a except that the woman cannot pay for FTPP.

Case 2a Infertility drug + twin gestation   A childless woman undergoing infertility treatment for 2 years becomes pregnant after taking perganol. She has been told that this drug might cause multiple gestation. At 8 weeks' gestation, ultrasound confirms the presence in utero of two fetuses, both of which appear healthy. One week later, the woman asks her physician to reduce the number of fetuses to one. Although the patient is informed that this procedure involves risk of losing the other fetus also, she persists in her request for FTPP, indicating that if this cannot be done, she will seek abortion of both fetuses, and 'try again' for another pregnancy.

Case 2b: Same case as Case 2a except that the twins are known to be male and female, and the woman asks the physician to target the female fetus.

Case 2c: Same case as Case 2a except that the woman asks the physician to target the male fetus.

Case 2d: Same case as Case 2a except that the woman has a triplet gestation and wants to have a singleton.

Case 3a Infertility treatment and high-order multiples   After having a daughter with the assistance of a fertility drug (metrodin), Bobbi McCaughey asks her doctor for similar assistance to have a second child. Six weeks later, ultrasound shows that she is carrying septuplets. Doctors present the option of FTPP as a means by which to optimize the chance of live healthy birth of at least one child. The option is rejected by the McGaugheys on grounds that it is morally equivalent to abortion.

Case 3b: Same as Case 3a except that fertilization occurs in vitro, allowing transfer of fewer embryos.

Case 3c: Same as Case 3a except that Mrs McCaughey is carrying quadruplets rather than septuplets.

ACTIVITY: What would 'producing the best children we can' suggest in each of these cases? Is this enough of a guideline, or do we need to incorporate other factors? For example, the effect on the five other children in the first case. You might want to make a grid in which you note, first, whether you would approve of FTTP (fetal reduction) in this case, and if so, why. Then look back over the factors you identified as ethically important in making such decisions. This could be the basis of a checklist for your own practice.

Section 5: Compliance in pregnancy

In the previous section, we used fetal reduction (or as Mahowald prefers to call it, fetal termination with preservation of pregnancy) as a practical sort of prism through which to view abortion, fetal and maternal rights, and the other 'big issues' of reproductive ethics. However, it has to be recognized that fetal reduction is only an issue in a small minority of pregnancies, as indeed is IVF itself.

ACTIVITY: What about 'ordinary' pregnancies? Do they also present ethical problems, and if so, what? Stop a moment to jot down the ethical dilemmas which may face clinicians dealing with 'normal' pregnancy.

You may have noted such issues as enforced Caesarean section, imposed by clinicians, or conversely, the mother's right to an elective Caesarean against the clinical judgement of her obstetricians. These are important issues, but only, of course, at delivery. Most of the debate on ethical and legal dilemmas surrounding pregnancy and childbirth has, in fact, tended to focus on childbirth.

Yet in terms of everyday practice some of these issues listed at the start of this chapter may look exotic but irrelevant. Human reproductive cloning attracted tremendous media attention in the late 1990s, after the creation of 'Dolly the sheep', but how important was it to the average practitioner? So-called 'therapeutic' cloning has been the object of much media 'hype', but at the time of writing, it has not yet resulted in any actual therapies. In this section, in line with our belief in the importance of 'everyday ethics' rather than just the headline-grabbing instances, we turn very explicitly to a more everyday sort of issue throughout pregnancy: compliance.

Non-compliance is the sort of problem which looks purely clinical, but actually turns out to raise more ethical dilemmas than we generally think. The first stage of solving ethical dilemmas is recognizing one when you see one, and elsewhere in this textbook we often ask you to think about the ethical aspects of what looks at first to be purely a 'technical' question: for example, in Chapter 6, we suggest that even 'routine' long-term care gives rise to many ethical questions for practitioners.

Once again, we will ask you to undertake a guided reading activity exploring the ethical issues in compliance, by Françoise Baylis and Susan Sherwin, respectively of the School of Medicine and Department of Philosophy at Dalhousie University, Halifax, Nova Scotia. Essentially, Baylis and Sherwin argue that 'noncompliance' is a value-laden term which prejudges the issue against the pregnant woman. Rather, they assert, we should think in terms of the woman's consent to or refusal of treatment at various stages of pregnancy. We already recognize that competent patients have the right to refuse consent at any stage of the treatment process; even once given, consent can likewise be withdrawn. This is now true in law of Caesarean section, where courts in both the US and the UK have made it clear that pregnant women enjoy the same rights in regard to treatment refusal as any other class of pregnancy. At least 'a subset' of non-compliant actions, Baylis and Sherwin argue, should also be considered legitimate treatment refusal. The task for ethically sensitive physicians to think hard about what sorts of actions are included in that subset.

As you read, think about the implications for clinical practice of Baylis and Sherwin's argument. If you disagree with their view, ask yourself, too, whether there are any limits to which women need not go in order to produce 'as good babies as we can'.

Judgements of non-compliance in pregnancy

Françoise Baylis and Susan Sherwin[4]

Medical knowledge regarding the ways in which women can actively pursue healthy pregnancies and the birth of healthy infants covers an increasingly broad spectrum of activities before, during and after the usual 9 months of pregnancy. In fact, depending upon the clinical situation, the number and range of activities are such that, if a woman were to take all obstetrical advice seriously, she would be faced with a daunting list of instructions ranging from mere suggestions to strong professional recommendations. Few women could (or would want to) fully adapt their lives to the entire range of advice from physicians, midwives, nurses, nutritionists, physiotherapists and childbirth educators, and generally this is not a problem. In principle, professional advice is something that patients can choose to follow or not – this is the essence of informed choice (Faden and Beauchamp, 1986). In some instances, however, failure to follow professional recommendations elicits pejorative judgements of non-compliance (Feinstein, 1990), and while these judgements are provoked by a failure to comply with specific advice, typically they are applied to the patient as a whole. Moreover, even if the patient ultimately consents to the recommended course of action, she may continue to carry the label of non-compliant because of her initial efforts to resist medical authority, and this labelling frequently has repercussions for her subsequent interactions with healthcare professionals.

[W]e suggest that a subset of the behaviours and choices that the language of non-compliance now captures are not inherently problematic. They ought not to be construed as non-compliance, but rather as informed or uninformed refusals. In our view, the only situations that are inherently problematic are those where the patient fails to comply with her own choices, which may or may not be consistent with directions from her physician. A commitment to provide respectful healthcare requires that these situations be dealt with in a way that enhances, rather than undermines, autonomy-respecting, integrity-preserving patient–physician interactions.

ACTIVITY: As Baylis and Sherwin say in the last sentence, their argument emphasizes patient autonomy, and views the pregnant woman's autonomy as no different from that of any other patient. Think about some 'tough cases' that might test that assertion. What about the pregnant crack cocaine addict, for example? Is her autonomy limited by her addiction? Or by the risk to the fetus of being born addicted? Even if it is, are we any more entitled to intervene against her wishes than we would be with a non-pregnant addict? Now continue with your reading of Baylis and Sherwin.

None the less, not all divergence from physician opinion will evoke the label non-compliant. For example, the term is seldom used when the behaviour in question is within a morally contested realm such as prenatal genetic testing. In the face of public and professional debates about the appropriateness of the genetics agenda, refusal of genetic testing is generally tolerated. Also, the label non-compliant is seldom used when patients demonstrate excessive enthusiasm for medical interventions deemed unnecessary. For example, patients who request Caesarean deliveries that their doctors do not consider medically required may have their requests refused, but they are unlikely to be seen as non-compliant. The same is true with patients who request/demand an amniocentesis in the absence of professionally accepted risk factors. Thus, it appears that failure to act in accordance with patient-specific medical advice is a necessary but not a sufficient condition for being so labelled.

ACTIVITY: What is the legal basis for viewing patients who 'request too much' differently from patients who 'refuse too much'?

There is no entitlement for a patient to demand a particular level of treatment in English law (*ex parte Hincks*, 1979), whereas there is a common-law right not to be subjected to unwarranted bodily interventions. Treatment without the patient's consent may be a battery; no treatment, even if the patient would have given consent, is not an offence. In this respect, pregnant women are no different from any other patient. So perhaps the anomaly which Baylis and Sherwin identify about 'excessively enthusiastic' patients not being labelled non-compliant is not really surprising. You will see, however, that they would be likely to explain these legal positions in terms of power and authority, rather than just accepting them at face value.

Now continue with your reading of Baylis and Sherwin.

Some clear patterns emerge regarding judgements of compliance and non-compliance. First, these judgements not only denote the existence of a doctor–patient (or healthcare professional–patient) relationship (or formal interaction); they also reflect certain assumptions about the nature of that relationship. Specifically, the framework of patient compliance and non-compliance implies a commitment to an implicit hierarchical structure within medicine, in

that these terms reflect an understanding of the doctor–patient relationship as inherently unequal. The labels compliant and non-compliant apply in cases where those with greater power have issued directives to those with less power, and these directives have either been followed or set aside. In marked contrast, those with lesser power can only make requests of those with greater authority. For example, patients who refuse to act in accordance with physicians' professional recommendations can be deemed non-compliant with medical advice. On the other hand, physicians who refuse to act in accordance with women's requests may be judged uncooperative, but not non-compliant. To be sure, it is possible for physicians to be labelled non-compliant, but in their case it is not for failure to respond to patients' demands, but rather for failure to comply with practice norms or professional guidelines, such as established protocols, prescription standards or research criteria (Cheon-Lee and Amstey, 1998; Helfgott *et al.*, 1998).

In addition, situating patient behaviours within a framework of compliance and non-compliance discourages development of the trust that is essential for a good doctor–patient relationship. In labelling a patient non-compliant, the physician is expressing his/her distrust in the patient's ability or motivation to make appropriate use of medical expertise. The term is pejorative and often functions as an expression of exasperation at the patient's 'irresponsible' behaviour. For her part, the patient may be sensitive to any moral judgements surrounding her behaviour. She may be wary of negative labels generally, and, in particular, worried about being labelled non-compliant and abandoned by her physician if she is judged unworthy. Hence, she may feel anxious about being fully honest with her physician. Rather than bringing her questions and concerns to the forefront, she may tell the physician what she thinks he/she wants to hear and may also seek to minimize the time spent with the physician in order to hide her 'negative' behaviour and avoid disapproving lectures.

In sum, the framework of compliance and non-compliance trades on the unequal, hierarchical nature of the physician–patient relationship, potentially denigrates patients, undermines trust, reduces patient agency and conflicts with goals of informed choice. Given these problematic implications, it is curious that the framework is so prominent in obstetrics and other areas of medicine.

ACTIVITY: In your experience, are judgements of compliance prominent in obstetrics? More or less so than in other areas of medicine? Could the framework of non-compliance be completely jettisoned? If not, why not? Now continue with your reading of Baylis and Sherwin, to see their answer to this question.

[E]ven though countless studies demonstrate that patients in all areas of medicine routinely diverge from medical directives and that judgements of non-compliance are common throughout medicine, these judgements take on a particular urgency in obstetrics. This is because a non-compliant patient is thought to be risking not only her own health, but also the wellbeing of the future child she is expected to be nurturing. Social stereotypes that demand that women be self-sacrificing for the sake of their (future) children judge women especially harshly if they fail to make all reasonable efforts to protect the health of their developing fetuses. It is one thing to be bad at caring for oneself. It is generally considered a far greater flaw for women if they are bad at caring for their (future) children. These judgements are not entirely external. Women tend to internalize the social messages of good mothering, and pregnant women may well feel guilt-laden if they suspect their own behaviour could harm their future children.

To better understand the problems that the compliance and non-compliance framework is meant to capture, and to help set the stage for an alternative approach, we review a fairly standard range of behaviours in which patients fail to follow the specific advice of their doctors. In identifying these behaviours, we are particularly interested in understanding whether patients and physicians agree about the nature of the problem. Our aim is to see if other responses might better address the perceived problem than the pejorative labelling represented by judgements of non-compliance, and to determine whether the situations might be better described according to alternative frameworks.

Deliberate refusals: value conflict As noted above, women sometimes make a deliberate decision to reject their physicians' advice because it runs contrary to their values. For example, a woman who has undergone infertility treatment and is carrying three or more fetuses may be advised to submit to selective termination in order to increase the chance of a healthy pregnancy, uncomplicated delivery and the birth of healthy infants. If she is adamantly opposed to abortion, however, she will reject the advice out of hand, as it is in direct conflict with her deep-seated values. As long as the choices that the woman is following are clear and accepted within the culture, she is unlikely to

be labelled non-compliant. Nonetheless, she may experience less support from her physician as tensions mount because of potential harms associated with her choice. In the abstract, most physicians will formally acknowledge a patient's right to make her own deliberate value choices; in practice, though, some will find it extremely difficult to demonstrate full respect for what they perceive to be poor choices.

Deliberate refusals: epistemological conflict In other cases, women may agree with the values that inform the physician's recommendation (e.g. promotion of their own health and that of their fetuses), but question the medical knowledge on which that advice is based. Medical knowledge is, after all, imperfect and continually subject to revision and re-interpretation. Consider, for example, how in the past 100 years medical advice regarding morning sickness has changed. In 1899, a pregnant woman might have been advised to take cocaine for nausea (10 minims of a 3% solution) and to sip champagne to prevent vomiting (*Merck's Manual of the Materia Medica*, 1899 edition). In the 1950s, tragically, thousands of women worldwide were advised to use thalidomide to control nausea in pregnancy, until the disastrous effect on the fetuses' developing limbs became evident.

Not only are there inconsistencies over time with respect to the information on which medical advice is based; there are sometimes also significant inconsistencies among physicians at any one point in time. For example, there is significant variation in rates of Caesarean deliveries, use of fetal monitors, and numbers of ultrasounds performed in different geographical centres. Not surprisingly, such differences in professional practice patterns undermine patient confidence in expert medical opinion.

A second reason for some women to doubt medical knowledge is evidence of past mistakes. In the 1950s, for example, women considered at risk for miscarriage were advised to take diethylstilbestrol (DES) to reduce the likelihood of miscarriage, even though research failed to establish its effectiveness at this task. The tragic consequences of such marketing include an exceptionally high frequency of genital cancers among the young adults whose mothers took DES while pregnant.

Finally, women may also doubt medical knowledge because they 'know' better, as when their lived experience (or that of a family member or close friend) contradicts medical dicta. A woman advised to exercise during pregnancy because this will help ease her labour may deny this claim based on personal knowledge, e.g. she may have experienced a long hard labour with her last pregnancy, despite having followed medical advice in favour of exercise. Similarly, a woman informed of the need for a Caesarean delivery may remember having a successful vaginal delivery after having been told once before of the need for a Caesarean.

In addition to any doubts that women may have about the validity of particular medical knowledge, there may also be disagreement with the (problematic) epistemological assumption held by many physicians that medical knowledge is preferable to other forms of knowledge and should always be privileged. As feminist epistemologists have argued, there are multiple ways of knowing; scientific knowledge is one form among many ... Experiential, and particularly, embodied ways of knowing provide other essential kinds of knowledge that cannot always be accessed through scientific methods. In the complex, embodied experience of pregnancy, women must depend upon both scientific and experiential forms of knowledge (Abel and Browner, 1998).

For many women an important test of whether their doctor values experiential knowledge is if the doctor is attentive to (and validates) her reports about her experiences throughout her pregnancy. To care well for their obstetrical patients, physicians need to listen carefully to women's descriptions of their bodily experiences. If this is a repeat pregnancy, for example, they should be very interested in learning what is different in this experience from that of the earlier pregnancies. Often, it is women's own reports that give the first indication of complications or difficulties in a pregnancy. Physicians who disregard women's reports or concerns about their embodied experience in favour of abstract scientific knowledge may find that their own advice is disregarded in turn because their patients do not believe it was based on all relevant information.

Deliberate refusals: distrust   Some women who intentionally reject medical advice do so not because of conflicting values, or problematic knowledge claims, but rather because of a deep-seated mistrust of physicians and the medical profession as a whole. There is some evidence, for example, that African–Americans who reject medical advice do so in part as 'a response to racially differentiated histories and sentiments concerning medical intervention and experimentation' (Rapp, 1998, p. 147). In some jurisdictions, women from ethnic-racial minorities are much more likely to be encouraged to accept sterilization as a form of contraception than are women who are part of the dominant social group (Lopez, 1998). Poor women, especially those dependent on welfare, are subject to intense monitoring and regulation by the state in

many aspects of their private life, and may assume that the physician is simply one more agent of the state, intent on extending the state's control ever further into their lives. Lesbian women may sense their doctor's disapproval of their plans to raise children in a non-standard family. And women with serious addictions, especially those with criminal records, may expect that the physician has only contempt for them and little concern for their welfare. Women from these various social groups have reason to see physicians as representing a culture that is hostile to them; hence they may distrust the physician's commitment to their well-being and that of their children. Under such pervasive conditions of distrust, it is difficult to see why women would choose to follow medical advice unless the value of doing so is made very clear to them.

ACTIVITY: Baylis and Sherwin are writing from a North American perspective. How might distrust between doctor and patient manifest itself in other cultures? Is it equally problematic in your own practice? It is also interesting to reflect on how 'politics' enters clinical practice this way, no matter how separate one may want to keep the two. Now continue with your reading of Baylis and Sherwin.

Failure of understanding   Failure of understanding also colours many decisions regarding prenatal testing where patients who are not scientifically literate may have difficulty deciphering the language. Consider, for example, the counter-intuitive use of the medical phrase 'positive test result' to denote a negative outcome. There are also patients who will have difficulty with statistical thinking and who may forgo or accept testing having misunderstood the risk of miscarriage or the risk of carrying a fetus with a chromosomal abnormality.

Inadvertent non-compliance   Medical attention often focuses on specific behaviours without considering the full range of concerns and constraints that structure patients' lives. Consider, for example, patients whose jobs depend on working long and unpredictable shifts. They may not eat properly, get adequate exercise or be able to keep their doctors' appointments. They may appear irresponsible to doctors who do not appreciate the lack of control these women have over their time. Similarly, pregnant women who work in unhealthy environments may not be able to change jobs and for financial reasons may not be able to quit working. They may be judged non-compliant if they have been advised that the workplace exposes the developing fetus to toxic substances. Another example of this problem is women who develop diabetes during pregnancy. They will need to learn to test their blood sugar frequently, to eat at regular intervals, to modify their diet significantly, and perhaps to administer insulin daily. They can agree with their physicians about the medical need for such adjustments, but still find that the stresses of daily life make adaptation to the recommended regimen very difficult. Further, their own conflicting emotions about having such a serious disease may foster ambivalent attitudes about fully acknowledging and addressing their state.

For other women, apprehension (possibly engendered by a failure of understanding) is another reason for diverging from recommended actions. For example, fear of amniocentesis, chorionic villus sampling and percutaneous umbilical cord sampling is often the reason for missed prenatal diagnosis appointments. In yet other cases, patients have difficulty explaining, even to themselves, the reasons for their failure to follow medical advice and feel very confused about their competence as future mothers. The underlying assumption with compliance and non-compliance judgements is that patients are purely rational beings who will follow medical advice if it is fully explained to them and they understand the likely consequences of their behaviour. Yet human beings are more complex than this simplistic picture suggests. Our actions reflect both conscious and unconscious motivations, and our reasons for action are not always transparent to us. The biomedical model suggests that experiences should all be subject to rational evaluation and control, but daily life makes it evident that the experience of pregnancy cannot be reduced to this model without losing important dimensions. Emotional and physical experience – yes, even 'intuitions' – need to be acknowledged as part of a patient's motivational structure.

Judgements of non-compliance in review In this schema, there is no place for the language of compliance and non-compliance – language that is imbued with the hierarchy of medicine and thus is fundamentally at odds with the commitment to promote agency and respect the autonomous choices of patients. Such language inappropriately obscures that which is important, namely the context within which, and the reason(s) why, a patient does not conform with medical advice. To fashion an ethically acceptable response to situations where patients do not follow medical advice, it is necessary to understand the patient's motivations and life setting, the legitimacy of goals other than the pursuit of health, and the limits of individual physicians and of

medicine more generally. Seeking appropriate targets for blame inhibits rather than facilitates this task. Enhancing the patient's sense of agency and control is more consistent with a commitment to respectful patient care and, moreover, helps to support the patient's own desires for achieving a healthy pregnancy.

ACTIVITY: As your final activity for this guided reading, make a list of the 'big' philosophical and ethical concepts and dilemmas which have been raised in what may seem the rather everyday, non-ethically charged area of non-compliance in pregnancy. For example, the question of the relationship between rationality and reasons for action arises toward the end of Baylis and Sherwin's article. Social justice, too, is an issue in judgements of non-compliance, as are autonomy and paternalism, and tolerance for multiculturalism as it affects women's trust in doctors from another culture. Underlying many of the other issues, one might argue, is the question of why pregnant women appear to be labelled non-compliant so easily, perhaps more so than other patients. Does this itself raise issues about justice and fairness? Why is it so, if it is so?

Section 6: A case study of high-risk pregnancy

In these later sections of the chapter, we have concentrated on 'everyday' ethical issues in preference to hypothetical situations or rare clinical events. Our reasoning here has been twofold.

We think it is important for you to see that there are ethical issues in what may look like routine decisions that can be made on a purely clinical basis. Thus we frequently begin by asking you to think about what might be ethically problematic in what looks ethically problem-free – for example, routine judgements of pregnant women as non-compliant. We prefer 'real-life' situations to the hypothetical cases beloved of many philosophers. For example, in the area of abortion, instead of fetal reduction, we could have used Judith Jarvis Thomson's famous 'violinist' hypothetical (Thomson, 1971), in which you are asked to imagine that you wake to find a famous violinist plugged into your circulatory system for 9 months. Although Thomson's compelling hypothetical case has generated an enormous literature, it leaves out childbirth in favour of pregnancy itself, and in our opinion this is a fatal omission (Dickenson, 1997). It is easier not to forget the full realities of the situation if one uses 'real-life' cases.

However, it is also important to remember that there are plenty of real-life situations which are far from routine. In the final part of this section on pregnancy and childbirth, we look at an anonymized case study illustrating the ethical problems of paternalism and autonomy which arose during a high-risk IVF pregnancy. The case study was written by Gillian Lockwood, an infertility specialist with an interest in ethical issues. It has the great merit of bringing together your earlier work on assisted reproductive technologies (Overall and Mahowald) with the issues about management of pregnancy and non-compliance raised by Baylis and Sherwin. Again, this section is designed as a guided reading exercise. As you read, we would like you to keep a 'log' of the ethical problems you identify at each stage of the clinical situation, and what you would advise the clinician to do at this stage. Ask yourself, too, whether the clinical team handled this patient's quite profound 'non-compliance' in the right way, refusing to view it judgementally as non-compliance but nonetheless setting limits to what they, as clinicians, felt called upon to do.

Problems of paternalism and autonomy in a 'high-risk' pregnancy

Gillian M. Lockwood[5]

Introduction

Renal transplantation, the treatment of choice for patients with end-stage renal failure, can correct the infertility due to chronic ill-health, anaemia and tubal damage generally encountered when these patients are managed by renal dialysis. Currently only one in 50 women of child-bearing age becomes pregnant following a renal transplant, and it may be that many more would welcome the chance of biological parenthood if their fertility problems could be overcome. The first successful pregnancy, conceived in 1956 following an identical twin renal transplant, was reported in 1963 (Murray et al., 1963).

Until recently pregnancy had been thought to present considerable hazards to the transplant recipient. However, some reviews (Sturgiss and Davison, 1992; Davison, 1994) have suggested that pregnancy in the graft recipient, unlike the rare pregnancy in patients undergoing dialysis, is usually likely to lead to a live birth, and the pregnancy may have little or no adverse effect on either renal function or blood pressure in the transplant recipient. The current medical consensus is that if, prior to conception, renal function is well preserved, and the patient does not develop high blood pressure, then only a minority of transplant recipients will experience a deterioration of their renal function attributable to pregnancy (Lindheimer and Katz, 1992).

It is inevitable that the rapid return to good health enjoyed by the majority of women following successful renal transplantation should encourage them to consider conception. Although only a small proportion of women with a functioning graft become spontaneously pregnant, modern Assisted Reproductive Technologies (ARTs), especially in vitro fertilization and embryo transfer (IVF–ET), could theoretically increase this proportion to near-normal levels. Pregnancy, especially if ART is required, clearly entails extra risks for the renal transplant recipient, but these are risks that, with appropriate counselling, the patient may be prepared and even eager to take.

In this paper, I shall discuss the ethical dilemmas involved in counselling renal transplant patients seeking pregnancy but requiring ART. This case concerned a couple with long-standing infertility by means of IVF–ET. The wife was a renal transplant recipient whose initial renal failure was due to severe, recurrent pre-eclampsia, a potentially life-threatening condition of late pregnancy causing raised blood pressure and renal complications, which can progress to cause fits and cerebro-vascular accidents [strokes]. It is associated with severe growth retardation of the fetus, and often, premature delivery.

A case of high-risk pregnancy

A 34-year-old woman (Mrs A) was referred to an IVF unit following 8 years of failure to conceive after a reversal-of-sterilization operation had been performed (Lockwood et al., 1995). She had been born with only one poorly developed kidney, but this was not known until, at age 20, she was investigated for very severe pre-eclampsic toxaemia (PET), which she suffered during her first pregnancy. Her baby was born very premature at 26 weeks' gestation, and he died shortly after birth from complications of extreme prematurity.

A second pregnancy in the following year was also complicated by severe PET, renal damage, premature delivery at 26 weeks' gestation and neonatal death. Sterilization by tubal ligation was offered and accepted under these circumstances, in view of the anticipated further deterioration of her renal function with any subsequent pregnancy. There was a significant further advance of her renal disease, necessitating the initiation of haemodialysis (a kidney machine) 2 years later, and a living, related donor renal transplant (from her mother) was subsequently performed. After the transplant, Mrs A remained well and maintained good kidney function on a combination of anti-rejection drugs, steroids and blood pressure tablets. At age 26, a reversal-of-sterilization operation was performed because she had become so distressed by her childlessness, but hysterosalpingography (a test to check for fallopian tubal patency) 2 years later, when pregnancy had not occurred, showed that both tubes had once again become blocked.

ACTIVITY: What ethical issues are presented at this point? For example, is it right to try to help Mrs A become pregnant, no matter how distressed she is about her childlessness, if it may harm her clinical condition? Is this part of the duties of a doctor? – conceived as responding to the patient's autonomous wishes. Or, is it actually antithetical to the duties of a doctor? – seen in terms of benefiting rather than harming patients, and with benefit primarily seen in turn as being to do with medical best interests.

You might also want to look at the autonomy chapter, and consider how reproductive ethics takes our concern beyond the patient alone. In the Lockwood case, it might be argued that patient autonomy is not the same as giving the patient what she wants – particularly because others in the family constellation also need to be considered. For example, Mrs A's mother now has only one kidney, because she has donated her other one to her daughter. Does this mean that Mrs A is in some sense not entirely free to risk the donated kidney on her high-risk pregnancy? If it gives Mrs A's mother some say, exactly how much and what kind of say?

Now continue with your reading of the case.

At the time that Mr and Mrs A were referred to the IVF unit, there were no case reports of successful IVF in women with renal transplants, but specialists were becoming increasingly reluctant to advise women with transplants against trying for a baby, as medical care for 'high-risk' pregnancies was improving dramatically. Following discussion with the Transplantation Unit and the high-risk pregnancy specialists, the IVF unit felt that an IVF treatment cycle could be offered to Mr and Mrs A as long as the risks of IVF–ET, over and above those attendant upon a spontaneous pregnancy in these circumstances, were understood and accepted by the couple and minimized, as far as possible, by the IVF team.

ACTIVITY: How would you characterize the solution taken by the IVF team to the dilemma identified in the last activity? One way to see it is in terms of informed consent to treatment. The IVF team seem to take the view that provided consent to treatment is genuinely informed, and that all risks are fully communicated to the couple, it is really up to the couple to decide. This is consistent with the view of the function of informed consent which one of us has argued for elsewhere (Dickenson, 1991, 2003), as transferring responsibility for ill-luck in outcomes from clinician to patient. (Of course, the team also view their duty as including maintaining good medical standards and minimizing risk; it would not be sufficent to say the couple had consented if the procedure was then performed negligently, in effect increasing the risks beyond the level to which they had given consent.) Now continue with your reading of the case.

An IVF treatment cycle was started using the normal drug regimen, but the patient was given a much lower dose than usual, with the aim of minimizing the effect of the hormone stimulation on the transplanted kidney. Two oocytes (eggs) were obtained, which fertilized normally in vitro, and the two embryos were transferred to the uterus (womb) 54 hours later. Mrs A's pregnancy test was positive 13 days after embryo transfer, and an ultrasound scan performed at 8 weeks' gestation showed a viable twin pregnancy.

Throughout the treatment cycle and during pregnancy, the patient's antirejection drugs (azathioprine and prednisolone) were continued at maintenance doses. Renal function was monitored closely throughout the treatment cycle and during pregnancy, remaining remarkably stable.

The pregnancy was complicated at 20 weeks' gestation by a right deep vein thrombosis, affecting the femoral and external iliac veins, and anticoagulation with heparin and warfarin was required. Spontaneous rupture of the membranes, leading to premature delivery, occurred at 29 weeks' gestation; the twins were delivered vaginally and in good condition three hours later. The twin girls were small for dates (at 1.48 and 1.19 kg) but were otherwise well, requiring only minimal resuscitation and respiratory support. After delivery of her babies, Mrs A remained well and her renal graft continued to function normally, with no change in immunosuppressive or antihypertensive (blood pressure) medication required.

ACTIVITY: Stop again to make another entry in your log. Does the favourable outcome indicate that the decision to treat Mrs A was ethically correct? Or is this judgement from hindsight? Consider some further evidence of the risks to health of both mother and child, presented by Lockwood.

Risks to the mother, the fetus and the neonate   Severe pre-eclampsia and eclampsia can result in irreversible damage to the maternal kidney, particularly due to acute renal cortical necrosis. Women who have recurrent pre-eclampsia in several pregnancies or blood pressures that remain elevated in the period following delivery (the puerperium), especially if they have pre-existing renal disease and/or hypertension, have a higher incidence of later cardiovascular disorders and a reduced life expectancy (Chesley et al., 2000). Pregnancy is recognized to be a privileged immunological state, and therefore episodes of rejection during pregnancy might be expected to be lower than for non-pregnant transplant recipients. Nevertheless, rejection episodes occur in 9% of pregnant women, occasionally in women who have had years of stable renal functioning prior to conception. More rarely, rejection episodes occur in the puerperium, when they may represent a rebound effect from the altered immunosuppressiveness of pregnancy.

Immunosuppressive (anti-rejection) drugs are theoretically toxic to the developing fetus; however, maternal health and graft function require continuation of maintenance immunosuppression. Women with impaired renal function are recognized to be at risk of giving birth prematurely, often to growth-retarded or small-for-dates babies. A large French study of women with pre-existing renal damage reported a prematurity rate of 17% and a spontaneous abortion rate (miscarriage) of 20%, as compared to prematurity and spontaneous abortion rates of 8 and 12%, respectively, in the normal population (Jungers et al., 1986). However, the long-term health effect of events in utero for the offspring of transplanted mothers is harder to quantify. There is animal evidence of delayed effects of immunosuppressive therapies and intrauterine growth retardation.

ACTIVITY: At this point, review your log of the ethical issues in the case, before reading Lockwood's discussion of them. As you read her analysis, you may wish to add other considerations, or perhaps her discussion may suggest counter-arguments to your own views, which you might want to consider. When you have finished, you should have a matched list of arguments for treatment, and corresponding counter-arguments against, together with an overall conclusion weighing up both pros and cons. Lockwood puts her analysis primarily in terms of paternalism and autonomy, but your arguments and counter-arguments may be structured differently. For example, having just read Baylis and Sherwin's discussion, you may be asking yourself whether Mrs A's decision to request IVF was in a sense 'non-compliant' with medical advice concerning her kidney condition. You will see that there is also a link to multiple embryo transfer for successful pregnancy in kidney recipients, so that your reading of Mahowald should have alerted you to the ethical complications here. You will probably also want to ask Overall's question, in a slightly different context: is it clear that IVF in this case would benefit the children who might be born as a result? Given that the babies were born at rather dangerously low birthweights, and that two previous pregnancies had resulted in stillbirths, this is a very real question.

Case discussion   The decision to accept the couple for IVF treatment posed significant dilemmas of both a technical (obstetric and renal) and an ethical nature.

The ethical aspects of undertaking IVF and embryo transfer in these circumstances are possibly harder to quantify and yet more contentious. It is recognized that even under optimum circumstances, at the most effective units, the probability of a successful pregnancy with a single treatment cycle of IVF–ET is only about 25%. Was it acceptable to expose Mrs A to all the risks of an IVF cycle that was four times as likely to fail as to succeed? Even where the IVF is successful in establishing a pregnancy, there is still the non-negligible risk that renal function may deteriorate. The patient may have safely delivered, but again become dependent upon renal dialysis. The Human Fertilisation and Embryology Act 1990 laid great stress on the importance of obtaining true informed consent from patients undertaking procedures such as IVF; it was particularly important that the patient and her husband were made aware of the risks associated not only with the failure of IVF–ET but also with its success.

Arguments that could be advanced against offering fertility treatment to renal transplant recipients, such as whether it is in the best interests of the patient to be helped to achieve a state as a result of which she may suffer chronic ill-health or even early death, have also been advanced against permitting 'old', i.e. post-menopausal, women to become pregnant through the technique of egg-donation IVF. In both instances, one could argue that as long as the risks associated with fertility treatment and pregnancy were thoroughly explained to and accepted by the woman (and her partner), then to refuse treatment on the sole ground that her health may deteriorate is unacceptably paternalistic on the part of the clinicians involved. Mrs A stated that if she had not agreed to the sterilization (which she claimed she had been placed under undue pressure to accept at the time she was diagnosed with renal failure), then she would not only have been able to, but definitely would have tried to, achieve a further pregnancy, as she did after the reversal of sterilization was performed.

The Human Fertilisation and Embryology Act 1990 [operative at the time this case occurred, prior to the adoption of the revised law in 2008] also places great emphasis on the 'interests of the child' who may be born as a result of procedures such as IVF–ET. This emphasis has been interpreted by some authorities as encouraging fertility units to feel justified in refusing treatment to women with significant health problems (or to post-menopausal women) as it would, so they claim, not be in the 'interests of the child' to be born to a mother with reduced life expectancy due to chronic ill-health or comparatively advanced age. Apart from the obvious rejoinders that society happily countenances men becoming fathers at an age when their life expectancy is reduced, and the medical profession's heroic efforts to assist women with serious health problems who become pregnant spontaneously, it is unquestionably in the interests of the child. After all, the child will only be born if his transplanted mother is offered fertility treatment, so that she should be offered such treatment even if he loses his mother at an early age or has to deal with the consequences of her ill-health, as otherwise he won't exist!

ACTIVITY: Compare the stances taken by Lockwood and Overall on the prospective child's interests. How do they differ? How would Lockwood's view affect her opinion of whether IVF treatment was right in this case?

Our answer is that Lockwood, who has elsewhere described herself as an ethical consequentialist, like John Harris, appears to believe that it is 'unquestionably' in the child's interest to be born. This would presumably be an argument in favour of IVF, although it assumes that existence is a benefit – a view with which many religions and world views, Buddhism for example, or the Greek tragic authors – would emphatically not agree. Overall, on the other hand, views the

question of the child's best interests as a nonsense, because there is no entity which can have best interests if the child is not born.

Your comparison of Lockwood and Overall has brought this chapter full circle, as have the issues of choice and vulnerability in this high-risk pregnancy. At the very start of this chapter we asked you to consider the implications of NRTs more broadly, and in particular for the women who undergo them. Lockwood's patient Mrs A was vulnerable not only because of her clinical condition, but because of her deep desire to overcome her childlessness. Her pregnancy was clinically riskier than a 'normal' pregnancy, but her feelings about riskiness and uncertainty mirror those experienced by both partners in the IVF context as well. New reproductive technologies have given hope to many couples, but they also create pressures and vulnerability which are not always acknowledged (Franklin and Roberts, 2006).

References and notes

1. For example, the criminalization of maternal substance abuse indirectly threatens the well-being of children, since the threat of criminal prosecution may deter pregnant women from seeking medical care (Blank and Merrick, 1995: 165).

2. Berkowitz, R. L., Lynch, I., Stone J. and Alvarez, M. (1996). The current status of multifetal pregnancy reduction. *American Journal of Obstetrics and Gynecology*, **174** (4), 1265–6.

3. Clinical texts usually define abortion as termination of a non-viable pregnancy; popular understandings tend to identify it with termination of fetuses; cf. Mary B. Mahowald (1982). Concepts of abortion and their relevance to the abortion debate. *Southern Journal of Philosophy*, **20**, 195–207.

4. Mahowald, M. B. (1993), *Women and Children in Health Care: An Unequal Majority*. New York: Oxford University Press, pp. 87–90.

5. For example, Berkowitz *et al.*, p. 1265; Evans *et al.*, p. 771; and the American College of Obstetricians and Gynecologists; cf. Rorty, M. V. and Pinkerton, J. V. (1996). Elective fetal reduction: the ultimate elective surgery. *Journal of Contemporary Health Law and Policy*, **13**, 55.

Notes

1. Adapted with permission from Christine Overall (2002), 'New reproductive technologies and practices: benefits or liabilities for children?' Originally appeared as 'Do new reproductive technologies benefit or harm children?' In *Ethical Issues in*

Maternal–Fetal Medicine, ed. D. L. Dickenson, pp. 305–21. Cambridge: Cambridge University Press.

2. Adapted with permission from Anna Smajdor, 'Is there a right not to be a parent?' *Bionews*, January 2008, www.bionews.org.uk.

3. Adapted with permission from Mary Mahowald (2002), 'The fewer the better? Ethical issues in multiple gestation'. In *Ethical Issues in Maternal–Fetal Medicine*, ed. D. L. Dickenson, pp. 247–60. Cambridge: Cambridge University Press.

4. Adapted with permission from Francoise Baylis and Susan Sherwin (2002), 'Judgements of non-compliance in pregnancy'. In *Ethical Issues in Maternal–Fetal Medicine*, ed. D. L. Dickenson, pp. 285–301. Cambridge: Cambridge University Press.

5. Adapted with permission from Gillian M. Lockwood (2002), 'A case study in IVF: problems of paternalism and autonomy in a 'high-risk pregnancy''. In *Ethical Issues in Maternal–Fetal Medicine*, ed. D. L. Dickenson, pp. 161–6. Cambridge: Cambridge University Press.

Genetics: information, access and ownership

Introduction

The continuing development of genetics has profound implications for the future of medicine. Since the first edition of this book appeared in 2001, there have been important advances in understanding some of the genetic factors in common disorders. Much genetic research ('genomic epidemiology') is intended to lead to a better understanding of biological mechanisms such as immunity, which will help to understand disease progression. An example would be research in malaria, using genetic variation in populations as a way into understanding mechanisms which may prove helpful in the development of a vaccine. In the medium to longer term, the impact is perhaps most likely to be felt in the development of more effective treatments for the major diseases, including the use of medicines tailored to fit an individual's own genetic profile ('pharmacogenetics'). Cheap and accurate sequencing techniques may conceivably allow everyone to know the full contents of their own genome, but that could be a double-edged sword, increasing the ethical, legal and social risks of genetic testing (Robertson, 2003).

What are these risks? And what are the practical ethical questions raised by genetics today? You have already encountered some of these issues in the previous chapter: for example, preimplantation genetic diagnosis. Here in Chapter 3 we will concentrate on the wider clinical aspects of genetics, outside the area of new reproductive technologies. In particular, we will focus on making decisions about genetic information, on rights in genetic data, and on the way in which knowing more about your genetic make-up actually increases both certainty and uncertainty.

We begin by focusing on the ethical issues surrounding the availability and use of genetic testing. The chapter opens with a short case about genetic testing for the BRCA1 and BRCA2 genes implicated in certain forms of breast and ovarian cancer. Genetics may seem to offer radically new and productive forms of knowledge about disease, but there are also important issues about vulnerability to be considered – just as we argued at the end of the previous chapter about the new reproductive technologies. Like NRTs, the 'new genetics' promises new powers to medicine but may sometimes leave patients, and indeed clinicians, feeling vulnerable rather than empowered, when their uncertainty is actually increased. Issues around certainty and false reassurance, together with questions of confidentiality and the right to know, are illustrated in the first case study, found on your CD-ROM.

This case is followed by a personal account of what it is like to live with the risk of inherited breast cancer. It is becoming increasingly clear that, like breast cancer, most genetically related conditions will turn out to be the result of a variety of factors, both genetic and environmental. This means that genetic tests for these conditions, when used presymptomatically, will give imperfect information about the likelihood of the condition occurring. This raises important ethical questions about the availability of such tests and the ways in which the results ought to be interpreted. As you read through this first section, consider what these ethical questions might be.

Following this first section, we go on to look at the ethical questions raised by those tests which provide information that is more certain, by means of two cases relating to Huntington's disease. Although you might think that certainty would be reassuring, it can have quite the opposite effect in some cases, for both the patient and family members. Is there a duty to share 'dangerous' genetic information with family members who may carry the same genetic mutation and risk developing the same disease? Because genetics is, by definition, about an entire lineage, the relevant consideration here isn't just the autonomous individual typically considered elsewhere in medical ethics, but the entire family. True, the weaknesses of the traditional autonomy-centred view of medical ethics may be thrown into relief by genetics, but then perhaps that is a good thing, requiring us to adopt a wider view of 'who is the patient'? (We'll return to these issues later, in the autonomy chapter.) If different family members have different views about what genetic information they want to know about themselves, who decides? It's all very well to say that the choice should be left up to the individual, but with many genetic conditions, one person's results may well reveal information about a related individual. That turns out to be the case in the Huntington's disease scenarios. Who 'owns' genetic information? The individual, or the entire family? We present you with a debate from the pages of the *British Medical Journal* on this crucial issue, and ask you to form your own opinion.

The question of who 'owns' genetic information is relevant not only at the level of the individual and his or her family, but also at the level of the wider society. With the development of genetic and tissue banks on a massive scale – for example, the recent UK Biobank, which will recruit 500 000 British citizens aged 40–69 to give samples – consent, confidentiality and ownership of genetic information are becoming important concerns for everyone. A high proportion of us will have donated tissue to a 'biobank', knowingly or unwittingly. What rights should we have to determine the uses made of that information? Is the traditional notion of informed consent a sufficient protection against uses we don't want to see? What about use of genetic information by insurance firms or employers? What about commercial firms who profit from our tissue? Or indigenous peoples who object to the use of their genome by Western biotechnology firms? In the third section of this chapter, we will ask how genetic data-banking affects ethical decision-making in clinical practice, examining examples from the UK, USA and Iceland. We will investigate the way in which developing countries have reacted against the attempt by Western researchers and firms to 'colonize' their often unique genetic resources. Beginning at the level of an individual family's story, this section moves to global issues about genetic databanking and the difficult question of who, if anyone, 'owns' the human genome.

Finally, in Section 4, we explore the common belief that we *are* our genes. If that is so, then genetics takes on a very special quality, compared with other medical and scientific disciplines – but *is* that so? Do our innermost beliefs and most significant actions just boil down to genetic factors? As the British bioethicist Ruth Chadwick has written, 'Are genes us?' (Chadwick, 1999a). You will be asked to come to your own view on this question, variously known as 'genetic determinism', the 'genetic mystique' or 'genetic exceptionalism'. The 'moral status of the gene', as the philosopher Mary Ann Warren calls it (Warren, 2002), is actually a great deal more complicated than the extreme view that our health, behaviour and even our thoughts are entirely genetically determined.

Section 1: Living with uncertainty

A case of breast cancer genetics

Please open scenario 2 on your CD-ROM, 'Genetic testing: breast cancer', and work through it, noting down your responses to the questions posed about clinical dilemmas as you go along. This case concerns a woman, Beth Brown, who receives a routine request to attend a breast cancer screening clinic. Believing herself to be at high risk of developing breast cancer because of familial patterns, and additionally concerned also for her own daughters, she asks her GP to refer her also for genetic testing for the mutations implicated in some breast cancers. The case raises practical ethical issues about patients' and practitioners' understanding of genetic testing, the right to know and genetic determinism, as well as the overall question of how someone like Beth can live with a degree of uncertainty which not even the most sophisticated genetic test can entirely dispel. The situation is further complicated by the fact that in cases where the test is carried out against the background of a family pedigree conferring high risk, a negative (i.e. 'good news') test result can fail to reduce risk sufficiently to take a woman out of a high-risk group and hence have no implications for screening/treatment. You will also find additional references for medical and legal information at the end of the scenario, together with a list of four key ethical issues we have identified in the scenario. You may wish to add others of your own to your responses. Also bear in mind that before you start playing the video clip at the outset of the scenario, you may wish to access the list of issues in the scenario, the list of further readings and/or the glossary from the Toolbar. The CD-ROM contains a rich variety of resources in addition to the scenarios themselves, including definitions of key medical and ethical terms.

When you have finished, please return to this text.

One of the most difficult features of genetic testing for most conditions is that the information gained is so often imperfect. For example, breast cancer is a multifactorial disease, and only about 10% of cases are thought to be due to an inherited risk. Also, a positive test for the BRCA1 gene indicates an 80% chance of developing breast cancer by the age of 65, but not an absolute certainty of it. Another factor which has important ethical implications is the fact that it is possible for the results of tests for BRCA1 to be either falsely negative or falsely positive. In the light of these facts, should a genetic test like this be marketed as soon as possible or only when there is a proven treatment? A testing kit for the BRCA1 gene is currently available on the internet. Do you agree that the BRCA1 test should be openly available for those who want to use it? If not, why not?

We would now like you to read the following account by June Zatz of what it is like to live with the risk of developing breast cancer after having come across the information by chance. Although her initial contact with information about her risk did not come about through a genetics test, her case has interesting parallels with Mrs Brown's. Ask yourself if there are particular ethical questions related to the availability of this kind of genetic information. What are the possible benefits and harms?

I am definitely having it done

June Zatz[*]

I remember in 1973, when I was 23 years old, sitting in the hairdresser's, reading some obscure American magazine. I came across an article about a 19-year-old girl from New York where every female on her mother's side had contracted breast cancer, going back two or three generations. A decision was taken that she have both breasts removed as this was the only way to ensure that she would not contract the disease herself. I was absolutely aghast when I read this article. This was the first time I learnt that breast cancer was hereditary. My mother, her two sisters and her first cousin had had breast cancer but I never really thought of it as being a threat to me. And the thought of a 19-year-old having such a drastic operation! I never discussed the article with anyone. It was after reading the article that the implications were clearer to me of contracting the disease. I dismissed as ridiculous the part in the article about the

operation, but I know that I stored it away in the back of my mind.

My mother had a radical mastectomy when she was 42 years old. As a result of the operation she was left with fluid in her right arm, which caused severe infections where she was bedridden for days. She had bouts of ill-health for years but in between she was a determined lady who never complained. She had a second mastectomy 13 years later followed by various operations and bouts of ill-health. After a benign tumour was removed from her liver when she was 58, her consultant warned my brother and me that 'cancer will get her sooner rather than later'. Her ultimate illness was when she was 66 years old, short and sharp – cancer of the spine – paralysis – painful death – even now, 7 years later, I cannot think of this period without immense pain.

My mother's younger sister developed breast cancer when she was 46, and after numerous operations and great pain died 2 years later when 48 years old. This was prior to the days of the hospice (where my mother died) and so my mother looked after her, but the pain was not well controlled.

My other aunt died when I was only 7 years old. My mother told me she had breast cancer in her early 40s, but also had a heart condition from which she died in her mid-40s.

ACTIVITY: Awareness of genetic risk can arise in many different ways. As this case shows, the trigger may be discussion in the media, the sharing of information in families or a clinical diagnosis. Most clinical geneticists agree that when possible, genetic testing should be preceded and followed by counselling. Should such counselling be compulsory? Or, do you think that those who wish to take a genetic test ought to be able to do so freely, whether or not they want to have counselling? What are the ethical implications of this question?

After finding out that breast cancer can be hereditary, I read everything I could get my hands on. Only once when in my mid-20s I attempted to bring up the subject with my mother, as I felt perhaps she could get advice for me from her specialist. But she just dismissed it and refused to discuss it. I never attempted to mention it again. My husband, however, got to know of my fears because I often imagined I felt a lump in my breast. Then I became depressed, lay awake at night imagining all sorts of things and, having two young children, I naturally worried about the children – what would happen if I weren't around for them? Throughout the years, I only ever went to the doctor twice when the 'lump' didn't seem to disappear and I was literally going round the bend. Even when at the doctor's I managed to conceal my true feelings, was very matter of fact, and he was never aware of the family history as I didn't tell him.

My mother died 7 years ago, when I was 37 years old. Within a few weeks of her death, I realized that I had to do something about my fears and get them out in the open. It was almost as though with her death this released me to discuss my fears out in the open. I wrote to my mother's oncologist detailing the family history and asking whether there was anything else I should be doing apart from self-examination.

This resulted in me being referred to an oncology clinic for regular monitoring, initially 6-monthly, then annually. These visits to the clinic I can only describe as horrendous. First of all there was the waiting area where females of all ages (many surprisingly young) were waiting to find out whether they had breast cancer or because they already had it. Then, in the cubicles while waiting to be examined, you could hear the registrar in the next cubicle talking to the patient and I knew from the conversation that all was not well. By the time I was due to be examined, I would be a wreck – then the mammogram; then the waiting a week for the result. After the result I would be elated, my first thought would be thank God, I will be around for another year. I would immediately calculate all my children's ages. This was what was of prime importance for me – I wanted to be around to see them into adulthood.

As I neared the age when my mother developed her first breast cancer, I became more fearful. Over the years I had read many articles and I did not feel that treatments were any more effective today than years ago, even if it were detected at an earlier stage. I felt that I would get breast cancer as my body was similar to my mother's in many ways – she had fibroids and a hysterectomy – she had gall stones and had her gall bladder removed. I had had both these operations by my late 30s.

My mind kept casting back to the article I'd read all those years ago about the 19-year-old who had both breasts removed as a preventative measure. I had never read of this again but decided it was time to pursue it further.

In the summer of 1991 I wrote to my oncologist asking if such an operation were possible. His answer took a fairly long time coming, mainly due to administrative procedures. While I waited for the reply, I was on tenterhooks: my feelings were that I would be told that I was crazy, that this operation could be done only in America.

Eventually when his letter arrived stating that yes, I could have this operation – I literally couldn't believe it – I read the letter over and over for days. Then I wrote another long letter with lots of questions. There followed several letters to and fro: a referral to a plastic surgeon to discuss reconstruction and a referral to a specialist cancer geneticist to discuss the genetic side of things.

It took me months to make up my mind definitely. After the second letter from the oncologist, I told my husband what I was investigating and he was horror-struck. He just could not understand why I should have both breasts removed when they were perfectly healthy. To him the logical thing was to wait and, if the cancer appeared, then it will have been caught early, then I should have a mastectomy. He didn't understand that, the way I saw it, it was too late by then. At this stage, however, I hadn't made up my mind and in fact because of my husband's attitude I put things on hold for several weeks. One day, however, I woke up early feeling such anger and resentment towards him – he and I had always until now agreed on major issues.

I discussed it with him again. This time I had a different attitude: he had made me feel selfish contemplating such an operation but what I said to him was: What about me, my fears; this is my life and who's going to look after me if I get cancer – will he nurse me? At the same time I said I hadn't yet made up my mind but I was going to continue my investigations whether he liked it or not. He listened and said he'd like to come with me when I next had a consultation with either the oncologist or the plastic surgeon. I refused as I knew he was still against it but said I'd tell him everything they said.

Some days I would wake up and say, 'I'm definitely having it done'. Other days I'd think I was crazy – I tried to imagine what it would be like without breasts, although there was the chance of reconstruction.

Gradually my husband came round to my way of things. The more information I gathered the more he understood what I could be facing. One day I said, 'I don't think I'll have it done', and then to my surprise he said, 'You should go ahead – I'd rather have you alive and well with no breasts'.

In April 1992 I made the decision to have the operation. Throughout the 6 months it took me to come to this decision I had several consultations with the three specialists. The clinical geneticist put me in touch with another lady who had had a similar operation. She had an almost identical family history to mine. I had a long discussion with her on the phone. It was invaluable to talk to someone who had been in my situation. She and her sister had had the operation and were greatly relieved that the chance of breast cancer had been removed.

The only people who knew about it were my husband, my two children and two friends, one of whom had a medical background and the other was a cousin to whom I'm very close and with whom I'd often discussed the 'family history'. I instinctively knew from the beginning that I didn't want anyone's advice on the matter, I wanted facts on which I could base my decision. The professionals were wonderful. Everyone was patient, answered my questions, was quietly supportive and never offered advice on what I should do. There's no way the outcome would have been as successful without their help and support. I should also point out that they were all males.

At the time my daughter was 18 years old and my son 16. They knew what was happening but my daughter could not understand my contemplating such an operation, so I didn't discuss it with her, and my son couldn't deal with it at all – perhaps due to his age and sexuality.

The plastic surgeon had discussed the breast reconstruction he would be performing, which involved a lengthy operation. At the same time as performing the mastectomies, he would remove fat and muscle from my stomach and use this to form new breasts. It was a complicated procedure and there was also a chance that it wouldn't work. I asked myself, could I cope with having no breasts? I'd decided not to have silicone implants because of recent bad publicity. I concluded that disfigurement was of secondary importance to the certainty of not getting breast cancer. Since 12 years of age I'd been surrounded by this disease and here was a way to get rid of it.

From the time of making my decision in April 1992 I never looked back once. Now I had to decide when to tell people because I'd be in hospital for 2 weeks and off work for a couple of months. I had lunch with a close friend and started to tell her. She was so aghast that I didn't finish telling her about the reconstruction. I couldn't wait to get away from her. She just couldn't hide her feelings. After this I told a few more people but got more or less the same reaction. I was furious and upset. The way I saw it I had made a very difficult decision and these supposed close friends were completely unsympathetic. They made comments like 'Do you know what you are doing?' or 'Why remove your breasts when you haven't got cancer?'

I told my doctor friend who had known from the beginning and she said, 'They're so busy trying to deal with their own feelings that they can't focus on you and provide support for you'. I realized just what a threat this seemed to be to other women – to have one's breasts removed. I told my husband I couldn't tell anyone else so he said to make a list and he would sit down and phone them. I gave him half a dozen names and he did it immediately as I didn't want these people to find out from others. Needless to say I received a few phone calls from people we'd not told, to say that they'd heard about it; again they were very unsupportive. Despite the lack of help I never faltered.

The operation was performed in September 1992. I was really quite ill, which was to be expected. The plastic surgeon was so attentive and kind that somehow, even though I felt very ill, so long as he was looking after me I knew everything would be OK. I was fortunate in that the reconstruction was successful. While lying in hospital I became obsessed with the imminent pathology result of both breasts. What if I'm too late and the cancer was already there? Prior to the operation I remember saying to the surgeon, 'Please cut everything out.' I didn't want any chances taken. It took about 10 days for the pathology results and when I was told that everything was OK, I just couldn't take it in.

After the operation people's attitude was how brave I'd been to have such an operation, but I didn't see it like that at all. I'd had the operation done through fear – fear of getting breast cancer.

I've never looked back since the operation. It's the best decision I made in my life or am likely to ever make.

This may sound odd, but it took about 6–12 months after the operation for the full psychological effects to be felt. I now read articles about breast cancer and watch programmes on TV without dread and despair. Something else that also became apparent was that prior to the operation I had never made any serious plans for the future – subconsciously I had thought I would die at a relatively early age from breast cancer. Now this inevitability had been removed along with my breasts. I now felt a person given their freedom, with a whole new quality of life.

Once the decision to proceed with the operation was made, my husband's support was invaluable. He is delighted that I will never get breast cancer, the bonus being that the reconstruction was successful.

With the advances in genetic knowledge, more women are going to be identified as having a high risk of contracting breast cancer. The dilemma that I faced will be much more common. I can only say that the radical surgery I decided on was for me by far the lesser of two evils.

The ethical questions raised by genetic testing are particularly difficult both because of the interpersonal/ intergenerational nature of the information provided and also because in many cases, as in the case of the BRCA1 gene, the information is statistical and not easy to translate into action. Not all genetic tests are like this, however. In the case of Huntington's disease, a positive test does mean that the test subject will develop the condition at some point and that their children will have a 50% chance of inheriting the gene. As we will be going on to see in the next section, such tests raise ethical questions of their own. You saw in the CD-ROM case that Mrs Brown's daughters, Rebecca and Laura, were contemplating taking the genetic test for the BRCA1 and BRCA2 mutations, regardless of whatever their mother decided about having the test herself. But if their results came back positive, that would have revealed information about their mother's status – so she would have known the truth whether she liked it or not. What does this aspect of genetics imply about an individual's right to know, or her autonomy? In the next section we will examine that question in greater detail.

Section 2: Living with certainty

A case of the right not to know

ACTIVITY: Please open scenario 4, 'Genetic testing: Huntington's disease', on your CD-ROM. (Again, bear in mind that the toolbar contains additional resources such as a glossary of unfamiliar terms, which you may wish to consult before viewing the scenario.) Work through the scenario and associated questions, which will take you about 40 minutes, and then return to this text.

This scenario concerns Henry, a 73-year-old man who was diagnosed with depression and then with atypical Alzheimer's disease. But Henry's symptoms were still not fully explained, and his dementia was now so severe that communication with him was effectively impossible. The family history, however, included members who had manifested jerky movements or dementia late in life. This suggested a possible genetic link.

In conversation with a researcher from a project on memory and ageing, the general practitioner involved in Henry's care learned that a new testing procedure could determine accurately whether Henry might have Huntington's disease (HD), an incurable progressive disease of the central nervous system. The testing procedure, based on the number of repeats of the gene for HD, would only be available if Henry was enrolled on the research project. (This is no longer the case as far as HD is concerned, but it may well apply for other conditions.) Henry's clinical team decided to request consent from his family to use the newly available genetic test and to enrol him in the research project. The family agreed, and Henry tested positive for Huntington's disease 10 days before his death.

But it turned out that Henry's family hadn't really understood the implications for themselves of allowing him to be tested. Huntington's is an autosomal dominant condition, meaning that Henry's children Ann and Peter would have roughly 50–50 chances of developing the condition themselves. Henry's wife Mary now wanted everyone in the family to be tested for HD, including her grandchildren (who would have a 1 in 4 chance of developing HD). Ann was willing to be tested herself, but Peter was adamantly against finding out his genetic status or allowing his wife Ruth to learn about Henry's test results, even though he and his wife already had two young children, and might have more.

ACTIVITY: How does Henry's case compare with those of June Satz and Beth Brown? Information and access issues seem crucial here, the cause of conflict within the family. How can they be resolved?

In contrast to the first section, on ethical dilemmas raised by the *uncertainty* more characteristic of genetic testing, Henry's case demonstrates the troubling consequences of a greater degree of *certainty*. Because Huntington's disease is an autosomal dominant condition (see the glossary on the CD-ROM), caused by mutations on a single gene rather than the many genes typically involved in other genetic conditions, the choice faced by Henry's descendants is particularly clear and stark. That does not necessarily make the ethical choices any easier, for example in the effects on Henry's grandchildren.

Should the eldest grandchild, Tom, have the right to know his genetic status even though he isn't yet 18? Or is it more important to protect the grandchildren's right to an untroubled, open childhood, and maintain the option for them to make their own choice about whether or not to be tested in the future? There is no cure currently possible for Huntington's disease, so on an ethical consequentialist basis, knowing one's diagnosis does no therapeutic good. (Consequentialists stress the importance of maximizing beneficial outcomes, and would probably say that truth-telling is not an absolute principle in itself.) Furthermore, the grandchildren may well not carry the mutation; should their young lives be clouded by fear of developing a condition that may never arise? Or is that an old-fashioned, paternalistic attitude? One of us has argued elsewhere that in a similar case involving a teenager, wanting to take control of one's future is particularly potent for adolescents, and that it is 'a perfectly valid and indeed very "adult" motivation for a young person to request genetic testing for an incurable adult-onset disorder' (Dickenson and Fulford, 2000, p. 205). We would now like you to read a version of this case and a commentary, which appeared in the *British Medical Journal* (Dickenson, 1999a).

The case of Alison

As a general practitioner, you are confronted with the case of Alison, an intelligent 15-year-old girl whose father has recently tested positive for Huntington's disease. His own mother died of the condition before Alison was born. Alison wants to know whether she, too, will develop Huntington's disease. Her parents, who have accompanied her to the surgery, support her wish. Alison's mother is herself contemplating genetic testing for the BRCA1 gene implicated in some breast cancers, following the death of her own mother and her elder sister from the disease.

You know that the clinical genetics unit which serves your patients will not test young people under 18, although Alison can have counselling. You point out that even those over 18 must undergo counselling before having the test, according to the unit's careful protocol. Alison thinks this over and replies: 'I can see the point of having some talks with the counsellor first. But if I do decide I want it, do I still have to wait another three years before I can actually have the test?'

Can children and young people consent to be tested for adult-onset genetic disorders?

Donna Dickenson[**]

Although many regional genetics units are evolving policies which do take young people's requests seriously, in the wake of policy recommendations from the royal colleges, the Nuffield Council[1] and the British Medical Association[2], it would still be unusual for a request like Alison's to be granted, where the disorder is of the magnitude of Huntington's disease. I will argue that the situation is anomalous in the light of law giving young people under 18 the right to consent to treatment, including testing. The argument primarily concerns consent, but it is also

important to note that an action in negligence could arise if Alison gave birth to an HD-positive baby which she would not have had if she had known her genetic predisposition.[3]

Professional guidelines Professional literature and guidelines on the predictive testing of at-risk children have often focused on the situation where parents request testing on the child's behalf, rather than the scenario in which the young person herself wants to be tested. In 1989 a research group of the World Federation of Neurology declared that children should not be tested for Huntington's disease on their parents' request. The age of majority remained the touchstone in the 1994 recommendations of a joint committee of the International Huntington Association and the World Federation of Neurology Research Group on Huntington's Chorea,[4] although that report added: 'It seems appropriate and even essential, however, that the child be informed of his or her at-risk status upon reaching the age of reason.'

In the same year, the Clinical Genetics Society working party[5] concluded that, although discussion and counselling could and should be offered to minors, "formal genetic testing should generally wait until the "children" request such tests for themselves, as autonomous adults'.[6] However, the working party did say that testing should wait either until the person affected is adult or 'is able to appreciate not only the genetic facts of the matter but also the emotional and social consequences'.

The legal position These documents mainly focused on younger children. The argument here is that English law already allows competent older children and adolescents to consent on their own behalf. There are two strands in this syllogism:

(1) Treatment includes diagnosis,[7] and therefore consent to testing is considered under the same rubric as consent to treatment.
(2) The general legal principle that 18 is the age of majority was modified in the Family Law Reform Act 1969 to allow young persons of 16 to give consent which would be as valid and effective as an adult's. Subsequent case law undermined the ability of young people under 18 to refuse consent to a procedure: in *Re W* [1992][8] the Court of Appeal held that where someone with parental responsibility gave consent to treatment on the minor's behalf, the young person could not refuse.

However, both Alison's parents and she give consent, and the young person's right to consent was reiterated in *Re W*. Alison is still only 15, whereas the dividing line in the Family Reform Act was 16 – also the age of the girl in *Re W*. But in the Gillick case[9] (involving a 15-year-old girl's consent to treatment) a function-specific, flexible test of competence was set down: whether the young person had 'sufficient understanding and intelligence to enable him or her to understand fully what is proposed'.[10] (This is assumed to be an English case, but in Scotland Alison would also probably be able to consent on the similar grounds that she had sufficient understanding of the issue to make a choice.[11]) Alison is likely to have a fuller understanding than many 15-year-olds of what genetic disorders imply. She is like the children with chronic cardiac or orthopaedic conditions studied by Alderson,[12][13] who discovered surprisingly high levels of familiarity with diagnostic procedures, cognitive sophistication about probabilities and prognosis, and strong personal values. Against 'the child's right to an open future',[14][15] we could argue that young people with a family genetic history like Alison's grow up fast.

ACTIVITY: What do you think about the empirical argument here that children who have had experiences such as Alison's tend to have a fuller understanding of the issues than their peers? Do you agree that this is or might be the case? One argument which might be made against this claim is that in some families, perhaps where the experience of family members such as parents living with and coming to terms with risk or disease has been particularly difficult, children may actually find it harder to make a balanced judgement. At the very least, families and children may be very different from one another. To what extent do you think that this issue is ethically important? Is there a significant difference between understanding the issues and having the moral maturity to make a decision?

Harm, best interests and paternalism   **Another** legal strand is the requirement to consider 'the ascertainable wishes and feelings of the child concerned (considered in the light of his age and understanding)' into the 'welfare checklist' that must be used in any case affecting his upbringing.[16] The Children Act 1989 also requires consideration of 'any harm which he has suffered or is at risk of suffering'.

Would a positive test inflict harm on Alison? Even if there is no possibility of treatment, there might be benefits in terms of control, ability to plan, and family solidarity. If this is true in Huntington's disease, where the disease is terrible, no cure is possible and onset is comparatively remote from adolescence, then it is all the more true of lesser conditions.[17]

Against findings of higher psychological morbidity in those who test positive,[18] some studies of both Huntington's disease and breast cancer tests report relief of uncertainty even on learning of a high-risk test result.[19] According to another study, 'a high-risk result merely exchanges the uncertainty of whether Huntington's disease will develop for that of when it will develop'.[20] However, Brandt[21] found no greater psychological morbidity for patients informed that they had tested positive than for those told they had negative status.

Against earlier expectations that up to three-quarters of those at risk of inheriting the Huntington's mutation would choose to be tested in order to relieve uncertainty, fewer than 10% of those with a Huntington's-positive parent have chosen to have counselling about the possibility of a test. Of those, only about two-thirds actually opt for testing.[22] So Alison's wish is unconventional; but one could argue that it may therefore be all the more personal and deeply considered, an 'authentic choice' of the adult sort which many developmental psychologists believe should be honoured in adolescents.[23]

ACTIVITY: Since this article was first published, Alison's wish has begun to be less unconventional: older adolescents have been requesting such testing for themselves and guidelines have increasingly recognised the autonomy of the young person (Borry *et al.*, 2006), although clinical geneticists are still significantly more in favour of undertaking a test if the request has been made together with a parent (Borry *et al.*, 2008). Do you agree with this emerging consensus?

Autonomy and paternalism   The Children Act also leaves scope for courts to find that the child's expressed wishes are not his 'true wishes', those that serve his best interests.[24] Possibly Alison's expressed wishes are not really her true wishes, but there is a risk of paternalistic condescension.[25] Paternalism usually favours treatment on the grounds of best interests, even in the absence of the patient's consent. Yet the paternalistic thing to do in Alison's case is not to override her refusal and impose treatment, but to override her consent and withhold the test.

Alison may seem too vulnerable to request testing, because of the very fact that she has recently learned that she is at risk for HD. But we are all by definition vulnerable at the time we are asked to consent to treatment: generally we are ill, or facing uncertain results about a possible diagnosis. Another argument against allowing adolescents to be tested is that they are subject to family influence: 14- and 15-year-olds asked to make hypothetical medical decisions frequently deferred to what they saw as their parents' wishes.[26] But studies of adults might equally well show that they did what they thought their spouses or children would want. In Alison's case, where both the young person and the family agree, we must be particularly careful not to impose a conflictual, individualistic model based on the premise that individual and family interests necessarily collide.

If the young person's values and identity seem reasonably coherent and secure, then her consent should be honoured. Conversely, identity only comes with making choices and having them enacted.[27]

Key messages

(1) Existing case law almost certainly allows competent young people under 18 to consent to testing for adult-onset genetic disorders; but many clinical genetics units operate a bar at 18.

(2) Rather than relying on an age-specific test of competence, genetics units, and referring general practitioners, need to think whether they are being paternalistic in denying the test to a competent minor.

(3) Good practice suggests that each case should be considered on its own merits, taking into account the seriousness of the disorder and balancing that against the emotional and cognitive competence of the young person.

ACTIVITY: What are the ethical issues raised by these two cases? Before proceeding any further, make a list of the questions you think have emerged from the Henry and Alison scenarios.

The CD-ROM suggests four principal ethical issues in the Henry scenario: the right to know, the right not to know, children's rights to request genetic testing, and the concept of an 'open future'. Although you might initially think that the right to know is just an extension of the right not to know, that's not so clear. After all, the 'right to know' is based on the notion of a rational, autonomous individual needing all the available facts to make up her mind. We don't usually think of rational, autonomous individuals as deliberately choosing ignorance. If there is a right not to know, it might have to be based on a different notion of autonomy altogether. How would that right be balanced against denying others the right to know?

Does Peter have the right to resist testing, even if his choice deprives his wife and children of their 'right to know' important information about the family's future or their own health?

What is the moral status of the right not to know? Ought there to be limits to this right? Combined with the intergenerational nature of genetic information, the right not to know poses serious ethical dilemmas – as does the right to know, which may imply forcing others who refuse to be tested to know their own status by implication. That would be the case if Peter's children tested positive for the mutation, once they are of an age to request testing. Should one or both of them test positive, it would mean that Peter also carried the mutation. (Even if both of them tested negative, however, that would not necessarily mean that Peter was in the clear.)

In the Henry case, a serious ethical problem was created by the right not to know combined with the intergenerational nature of the information. As one of us has suggested elsewhere, genetic information may be more appropriately viewed as a 'joint account' held by a family as a whole, rather than an individual. 'Is it "personal" information, which a patient may sometimes have an obligation to share with other members of [the] family – for example, if its release will enable them to avoid serious harm? Or is it essentially familial information, drawn from a kind of joint account, which a patient may sometimes have a right to withhold from other family members – for example, if its release would cause harm to the patient?' (Parker and Lucassen, 2004, p. 165).

These issues arose again in a debate which appeared in the *British Medical Journal* in 2007 on the question 'Should families own genetic information?', between Anneke Lucassen, a consultant with the Wessex Clinical Genetics Service in Southampton, and Angus Clarke, a consultant clinical geneticist at the University Hospital of Wales in Cardiff. For both authors, this is a crucial question in genetic medicine, which frequently involves an entire family constellation rather than the archetypal doctor–patient dyad. As the evidence base in genetic medicine improves and increases, for example in familial screening for bowel cancer, the question becomes all the more acute.

As Lucassen writes, 'The genetic code is held inside the cells that make up a person's body. The genetic material, cells and body might be seen to belong to that person, but does the genetic information deduced from this code belong (solely) to the individual?' (Lucassen, 2007, p. 22). There is a particularly poignant dilemma, as the Henry case demonstrated, when a genetic test on one person tells us crucial information about the genetic code of other persons, who may well be unaware of their genetic inheritance. Even if we want to recognize a right to privacy for the person being tested, do we necessarily want that right to count more heavily than the harm to others which could result from respecting confidentiality?

Confidentiality, however, is not an absolute duty: there are statutory and professional guidelines setting out exceptions. In Lucassen's view those exceptions should extend to the case 'where genetic information points to an intervention that would decrease the morbidity or mortality from a disease, [and where] taking an individual ownership stance could lead to harm to others' (Lucassen, 2007, p. 22). She also believes we should consider reciprocity: most people only gain access to genetic testing because they have been given information (perhaps informally) about their relatives' ill-health. Therefore, she thinks, they have an obligation to make their information available to other family members.

For these reasons, Lucassen is sceptical about viewing personal genetic information as effectively the sole property of the person being tested; rather, it should be seen as jointly held between the individual and and family. She notes, 'The Human Genetics Commission's 2002 report (Human Genetics Commission, 2002) suggested that "genetic solidarity" and altruism should be promoted, and ... the joint account model argues that since genetic information is shared by more than one person, the conventional model of confidentiality should be reversed: the genetic information should be available to all "account holders" (family members) unless there are good reasons to do otherwise' (Lucassen, 2007, p. 23). This stance would mean that clinicians should presume that family members have a right to relevant genetic information from other members, unless proven otherwise. Effectively, that would also reverse the presumption behind informed consent, that it has to be actively given rather than assumed. An interesting parallel might be the the 'opt-out' model of organ donation, which is used in many European countries and which the British Medical Association would like to see adopted in the UK. In that system, it is presumed that an individual gave her consent to having organs removed for transplantation after death, unless she signed a form 'opting out' during her lifetime.

You might say, of course, that overriding the explicit wishes of a *living* patient (not to have genetic data revealed to others) is different from presuming the consent of a dead person (to have organs removed for the use of others). Perhaps you might think no harm is done to the dead person, at least not in any physical sense. But actually we do respect the wishes and autonomy of the dead – that is the entire basis of our system of wills and legacies, after all. A better distinction might be that there is no equivalent to 'opting out' in what Lucassen proposes, except in that rather vague last phrase 'unless there are good reasons to do otherwise'.

In contrast, Angus Clarke argues that, 'Although genes will often be shared within a family, most specific items of genetic information will have been generated by examining or testing an individual. Such information will, inevitably, belong more strongly to that person than to his or her relatives.' (Clarke, 2007, p. 23) However, he too is concerned about situations where that individual fails to pass on vital information to other family members, particularly when the person tested actually forbids health professionals to do so. In similar cases arising in other medical areas, health professionals may well have a duty to warn others even if the person affected wants to keep their status secret: for example, the law requires doctors to disclose information about infectious diseases, or, in relation to driving, information about epilepsy or other conditions that might endanger fellow road users.

Is someone like Peter, in the Henry scenario, a danger to others in this sense? In one sense, the parallel doesn't seem to work: by refusing to have himself tested for the Huntington's mutation, Peter is not posing an immediate threat to anyone else's health and safety, in the way an epileptic or alcoholic driver might. On the other hand, if Peter were to have another child with his wife Ruth, without having had the genetic marker test to determine whether or not he is 'clear' of Huntington's disease, his actions do seriously endanger that future child. Clarke, too, is concerned with the adequacy of such parallels, asking:

> Are genetic disorders sufficiently similar to infectious diseases – gonorrhea, syphilis, HIV – that doctors have a similar duty to enforce disclosure by patients or clients to other members of the family? I would argue that they are not, even when we agree that disclosure would be highly desirable. The harm done by a failure to disclose will usually not entail an immediate and grave form of damage. While

effective therapies are not available for most genetic conditions, the preventable harm to be avoided will often be the birth of a child with some physical or mental impairment or disease.

(Clarke, 2007, p. 23)

Taken to an extreme, Clarke thinks, the joint family model of owning genetic information would lead to absurd and impractical lengths. 'Should the individual who has been tested first be able to forbid the laboratory from using its knowledge of the mutation(s) when testing other members of the same family? This would be an absurdity, forcing laboratories to issue incorrect reports out of some formulaic or bureaucratic sense of respect for privacy, when the relevant personal information is already known by all concerned' (Clarke, 2007, p. 23). Indeed, Clarke argues, there might be a better argument for genetic information to be construed as belonging to the laboratory or health service that generates it, rather than either the individual or the family.

Section 3: Genetic databases and biobanks: who owns your genes?

Clarke argued that perhaps neither the individual nor the family should be viewed as owning genetic information: there might be a better argument for saying that ownership should rest with the clinical laboratory or the health service. However, Clarke, and to an even greater extent Lucassen, seem to think that genetic information also does naturally 'belong' to the individual from whom the DNA swab or other tissue was taken in performing the genetic test. We will see in this section that on the contrary, neither tissue nor genetic swabs 'belong' to the patient, because in our common law we do not own our bodies or any parts of them. That legal fact has allowed laboratories, hospitals, biotechnology firms, universities and health services to build up large holdings of tissue and genetic samples – databanks and 'biobanks' – affecting most of us, but not necessarily with our knowledge. Effectively, Clarke's recommendation already holds: neither the individual nor the family 'owns' genetic information. Does that matter, and if so, why? One reason why it does matter is that patients and their families are directly affected by it, as the following case study will show (adapted from Dickenson, 2008).

The case of Debbie and Daniel Greenberg

Debbie and Daniel Greenberg had lost two children to the rare but fatal genetic condition Canavan disease,

a degenerative brain disorder which primarily affects people of Ashkenazi Jewish descent. As with the commoner genetic condition cystic fibrosis and other recessive conditions, and unlike autosomal dominant disorders such as Huntington's disease, parents can carry one copy of the gene without knowing it, because they will have no symptoms themselves. But if two carriers have children, each child has a one in four chance of inheriting two Canavan's genes and developing the fatal brain disorder.

After the deaths of their children Jonathan and Amy, the Greenbergs contacted a genetic researcher, Dr Reuben Matalon, and urged him to begin research into the genetic basis of Canavan disease. They hoped he and his colleagues could develop a genetic test which could prevent other parents from suffering as they had done, by identifying carriers of the condition and giving them the chance to decide on having their children through IVF and preimplantation genetic diagnosis. With the aid of over 160 other affected families, the Greenbergs founded a genetic tissue and data bank, working collaboratively with Dr Matalon over a period of 13 years and contributing not only post-mortem tissue from their children, but also their time and financial support. 'All the time we viewed it as a partnership', Daniel Greenberg said.

They were mistaken. Without the Greenbergs' knowledge, the hospital at which Dr Matalon worked took out a comprehensive patent in 1997: US patent number 5,679,635, covering the gene coding for Canavan disease, diagnostic screening methods, and kits for carrier and antenatal testing. Two years later the hospital began to collect royalties for the patented genetic test, claiming that as a non-profit-making body – ironically enough – it needed to recoup its outlay on research. The genuinely charitable Canavan Foundation had been sponsoring testing for all couples of Ashkenazi Jewish descent who requested it, but now it could no longer afford to do so. Furthermore, the hospital imposed restrictions on which laboratories were allowed to administer the test, limiting access for many patients. Children who would suffer from Canavan disease were now being born unnecessarily, to a short life of suffering – precisely the outcome the Greenbergs had hoped to avoid for other families. In fact, it would have been better if they had never taken the initiative to get research started on the disease that killed their children. Now doctors were even being barred by the terms of the patent from diagnosing Canavan disease through more traditional methods not involving genetic testing.

In October 2000, the Greenbergs and other Canavan parents filed a lawsuit in a US court, alleging lack of informed consent to the further uses that had been made of their children's tissue. In addition to the consent issue, however, they argued that they had a right to determine what uses were made of the tissue and data which they had laboured to collect over so many years. This was very directly a case about who 'owns' genetic information: the patient, patient's family, researchers or hospital? The Greenbergs also complained that Dr Matalon and his colleagues were in breach of their 'fiduciary duty' of care, and that they had enriched themselves at the families' expense. They argued that if they had known that Matalon and the hospital intended to patent and commercialize the discovery, they would never have contributed time, money and tissue samples. Matalon's taking out a patent was common enough – some one in five of all human genes is now the subject of a patent – but on the other hand, the researchers who discovered the genetic basis of cystic fibrosis deliberately eschewed restrictive patents and licensing agreements on their discovery.

ACTIVITY: What do you think would be the likely outcome in this case? Why? How much does your answer rely on your understanding of whether you own your body, including your genetic data?

Three years later, the case was settled, largely in Matalon's favour. The Greenbergs lost their claim that no informed consent had been given, because neither they nor the other Canavan families were Dr Matalon's patients. This was not a one-to-one therapeutic relationship, and so neither informed consent nor the duties of a doctor had been breached, according to the court judgement. Medical law, which does tend to focus narrowly on the doctor–patient dyad, was too rigidly individualistic to take the weight the Greenbergs wanted to place on it. The only point on which the families won was the 'unjust enrichment' claim, but not because Matalon had taken what was rightfully theirs: the court accepted that the hospital was the rightful owner of the patent, and that the patent was itself lawful. All the court did was to impose a set of minor restrictions on its use – so that other researchers could have access to the genetic information – and to award the families a very small sum in settlement of the 'unjust enrichment' claim. In return for these concessions, the Greenbergs and the other families had to agree not to challenge the hospital's ownership of the patent.

Why did the court take this stance? Isn't it obvious that you own your body, and the genetic data generated from it? You might be surprised or even shocked to learn that the law does not in fact view the person from whom the tissue was taken, or that person's family, as its owner. Instead genetic swabs and other forms of tissue were traditionally seen as *res nullius*, no one's thing. Formerly that didn't matter, because normally tissue was only excised from the body if it was diseased. The patient had no further interest in it. But with the advent of modern commercial biotechnology, that position has radically changed. Genetic data, DNA and other tissue that can be used in creating a cell line or cloned for a patenting application now has enormous value.

In the debate between Anneke Lucassen and Angus Clarke, the question to be answered was 'should families *own* genetic information?' Actually, in legal terms, neither individuals nor their families own genetic information, or genetic material taken from their bodies. It would be better to phrase the debate, which is certainly a genuine one, in terms of claims or rights to access information and to prevent others from accessing it, rather than ownership. The rhetoric of ownership is powerful but incorrect.

How much does that matter? We have seen that in the Greenberg case, families at risk of producing children with two copies of the Canavan-linked gene were disadvantaged if they couldn't afford the fees imposed by the patent holders, the hospital where Matalon was employed. In other cases, including in fact a US patent on the BRCA1 and BRCA2 genes which figured in the CD-ROM scenario, patent holders have attempted to do the same. Whilst the European patent on these genes was rejected by the relevant courts, Myriad Genetics, which holds a US patent on these genes, had successfully defended its right to impose a charge for diagnostic testing at the time of the Greenberg judgement (although in March 2010 a US district court invalidated the patents, a ruling against which Myriad is appealing.) So one answer is that everyday practice – because breast cancer is certainly an everyday condition – *is* already being affected.

Another way in which the question of 'who owns your genes?' matters has to do with a slightly different issue, genetic and tissue biobanks. Many of us will have provided tissue to biobanks at some point, knowingly or unwittingly. The former case includes UK Biobank, which began in 2007 to collect genetic samples from 500 000 individuals aged between 40 and 69 for the purposes of large-scale epidemiological research. UK Biobank describes itself as merely the 'steward' of those samples, but in fact participants retain few rights over their donated tissue, once they have given their initial consent (Brownsword, 2006).

Biobanks created from scratch with the consent of the donors, like UK Biobank, are vastly outnumbered by biobanks formed of existing material, created without explicit consent in many cases. In 1999 a 'conservative estimate' put the number of stored tissue samples in the USA at over 307 million, from more than 178 million people (Skloot, 2006). At that time the quantity of samples was thought to be increasing at a rate of over 20 million a year. In the UK, the Retained Organs Commission, appointed in the wake of the Bristol and Alder Hey hospital scandals concerning tissue stored from dead children without their parents' consent, also uncovered large tissue banks at many other hospitals and academic institutions, held without patients' knowledge. The Alder Hey collection, which included organs and even an entire brain from an 11-year-old child, was contentious not only because it was secret, but also because of the emotional significance of retaining dead children's organs. Other biobanks might at first seem less contentious – for example, those only containing DNA, tissue blocks or slides. In the UK, the Human Tissue Act 2006 now regulates these practices more effectively, although other issues remain – often at a broader societal level rather than at the level of the individual practitioner, but no less real for that.

There are serious ethical questions about consent, confidentiality, the involvement of commercial firms, and public interest in the creation of national genetic databases. For example, should participants be able to withdraw consent to the use of their tissue, once given? This is a central issue in birth cohort studies, tracking individuals over a lifetime: even if their parents gave consent on their behalf when they were infants, subjects might want to 'opt out' once they are old enough to decide for themselves. Here, and in genome-wide association studies, there are issues about the use of archived samples: for example, whether a new consent should be obtained, or whether approaval by an ethics committee or the ethics oversight board of the study is sufficient.

The UK Biobank does now allow the right to withdraw, but in the original biobank, Iceland's deCODE, withdrawal was not allowed, and participation was on an 'opt-out' basis: you were assumed to be willing to take part unless you explicitly stated otherwise. In fact, in the end the only databank that was actually created was of those Icelanders who had opted out (Sigurdsson, 2001). Nevertheless, the Icelandic genetic databank throws into relief many questions of continued relevance: for example, security remains a major issue in the wake of several major losses of personal data by government bodies in the UK in early 2008, and commercial involvement is more of an issue now than ever, even though deCODE actually filed for bankruptcy late in 2009.

Even when the Icelandic database looked like a very promising concern, the British bioethicist Ruth Chadwick raised important and troubling issues about its operation in an article called 'The Icelandic database: do modern times need modern sagas?'. As she wrote, 'Debate about issues of informed consent, privacy, scientific freedom, benefit, and commercial monopoly is vigorous. The question at issue is whether the rules being applied to the database can deal with the issues raised. A debate that focuses on traditional principles risks ignoring new challenges brought about by advances in medical technology. If the role of commercialism is to be assessed and defined appropriately ... are the rules out of date?' (Chadwick, 1999b, p. 441)

Since Chadwick wrote of her concern that traditional medical ethics concepts like informed consent might be insufficient to deal with biobanks – whether modern times need modern sagas and concepts – there has been survey evidence bearing out her disquiet. It has been said that the governance framework for UK Biobank, and presumably also other similar banks, is indeed weighted too heavily towards individual informed consent (Brownsword, 2006), failing to take into account the needs of the wider community. Interviews from a number of focus groups underlined this concern (Levitt and Weldon, 2005), with participants asking why they couldn't exercise some 'downstream' control over the uses to which their tissue was going to be put – so that trivial or unethical uses coujld be ruled out. After all, some interviewees remarked, they had to continue providing medical and 'lifestyle' data to UK Biobank; why couldn't the biobank reciprocate by telling them what uses it had made of their contribution?

As it stands, recipients have an all-or-nothing choice: either donate tissue and accept whatever uses of it Biobank wants to make, or don't donate at all. The Scottish medical lawyer Graeme Laurie – now actually chair of the UK Biobank ethical governance board – wrote in an earlier article that such a limited notion of informed consent would actually *dis*empower patients (Laurie, 2004). It will be interesting to see if the UK Biobank can devise forms of ongoing consent that do *em*power patients. Levitt and Weldon suggest that without such genuine collaboration, the public will quickly lose trust in genetic databases, particularly if they come to be seen as vehicles for private biotechnology corporations to access large pools of genetic data. In the USA private companies have paid up to $200 million for access to biobank research on particular disorders and have sought to protect their investment by imposing restrictions on publicly funded researchers wishing to use the same data (Andrews, 2005). By contrast, in other countries, notably France and Tonga, public outcry has led to rejection of proposals to 'mine' genomes of local populations by setting up large genetic databases for commercial firms to use (Dickenson, 2007). There is also a growing body of work pointing out that the universal resource of the human genome is being 'enclosed' for private use, much as common agricultural land was enclosed in the eighteenth and nineteenth centuries in England and Scotland, with the loss of commoners' rights (Boyle, 1996; Dickenson, 2008).

On a more commonplace but deeply worrying level, what about the risks of disclosure of genetic information to third parties like insurers and employers? We saw in the Greenberg case that conventional medical ethics developed in the context of the individual doctor–patient relationship – so that some of its core concepts, like consent, autonomy and confidentiality, do not readily extend beyond that one-to-one relation (Williams, 2005). By definition, genetic databases and biobanks concern large numbers of donors, and a wide range of potential uses of their tissue – not all of them foreseen at the time of the donation, taking us back to the point about whether donors should have ongoing rights to determine those uses. None of those donors is in a conventional doctor–patient relationship with the administrators of the database or biobank. So how can conventional medical ethics prevent abuses of their rights?

And what happens if personal genetic data are leaked, not necessarily deliberately, to bodies outside both the doctor–patient context and the database or biobank itself? Several years ago the US bioethicist

Dorothy Nelkin devised the notion of a genetic *lumpenproletariat*, the lowest social level, who would be unable to get jobs or insurance because of unfavourable genetic profiles revealed to their employers or insurers (Nelkin, 1994). In the USA and in European insurance-based systems, being refused health insurance on a genetic basis could be a matter of life and death, so the concept of genetic 'untouchables' seems as crucial as ever – perhaps more so. Insurance firms in the USA have in the past refused cover even to carriers of genetic conditions, who are not affected themselves (British Medical Association, 1998).

Insurers, pension providers and employers have an interest in getting as much information as possible that may predict the future health of those they insure and employ, but that is rarely in the interests of the individual concerned (Archer, 2002, p. 96). There is a conflict of interests between the corporate body's need to consider the true extent of their contractual liability, and the privacy, confidentiality and right to non-discrimination of the individual. In such clear-cut if atypical cases as Huntington's disease, insurers could also argue that there is a wider social interest in reducing the level of premiums for everyone else if individuals who will definitely develop the condition could be identified and required to pay a higher premium. But is that fair or just? Does it not contradict the principle of solidarity or equal access to healthcare among all recipients of healthcare in a national insurance-based system? Taken to its logical extreme, it might even justify compulsory genetic testing for serious disorders, which is widely condemned: for example, the Dutch law on Medical Examinations of 1997 states that no one may be tested for untreatable genetic conditions. Many countries, including the UK, France and Germany, have at various times enacted a moratorium on the use of predictive genetic testing by insurers, but a moratorium is by definition temporary.

Genetic databases are not the only case in which questions about privacy and confidentiality in insurance and employment arise, of course, although they make them more prominent because of the large numbers of individuals affected.

ACTIVITY: Think about how questions of insurance and employment would impact on the case of Henry, from the CD-ROM. If his daughter Ann does the 'responsible' thing and has herself tested, suppose she loses her job or health insurance? After all, in applying for insurance, applicants are supposed to exhibit 'good faith', informing the insurer of all known conditions; if they fail to do so, their insurance can be revoked. Conversely, would Henry's son Peter, who doesn't want to be tested, be justified by fears for his employment or health insurance? How would those economic considerations weigh against the questions about the third generation's 'right to know' or, conversely, their 'right to an open future'?

Section 4: Are genes us? Genetic identity, social justice and the moral status of the gene

It is frequently thought there is something 'special' about genetic explanations for illness, genetic testing and the other concerns of this chapter. The term often used to describe this view is 'geneticization', coined by the Canadian–American sociologist Abby Lippman in 1992 to refer to the ever-growing tendency to define medical conditions and physiological behaviours as wholly or in part genetic in origin. In many people's eyes, genetics seems to exert an unusual power – or, conversely, to raise very profound fears

For example, when the Tongan nation were targeted for a genetic database on diabetes research, to be owned and administered by the Australian biotechnology firm Autogen, the leader of a popular resistance movement argued that 'we should not sell our children's blood so cheaply' (Senituli, 2004). The Tongans were not literally being asked to sell their children's blood, but there was a widespread sense that their national and individual identities, encapsulated in the genome, were threatened by being made a commercial object of trade. Senituli's influential article, titled 'They came for sandalwood, now the b . . . s are after our genes!', summarizes the Tongans' cultural and political resistance against Autogen, which eventually dropped the project altogether. Although many other indigenous populations are also opposed to genetic testing and genetic data-mining (Mgbeoji, 2007), the sense that genes are somehow special or sacred is by no means limited to Third World countries. In their classic book *The DNA Mystique*, Nelkin and Lindee asserted that even in the Western industrialized world, our DNA has become the equivalent of the Christian soul: the sacred essence of the person and of human existence. It has assumed, they claim, a cultural importance transcending the more humble role of the building blocks of life or the blueprint for how to make a human (Nelkin and Lindee, 1995).

Is our human essence really determined by genetic composition? In another article, 'Are genes us?', Chadwick has asked this very question. If that query seems abstract or rhetorical, on the one hand, it may also have very practical ramifications to the extent that patients and families *do* believe that genes have a special status (Chadwick, 1999a). The popularity of television programmes on exploring genealogy, or the tendency of the popular press to use 'it's all in the genes' as a mantra, might well predispose people to believe in something like 'genetic exceptionalism'. True, many authors have denied that there is any special 'moral' status about genes (e.g. Warren, 2002). But to the extent that doctors, pharmaceutical firms and patients prioritize genetic explanations, accepting 'the DNA mystique' whether unconsciously or consciously, there are very direct effects on healthcare provision. One such effect – a major one – has to do with equality and inequality in healthcare provision.

> **ACTIVITY:** Stop a moment and think of how acceptance of illness as mainly determined by genes could affect decisions about which treatments to fund, and how funding should be distributed. How could it affect your own practice, if you are a practitioner?

A particularly sensitive area here has to do with genetics and race. Think back to the Greenberg example. It has long been known, for example, that certain genetic conditions are associated with particular 'racial' groups: Canavan disease occurs mainly in families of Ashkenazi Jewish extraction, whereas sickle cell anaemia is most prevalent in African-descended people (e.g. African–Americans in the US or Afro-Caribbean people in the UK). Cystic fibrosis predominantly occurs among 'white' European-descended populations – and we have put 'white' and 'racial' in inverted commas for reasons you should easily be able to guess. It begins to look as if we're not very far from eugenics and 'scientific racism' when we start talking about whether race correlates with, or even causes, certain diseases.

Whether or not such associations are inherently objectionable, there is certainly a risk that genetic conditions associated with small minority ethnic populations will receive a lesser share of national health funding and that pharmacogenetic prescribing will become 'stratified' by ethnic background, raising important issues about ethics and social justice (Smart *et al.*, 2004). In an era when pharmacogenetics – drug regimes tailored to certain genetic profiles – is thought to promise great things, it is entirely possible that pharmaceutical firms will decide it is not worth their while to prioritize treatments which would only have a limited market among a very small racial minority (Holm, 2008).

As disease prevention comes to be associated with targeting certain 'defective' *individual* genes, the wider focus of health prevention in the *community* can easily be overlooked. Most of the great public health successes of the nineteenth century, such as the improved sewerage systems which radically lessened the incidence of cholera, were aimed at entire populations. (Genetics was of course largely unknown.) If anything, the populations thought most at risk were the poorest slum-dwellers, but there was a wider benefit for all classes in society, with an overall rise in life expectancy. That is also true of vaccination against diseases such as smallpox, where a high and reliable level of protection can only be achieved with population-wide measures. Once we begin to think instead of disease as something for which an individual's particular genome is 'responsible' –with the individualization of healthcare regimes and the focus on individual genetic profiles – that wider sense of social solidarity may be at risk.

But if genetic-based therapies can provide cures for particular populations, meeting the criteria of evidence-based medicine, doesn't that have to be a good thing for those groups? The promise of genetic engineering and genetic enhancement may well have been overstated, but pharmacogenetics is already producing some results. In 2007 the US Food and Drug Administration approved the first racially profiled pharmaceutical, a drug targeted at African–Americans with hypertension. Such therapies aim to cut the costs of prescribing therapies less likely to 'fit' a particular subgroup and to improve the effectiveness of treatment. What could possibly be wrong with that?

Racially profiled treatments have actually been criticized on several counts:

(1) There is already a misconception that someone who has 'the gene for' a certain condition will inevitably develop that condition. Huntington's disease is one of a comparatively minuscule number of conditions where a single gene codes for a particular condition with a great degree of certainty. Already genes are erroneously linked in the mainstream press to all manner of conditions, including sexual orientation, narcissism and even voting behaviour (Brooks and King, 2008). If those false beliefs are reinforced by prejudices about race, they could be even more dangerous.

(2) In most cases genes may *predispose* individuals to develop certain diseases, but not *determine* that they will definitely manifest those conditions. Environmental factors, including unbalanced diet, lack of exercise, pollution, workplace stress, poor housing and effects of social deprivation, may well count more heavily. If we lose sight of that basic insight, believing instead that we simply *are* our genes, then research on the environmental determinants of disease will take a back seat. Obviously, this threat is particularly serious when racial minorities already suffer worse social conditions than mainstream ethnic groups. That injustice could well occur at a global level as much as within one country (Holm, 2008).

(3) Race is as much a social concept as a biological one, arguably even more so (Brooks and King, 2008). That insight is not limited to minority ethnic populations within a larger national group: it has been shown that the Icelandic database was mistakenly believed to be uniquely valuable because Icelanders were thought to be a remarkably homogeneous population, who had not experienced the waves of successive immigration typical of other European countries. In fact, it was discovered, Icelanders are no more biologically homogeneous than Turks. They merely had a social concept of themselves as a unified 'race' (Rose, 2001).

Like the concept of race, the notion that genes straightforwardly determine our illnesses and our behaviours is very simplistic. Why then are we sometimes attracted to it? No doubt the hope of finding a genetic basis for every major disease looks attractive to many because it promises greater control over those diseases. Yet the philosopher Ronald Dworkin has also argued that the mapping of the human genome and the possibility of genetic engineering are unsettling because they may allow us to control *too much*. We actually need our genetic basis to be random and beyond human control, he asserts (Dworkin, 2000).

Dworkin draws a parallel between the sudden intensification of moral debate brought on by the new technologies in medicine that enabled doctors to 'play God' in extending or curtailing life, and the possibility of 'similar though far greater moral dislocation' occasioned by the mapping of the human genome and the possibility of genetic engineering (Dworkin, 2000, p. 444). He thinks we need our genetic basis to be random and beyond our total control because if we can control our genetic inheritance completely, then we can control too much. The crucial moral boundary between chance and choice is, to Dworkin, 'the spine of our ethics, and any serious shift in that boundary is seriously dislocating' (Dworkin, 2000).

The moral status of the gene is ambivalent. Geneticization, in its full-blown variant, suggests that we can control too little: that in the end, we are not responsible for very much at all. If all our behaviours are entirely 'in the genes', including the very possibility of making moral choices, then the notion of right and wrong ethical standards is radically undermined (Dickenson, 2003). As a Nuffield Council on Bioethics document put it, 'in the context of behavioural genetics, the concern is that we do not choose our genes, then insofar as our genes influence our behaviour, we are not truly responsible for those aspects of our behaviour: we are at the mercy of our genetic inheritance' (Nuffield Council on Bioethics, 2001, section 6).

So, in the end, are genes us? Can we simply be reduced to the totality of our genes and the interaction between them – the view sometimes called 'genetic reductionism'? Chadwick locates the modern tendency to say 'yes' to that question in an older, longer-standing debate about what constitutes the person. Consciousness, the soul, the brain, even the pituitary gland (in the philosopher Descartes) – all these have been candidates for the essence of human identity long before modern genetics came along.

By contrast, Chadwick begins from a view of personhood as self-awareness, which argues against equating the person with the genome. As she writes: 'The idea that we could hold up a disk containing our genetic profile and say "That's me", as has been envisaged by some genome scientists, does not take this into account. On the self-awareness account, it is the capacity to give voice to the statement "That's me" that is crucial, not the information itself' (Chadwick, 1999a, p. 185).

If the genetic profile is not sufficient to constitute the person, however, it is certainly a necessary 'blueprint', Chadwick notes – so that a weaker form of determinism is suggested. The genome would then be seen as identifying the person in the same way a fingerprint or an iris scan does, but we still would not

say either of them simply *is* the person. As one of us has argued elsewhere, even if we accept the metaphor of the genome as a blueprint for constructing a human being, 'construction depends on things other than the blueprint: the quality of the materials (i.e. the quality of healthcare and nutrition in childhood), the dedication of the workmen (i.e. the parents or other caregivers), and random factors like the weather (i.e. accidents and other environmental factors that affect our development)' (Dickenson, 2003, p. 169).

A further weakness in the 'genes are us' view is that it largely ignores relationships with others. Our interactions with others may be influenced by genetic components in our personalities, but not solely by them. The narrative of anyone's life cannot simply be predicted from the outline set forth in our genes. Studies of identical twins, raised both separately and together, show that personality and behavioural traits are not entirely determined by having the same genome. Identical twins raised separately only correlate to the degree of 0.75 (with 0 being no relationship and 1 a perfect relationship), but even identical twins raised together only correlate to the degree of 0.87 (Dickenson, 2003, p. 175). And as Chadwick points out, no one would claim that identical twins are the same person, even though they share the same genome.

ACTIVITY: Stop a moment and think about your own response to this question of what constitutes the person. What makes you 'you'? How far does your understanding of your own identity depend on a genetic basis, including such obvious factors as your height, your eye or hair colour, or your sex? This would be a good occasion to write a short paragraph in a learning diary, summarizing your reactions to the content of this chapter in relation to the question of geneticization.

To conclude, we think the answer to the question 'are genes us?' is 'only to a limited extent'. Even asking the question, we would add, betrays a very individualistic and self-centred point of view. Reducing the person to the genes ignores the impact that others' personalities and actions have on the narrative of our lives. While that impact may or may not give others – for example, family members – rights over our personal genetic information, as Lucassen and Clarke debated, it does suggest that the interaction between ourselves and others is not wholly determined by our genes. The whole of the person's narrative is greater than the sum of the genetic parts. And that narrative will be full of ethical choices, far removed from genetic determinism. Even if genetics shifts the boundary between chance and choice, as Dworkin claimed, that isn't the same thing as eliminating choice altogether. The sort of extreme genetic determinism that denies all power of choice is ultimately paradoxical, because I have a choice about whether or not to accept genetic determinism.

It may be bit speculative, but perhaps the appeal of genetic determinism is that it seems to offer some hard-and-fast certainties in a field where uncertainty is the norm. As Jackie Leach Scully and her colleagues have written about their study of patients like Henry's family, making decisions about testing for Huntington's disease and other genetic conditions, 'all genetic testing has predictive fuzziness – it generally does not remove uncertainty about the course or severity of the disease' (Scully *et al.*, 2007, p. 209). We would like to end this chapter with their philosophical reflection occasioned by the probabilistic, 'fuzzy' nature of genetic testing:

> Beyond the test lie multiple possible futures, some of which will be closed off by the test result, while others remain open because of the uncertainty. Because of this orientation, genetic tests force people to imagine their future(s). In the present in which a decision is made, it is also obvious that at some point in the future, this event will be history. When the patient asks, 'How will I live with this decision?', she is struggling to make an assessment of a past which has not yet happened
> (Scully *et al.*, 2007, p. 209).

References and notes

* Reproduced with permission from June Zatz, 'I am definitely having it done', from *The Troubled Helix*, ed. M. Richards and T. Martineau, pp. 27–31. Cambridge: Cambridge University Press, (1996).

** Reproduced with permission from Donna Dickenson (1999), 'Can children consent to be tested for adult-onset genetic disorders?' *British Medical Journal*, **318**, 1003–5.

1. Nuffield Council on Bioethics (1998). *Mental Disorders and Genetics: The Ethical Context*. London.

2. British Medical Association (1998). *Human Genetics: Choice and Responsibility*, p. 68. Oxford: Oxford University Press.

3. Nuffield Council on Bioethics (1998). *Mental Disorders and Genetics: The Ethical Context*. Appendix 2, 'The use of genetic information in legal proceedings', p. 3.

4. IHA and WFN Guidelines for the molecular genetics predictive test in Huntington's Disease (1994). *Neurology*, **44**, 1533–6.

5. See Note 1.

6. Ibid.

7. Family Law Reform Act 1969, s. 8 (2).

8. 4 All ER 627.

9. *Gillick* v. *W. Norfolk and Wisbech AHA*, 3 All ER 402.

10. Ibid., 423.

11. Age of Legal Capacity [Scotland] Act 1991, s 2 (4).

12. Alderson, P. (1990). *Choosing for Children*. Oxford: Oxford University Press.

13. Alderson, P. (1993). *Children's Consent to Surgery*. Buckingham: Open University Press.

14. Davis, D. S. (1997). Genetic dilemmas and the child's right to an open future. *Hastings Center Report*, **27**(2), 7–15.

15. Wertz, D. C., Fanos, J. H. and Reilly, P. R. (1997). Genetic testing for children and adolescents: who decides? *Journal of the American Medical Association*, **272**(11), 875–81, at 878.

16. S. 1 (1) (3).

17. Cohen, C. (1998). Wrestling with the future: should we test children for adult-onset genetic conditions? *Kennedy Institute of Ethics Journal*, **8**(2), 111–30.

18. Bloch, M., Adam, S., Fuller, A. *et al.* (1993). Diagnosis of Huntington's disease: a model for the stages of psychological response based on experience of a predictive testing program. *American Journal of Medical Genetics*, **47**, 368–74.

19. Wiggins, S., Whyte, P., Huggins, M. *et al.* (1992). The psychological consequences of predictive testing for Huntington's disease. *New England Journal of Medicine*, **327**, 1401–5. Lynch, H. T. (1993). DNA screening for breast/ovarian cancer susceptibility based in linked markers – a family study. *Archives of Internal Medicine*, **153**, 1979–87.

20. Scourfield, J., Soldan, J., Gray J., Houlihan, G. and Harper, P. S. (1997). Huntington's disease: psychiatric practice in molecular genetic prediction and diagnosis. *British Journal of Psychiatry*, **178**, 144–9.

21. Brandt, J. (1994). Ethical considerations in genetic testing: an empirical study of presymptomatic diagnosis of Huntington's disease. In *Medicine and Moral Reasoning*, ed. K. W. M. Fulford, G. Gillett and J. Soskice, pp. 41–59. Cambridge: Cambridge University Press.

22. Richards, M. (1998). Annotation: genetic research, family life, and clinical practice. *Journal of Child Psychology and Psychiatry*, **39**, 291.

23. Leikin, S. L. (1989). A proposal concerning decisions to forgo life-sustaining treatment for young people. *Journal of Pediatrics*, **108**, 17–22. Weir, R. F. and Peters, C. (1997). Affirming the decisions adolescents make about life and death. *Hastings Center Report*, **27** (6), 29–40.

24. Dickenson, D. L. and Jones D. P. H. (1995). True wishes: the philosophy and developmental psychology of children's informed consent. *Philosophy, Psychiatry and Psychology*, **2**(4), 286–303, at 289.

25. Dickenson, D. L. (1994). Children's informed consent to treatment: is the law an ass? [guest editorial]. *Journal of Medical Ethics*, **20**(4), 205–6.

26. Sherer, D. G. and Repucci, N. D. (1988). Adolescents' capacities to provide voluntary informed consent. *Law and Human Behaviour*, **12**, 123–41.

27. See Note 20.

Chapter 4

Medical research: participation and protection

Introduction

During the Second World War, Nazi doctors conducted some of the most horrific experiments imaginable in the name of medical research. An example is the experiment in which healthy people were thrown into freezing cold water in an attempt to see how long pilots who bailed out of aeroplanes into the sea could be expected to survive.

After the war, the international community responded to these and other atrocities carried out in the name of medicine by creating the Nuremberg Code, which you will find reproduced in an appendix at the end of this chapter. This was the first internationally agreed ethical code concerning the conduct of clinical trials. The code has since been superseded to some extent by the World Medical Association's Helsinki Declaration (first drawn up in 1964 and revised several times since, most recently in October 2008). It has also been supplemented, in relation to research in developing countries, by the guidelines of the Council of Medical Organizations of Medical Sciences (CIOMS) and the World Health Organization (WHO). None the less it is still an extremely powerful reminder of the horrors which have been and could be carried out in the name of medical advance.

But what are the most serious issues regarding medical research today? Some commentators suggest that less obvious developments related to the commercialization of modern medicine now pose a greater everyday threat than atrocities. They point to the way in which research agendas may be influenced too heavily by commercial interests, particularly those in the First World, at the expense of the global poor – citing, for example, recent research into a vaccine for meningitis which was developed for a serotype not found anywhere in Africa, where the medical need is arguably the greatest (Beauchamp, 2009). Market forces in genetic research are likely to take us down the path of treatment for common but trivial disorders like male-pattern baldness, rather than serious conditions with a limited patient base (Frankel, 2003). Other developments of concern include restrictions on researchers from patents on genes and corresponding licence fees (Andrews, 2002), or the potential development of a new 'underclass' of research subjects who gain their main employment from participation in research trials (Elliott and Abadie, 2008).

Notwithstanding actual and possible abuses of medical research, it remains the case that advances in medicine and the knowledge gained through medical research have been at the heart of many of the most significant developments in the improvement of the human condition. Medical research and the advance of medical understanding represents what is best about human endeavour and has been directly responsible for some of the most profound improvements in human wellbeing, particularly in the past two centuries. It seems certain that medical research will play an increasingly important role in the improvement of human wellbeing in the future too. But the undisputed benefits of medical research must be balanced against potential harms to research subjects. This tension underpins many of the ethical questions which we will examine in this chapter, which begins by putting the research subject's perspective first, through examination of a fictionalized case study.

In this chapter we shall be exploring the ethics of medical research in a range of different settings by means of the following unifying activity.

ACTIVITY: As you read through this chapter, we would like you to build up your own research ethics checklist, which will provide a useful tool for the identification of the ethical questions raised by a particular piece of medical research. In order to do so, we would like you, as you work your way through the chapter, to make a list of questions you feel it is essential to ask oneself as a research subject, a researcher or as a member of an ethics committee charged with assessing whether a piece of research is ethical or not. This checklist will also form the basis of the final activity in this chapter. At the end of each section, we will make a note of some of the questions which occurred to us. Add these to your list if you think they are relevant.

Section 1: The research subject's perspective: a case study

Please open scenario 1, 'Research: patient participation in drug trials,' on your CD-ROM. (Again, please bear in mind that the toolbar contains additional resources such as a glossary of unfamiliar terms, which you may wish to consult before or after viewing the scenario.) Work through the scenario and associated questions, which will take you about 40 minutes, and then return to the text.

We have begun with a case taken from a real-life instance, aimed at illustrating the difficulties patients may encounter when deciding whether to give their informed consent to participate in a research trial. This scenario concerns Jan, whose attention is caught by a newspaper advertisement requesting people willing to participate in a drug trial for a syndrome called 'generalized anxiety disorder.' It is based on an actual case from Finland, which seems particularly appropriate as the birthplace of the Helsinki Declaration.

This scenario concentrates on five key issues regarding the patient's perspective on medical research:

- Informed consent and criteria for determining research subjects' understanding of the risks and purposes of the trial;
- Placebo use in randomized clinical trials, the 'gold standard' of evidence-based medicine;
- Risk and adverse consequences of both participation and non-participation in clinical trials;
- The 'medicalization' of ordinary life, epitomized in this scenario by the dubious syndrome being studied in the trial, 'generalized anxiety disorder';
- The doctor–patient relationship in medical research and how it may conflict with that relationship in the clinical setting. In clinical medicine the patient's best interest is the doctor's

priority, but the research subject is not actually a patient and may derive no therapeutic benefit from the trial. Indeed, in Phase I trials, where the objective is to study potential side effects of the treatment, the participant runs the risk of harm rather than benefit. Those subjects assigned to the placebo arm of a clinical trial will receive no clinical benefits except possibly psychosomatic ones – another issue in Jan's case.

One point which does not come up in the scenario, but which is very relevant to a drug treatment for a 'condition' which affects a very large 'market', is the issue of drug company funding for clinical trials (Angell, 2000), relating back to questions about commercialization of research. A systematic review of the literature published in the *British Medical Journal* concluded that 'Research funded by drug companies was less likely to be published than research funded by other sources. Studies sponsored by pharmaceutical companies were more likely to have outcomes favouring the sponsor than were studies with other sponsors' (Lexchin *et al.*, 2003).

ACTIVITY: As always in the CD-ROM, you were asked to enter preliminary responses on these and other issues during the course of studying the scenario. Take a moment now to read through your initial responses (which you can print up while using the CD-ROM) and to elaborate on any points that seem sketchy. In Section 2 of this chapter, we will concentrate particularly on informed consent to participate in clinical trials.

Before that, however, we would now like you to go on to consider the extent to which it is possible to come up with a workable set of ethical principles of medical research. We would like you to do this by means of a guided reading exercise based on a paper by K. W. M Fulford. In his paper on the principles of medical research, which follows, Fulford discusses the problems raised by the ethical review of medical research and proposes a framework for such review. We would like you to read his paper and, as you do so, to attempt to identify any further additional questions it suggests that it might be useful to ask researchers. Add these to your checklist. Note that Fulford is principally concerned with research in psychiatry. How would these principles apply to other types of research?

The principles of medical research

K. W. M. Fulford

Is this good research?

What is most important is often what is left out. What is said may be important. But what is not said, the gaps and contradictions in the proposal, are often particularly significant ethically. This is not because researchers set out to deceive themselves or others. It is because the imperatives that drive research push one to think about a given project from a particular point of view. We have found a structured framework provided by the following four principles particularly helpful in opening our eyes to aspects of a situation we had neglected. (Fulford and House, 1998)

(a) Knowledge: the proposed research should be likely to produce an increase in knowledge directly or indirectly relevant to patient care.
(b) Necessity: it should be necessary for the research to be carried out with the subjects proposed rather than with some less vulnerable group.
(c) Benefits: the potential benefits arising from the research should outweigh any inherent risks of harm.
(d) Consent: research subjects should give valid (i.e. free and informed) consent to their participation.

ACTIVITY: How well does the case study in the CD-ROM fit these principles? It might be argued that the first criterion is particularly shaky in this instance, given the dubiousness of 'generalized anxiety disorder' as a genuine illness. What about the other criteria? And is there reason to think that psychiatric conditions like 'generalized anxiety disorder' will have more difficulty meeting these criteria than treatments for somatic illness? (You may have picked up the difficulty of establishing whether Jan's feelings about whether he is getting better or worse are purely subjective.) As a clinical psychiatrist, Fulford is well aware of this difficulty and discusses it at further length under the four headings below.

(a) Knowledge: The 'corpus of knowledge' is less well established in psychiatry than in other areas. This is due to scientific difficulty rather than scientific inadequacy. All the same, the lack of consensus in psychiatry is problematic. Against this, psychiatry offers the advantage that much of its research is close to the clinical coal face: the relative lack of mature theories of brain functioning means that the gap between research and clinical practice is much smaller than in, say, biochemical research on neurological disorders.

(b) Necessity: This principle implies a rough hierarchy: that in vitro preparations be used in preference to animals, that animals be used in preference to healthy subjects, and that healthy subjects be used in preference to patients. This principle, too, presents particular problems for psychiatric research. This is essentially because many forms of psychopathology are uniquely human experiences. There are animal models for, say, some forms of obsessive–compulsive disorder; but even here the gap between animal model and human counterpart is considerable (it includes, for example, the whole question of the meaning of the phenomena for the individual concerned; and when it comes to symptoms like thought insertion, which require the capacity for second-order thinking, animal models are simply not available).

The principle of necessity is also important between different groups of patients. For example, in dementia research it is important to work where possible with subjects who still have capacity for consent, or, in general, to work with patients who are not being treated under the Mental Health Act or are in prison. However, notwithstanding the principle of necessity, it is often important in psychiatry actually to involve the most vulnerable groups (i.e. those with serious mental illness) to ensure that their voice is heard.

(c) Benefit: The calculation of the balance of benefits to risk is complicated in psychiatry by both empirical and evaluative factors. Empirical factors include the lack of an agreed 'corpus' of knowledge noted above. Perhaps even more significant, though, is the diversity of values by which, as we have several times emphasized, psychiatry is characterized. This is important for both sides of the equation: what is an unacceptable risk to one person, may be entirely acceptable to another; what is a clear benefit to one person may be a disbenefit to another.

It is important to be aware just how risk-laden non-invasive techniques like interviewing may be. The standard paradigms of high risk in research are patients being given a new drug or subjected to an 'experimental' operation. Far less calculable, though, are the effects of being asked a series of probing questions, or merely of being 'recruited' into a trial in the first place. Randomization, too, the basis of modern research methods, may be a highly adverse experience where subjects feel that they or their relatives have been denied standard treatments.

ACTIVITY: Consider how the CD-ROM treated the risks of both being recruited and not being recruited into the trial: in one outcome, for example, Jan is deeply troubled by having been excluded from the trial. Since those who are not recruited have no further contact with the research team, it is difficult to see how the potential risks to them can be measured and taken into account. What could ethical review committees do to ensure that the interests of those rejected for the trial are also considered? The CD-ROM also considers one corollary of randomization, the effects on the placebo group of not being given the drug which they may have been expecting to receive when they signed up for the trial. Is it unethical to ignore the interests of the placebo group in the name of 'gold standard' research? Again, what measures can research ethics committees take to ensure that patients fully understand that they have an equal chance of not receiving the treatment? This leads us into the final principle suggested by Fulford, informed consent.

(d) Consent: Both limbs of the consent formula – freedom of choice and information – may be problematic in psychiatric research.

Constraints on freedom of choice may be external or internal. External constraints arise from the unequal power relationship between doctors and patients. Pressure to take part in research is rarely overt, but concerns for one's treatment, or inducements, may amount to strong covert pressures. Patients who are being treated on an involuntary basis, and mentally abnormal offenders in prisons or other institutions, are particularly vulnerable in this respect.

Internal constraints on freedom of choice are generated in a number of ways by different kinds of psychopathology: people who are depressed, or suffering from long-term schizophrenia, are sometimes unduly compliant; obsessive–compulsive disorders may involve a pathological inability to make up one's mind; and patients suffering from psychotic disorders may have aberrant (and often concealed) motivations. A psychotically depressed man, for example, agreed to take part in a research project which involved having some blood taken. He appeared to understand what was being asked of him and to be fully capable of consenting to this procedure. Subsequently, however, it was discovered that his interpretation of the situation had been that he was to be executed. He welcomed this because his profound delusions of guilt led him to believe that he deserved to die and that everyone around him would be better off if he were dead.

Psychopathology may also generate problems for the information limb of the consent formula. Thus, patients with dementia may be unable to retain or recall even quite limited amounts of new information. Depression slows information processing. Anxiety may block it altogether. Hypomania involves marked distractibility.

Problems of this kind, furthermore, complicate the general problem in research ethics of how much information is required for consent to be valid. In clinical work in the UK, practice is still governed legally by the 'prudent doctor' standard (originally set by the 'Bolam' test, *Bolam* v *Friern Hospital Management* Committee [1957] 1 WLR 582). Even in clinical work, though, law and practice are moving towards a 'prudent patient' test. In research (e.g. General Medical Council, 2008) this is already the norm (reflecting the more exacting standards arising from the difference of intent between research and clinical work). Thus the Royal College of Physicians suggests that 'any benefits and hazards' must be explained to research subjects (Royal College of Physicians, 1990). The standard set by the Royal College of Psychiatrists' Guidelines is 'important' risks, what is 'important' being a matter for a research ethics committee, which should 'apply common sense to decide what level of risk would be likely to affect a reasonable person's decision' (Psychiatric Bulletin, 1990). This is helpful advice, then.

ACTIVITY: As we come to the end of this first section of the chapter, we would like you to stop for a few moments and take a look at the checklist you have been constructing as you read the case. Is there anything you feel ought to be added to the list at this stage? Remember that the checklist is to be framed as a set of questions one would ask oneself when assessing the ethical implications of a piece of research.

Below is a list of some of the questions we came up with.

- Is the proposed research going to offer some benefit? Is it going to answer the proposed question? Is this an important question?
- Is it necessary for this research to be carried out on human subjects? Could the answers be gained in the laboratory, or by animal studies?
- What is the balance of harms and risks likely to occur as a result of the research?
- Is there a Patient Information Sheet? Is this clear and accessible to the research subjects who will be asked to participate in the study?

- Are the subjects going to be asked to give their consent? Will this consent be valid? Is there a consent form? Is it clear (as above)? Who will be asking the potential subjects for their consent?
- Is it clear to the subjects that they can withdraw from the study at any time and that this will not affect the quality of their treatment?
- Does it make it clear that the subject can refuse to participate and that this too will not affect the treatment received?

Section 2: Valid consent, mental capacity and best interests

A case of genetic research

The research ethics committee of a major teaching hospital receives a proposal from researchers associated with a major migraine clinic asking for permission to do gene tests on their clinic patients and their families. The researchers are particularly interested to discover whether one variant of a gene called ApoE is associated with migraine.

Most of the patients at the clinic are young. The clinic has an excellent reputation and good loyalty from its patients. Indeed, the research ethics committee knows that the researchers concerned are one of the teams in the hospital with an international reputation for excellent research.

A problem arises, however, because the team mentions in its application that, in addition to its suspected association with migraine, variants of the ApoE gene they wish to study may also be associated with early-age onset of Alzheimer's disease. Because of this potential link, they suggest that they should keep the genetic information they obtain to themselves and not advise the patients and families.

They say, rightly, that the implications of having the ApoE allele are not completely clear, and in any case they have neither the time nor the money to organize counselling. They also say that their study is very much related to migraine, and that if there is a risk of Alzheimer's disease, the onset will be many years in the future, and telling people would only create unnecessary worry.

ACTIVITY: The question of just how much information is reasonably required for the subject to have given his or her valid consent is an important question. What is it to be 'reasonably informed'?

In a nutshell, a proper consent is a clear, open, intentional – and, we might usefully add, true – statement by the subject that he understands what he is about to do and that he freely chooses to do it. This is possible only where two conditions have been met: first, his choice must be based on his possessing and understanding all the information which is relevant to making the choice; and second, the choice must have been made freely, without pressure. There are, of course, difficulties in knowing quite how much is 'all that is relevant' and in knowing quite what is to count as pressure [. . .] But unless it can reasonably be said that the two conditions have been met, then a proper consent has not been given.

(Evans and Evans, 1996, pp. 78–9)

As Evans and Evans point out above, one of the most fundamental principles in the ethics of medical research is that no one should be enrolled onto a research study without their explicit consent. This clearly means a great deal more than that they have simply said 'I agree' or have signed the bottom of a consent form. In this section we shall be exploring the ethical issues which arise in relation to the question of consent in medical research. Start by reading an extended extract from a paper by Richard Ashcroft in which he addresses the role of informed consent in medical research. He investigates the extent to which the concept of 'explicit informed consent' can act alone as a criterion of ethical research on human subjects and looks at the types of situations in which the criterion may have to be modified, for example in situations where potential research subjects are incapable of providing explicit consent and yet research on them seems to be ethical under certain circumstances. Ashcroft begins somewhat as Fulford did, by trying to develop some general principles of research ethics.

Autonomy and informed consent in the ethics of the randomized controlled trial: philosophical perspectives

Richard Ashcroft[**]

Introduction

There are two central principles in human experimentation ethics. The first is that the experiment should be scientifically sound and present a fair proportionality of risk to benefit to the subject. This is uncontroversial, although it can be difficult to spell out this principle in detail in practical situations. The second principle is that no one should be enrolled into an experiment without their express, informed consent. In what follows I examine the arguments used to defend this second principle, and the arguments used to defend departures from it (including the ways departures are sometimes tacitly brought about sans argument). I do not discuss the legal context of the consent doctrine, which is not specific to clinical experimentation, and which is in any case well known. Nor do I discuss in depth the arguments about consent by minors or the mentally ill.

The randomized controlled clinical trial is a type of experiment on human subjects. As such, it falls within the domain of the 'Nuremberg Code', and the 'World Medical Association Declaration of Helsinki'.[1,2] Both of these codes were framed with the Nuremberg War Crimes trials in mind, and sought to specify minimal conditions on human experimentation, such that basic human rights should be protected and respected in all experiments which use human beings as subjects. The aim of these codes is essentially protective; and the philosophical premise of the rights which are described – or perhaps stipulated or constituted – by these declarations is individualist.[3,4] In other words, each individual's wellbeing and integrity takes precedence over the interests of the social body, especially the fraction of the social body which is the state.[5,6] This is, of course, directly targeted against totalitarian doctrines which hold that on certain occasions, or for certain groups of subjects, the interests of the state (or the remainder of the social body) are taken to be rights, and to take precedence over those of the individual subject.

I will concentrate discussion on the Nuremberg code's provisions, because it is the simplest, clearest and oldest relevant code on ethics of experimentation. The later Helsinki codes preserve substantially the same position, but devote much more attention to explaining the notions of risk and benefit, which clarifies some considerations about fair risks for incompetent subjects. Arguably, the Helsinki codes weaken the force of the Nuremberg principles, however, and for clarity about the stakes in the debates on consent I concentrate on their original expression in the Nuremberg code.

ACTIVITY: It is clear that the Nazi experiments involved a gross violation of individual human rights, but to what extent do you think it is true to say that individual rights should always take precedence over the public interest or benefit? That statement would be questioned by many utilitarian ethicists, for example, who focus on the beneficial or adverse outcomes to be gained rather than on individual rights.

Taking the case above, for example, it might be the case that informing the research subjects about the link with Alzheimer's would mean that no one would be willing to take part in the research. This would be an adverse outcome which, in a utilitarian framework, might offset the individual subject's right to be fully informed.

Are there situations or types of research in which you consider the informed consent of research subjects to be less important or to be outweighed by the public interest in the research? What, for example, about research involving linking a great many patient records? How would you go about deciding whether and to what extent informed consent was required in such research?

Voluntary consent   The first principle of the Nuremberg code states that for research to be ethical, 'the voluntary consent of the human subject is absolutely essential'. In other words, each and every subject in the experiment must give their voluntary consent to be part of the experiment. As this stands it is very unclear what is required; is it enough to say to a subject 'would you like to take part in an experiment?' without saying any more? And would an affirmative reply constitute consent in the required sense? Not yet, because the test of voluntariness may not be passed. And as this test of voluntariness is the nub of the matter, we cannot leave it with the investigating physician's own satisfaction that the patient (or healthy volunteer) has consented voluntarily. Indeed, remembering that the Nuremberg Code has a legal dimension as well as an ethical one, some criterion assessable by a third party is required.[7]

Not only is the principle much more vague than its simplicity seems to imply, it also has some medically puzzling features. It seems to rule out any experimental procedures where the normal condition of the subject is such as to rule out voluntary, or even involuntary consent. Under this test, no experiments seem possible in emergency medicine, in perinatology, in psychiatry or clinical psychology, and probably in most paediatric medicine. Arguably, it disallows any research on pregnant women, not because the women cannot give consent, but because the foetuses cannot.[8] The principle is quite explicit: and so-called proxy consent is no consent at all.[9,10]

Premises of the consent requirement   Let us examine now the premises of the argument for voluntary consent. In the first place, we took it that the principle of voluntary consent is a moral rule. Next, the principle takes as read the principle of individualism as mentioned at the outset. Thirdly, there is a clear distinction between experimental and other sorts of medical care.[11,12,13] Fourthly, there is the presumption that human subjects need protecting.[14]

If we want to avoid the conclusion that much medical research will become impossible if we grant the principle of voluntary consent, then we will need to weaken or discard one or more of these premises. Before we do this, let us reflect on what this principle does not say.

Nothing philosophical is asserted about voluntariness or autonomy or personhood: but it is clear that each human subject – whatever we take that to mean – must voluntarily consent to taking part in the experiment, whatever voluntary consent is.[15,16,17] The words here have – at least – their common-sense meaning. So an unconscious patient has not consented, for example.[18,19,20,21] Nor has a member of a football club consented to participate, simply because his club chairman has indicated that his club as a corporate body will participate in the experiment. Only human subjects are mentioned in the principle, and whatever a collective is, it is not a human subject.

The principle makes no claim to sufficiency. We can easily imagine 'experiments' where a number of human subjects voluntarily consent to take part, but we would not (as outsiders) regard these experiments as ethical. The authors of the Nuremberg Code reflect this point, by following the principle of voluntary consent with a series of nine other principles. The bulk of these concern experimental risks and scientific utility and competence. The final two principles state the right of the subject to leave the experiment at any time (subject to a condition which I will discuss later) and the obligation of the researcher to terminate the experiment if the experiment becomes, in its process, dangerous to the subject. This last principle, stating the investigator's duty to terminate an experiment early under certain conditions, will prove troublesome when we look at randomized controlled trials.

ACTIVITY: How did the question of leaving the trial arise in Jan's case? And why might the subject's right to quit a trial early prove a problem for experimenters? One problem that occurs to us is the need to maintain roughly equal numbers in the experimental and control arms. If more people leave the experimental side than the control group, for any reason, that balance could be undermined.

The final element about which the Nuremberg Code is silent is the element which the Helsinki Declaration faces directly: the nature of specifically medical obligations to patient subjects in biomedical research. Nothing in the Nuremberg Code is intended to have specific relevance to this issue. This is slightly puzzling because the Nuremberg Code is addressed to the medical profession and speaks of 'Permissible Medical Experiments'. But nothing is said concerning the experimenter's obligations vis-à-vis the Hippocratic code of medical ethics (or indeed any other vademecum of medical obligations, responsibilities and purposes). The authors of the Code state that most experiments, to the best of their belief, do 'conform to the ethics of the medical profession generally'.

Note at this point that medical ethics is conceived not on an individual basis but a collective one: the duties of the doctor are framed as elements of a professional ethic, not as duties analytically derivable from the concept of medicine. There is something of a tension in later developments of medical ethics between perspectives which emphasize the collective and traditional, or socio-legal, foundations of medical right, and those which emphasize supposedly self-evident principles of medical good practice (substantively or procedurally justified).

The question of the relationship between the principle of voluntary consent and the ethics of routine medical practice is open, so far as the Nuremberg Code indicates. It may be that the principle of voluntary consent is an additional and independent principle which supplements those of medical ethics in experimental contexts. Or, it could be that the principle of voluntary consent is logically independent of the ordinary principles of medical ethics, and the possibility exists that the two sets of principles will conflict in some situation. Or, it could be that the principle of voluntary consent applies in all experimental situations involving human subjects, and the principles of medical ethics amplify and supplement this principle in just those cases where the experiment has some medical significance: for instance where the human subject has been enrolled into the experiment qua patient.

Most of the experiments (or pseudo-experiments) which the authors of the Code had in mind were experiments of no direct medical merit for the subjects (not all of the experiments were medically uninformative, although many were, and there has been some debate about whether the use of the results of these experiments was legitimate, given the way in which the results were obtained). And many were of no direct medical relevance at all, being natural-historical or physiological in character. As such, these experiments could not be considered part of normal or innovative medical care. The point of the principle of voluntary consent was to ensure that experiments of this kind were legitimate, subject to consent. Naturally, in many cases the conduct of these experiments would require medical help to be on hand, or indeed that the investigator be a medical professional. Whether all such experiments had to be carried out under the scrutiny and professional ethics of the medical profession is probably an issue in disciplinary politics rather than law or ethics. So, as far as ethics is concerned, we can rule out the first possibility that human experimentation is a specialized branch of medicine, and should be governed by medical ethics as supplemented by the principle of voluntary consent. On the other hand, we can accept without further comment the argument that the principle applies to all human subject experiments, but needs supplementing with the ethics of medical care when the experiment is carried out using subjects who are patients (even if their patienthood has nothing to do directly with the topic of the experiment). Or can we?

ACTIVITY: Ashcroft raises an interesting question here about the relationship between the ethics of medical research and the ethics of medicine more broadly. To what extent does the principle of respect for voluntary consent conflict with other ethical demands in medicine, and in such situations, what ought to be done?

Is consent consistent with beneficence?   The second possibility (having dismissed the first and accepted the third) is that the principle of voluntary consent conflicts – either always or on occasion – with sound medical ethics. We saw that the raw principle seems to conflict with medicine in some common cases (children, the mentally incompetent, etc.). Many writers have argued that medical experiments – especially the randomized controlled trial – involve a conflict of principles, or, on many accounts, of roles.[22,23,24] The role conflict they have in mind is the conflict between the investigator as doctor and the investigator as scientist; and to complicate matters further we could balance that with a conflict of roles between the individual as patient and the individual as subject.

Does duty override consent?   Given the protection-oriented nature of the Nuremberg Code, it is natural to emphasize the duties of the investigating physician and the rights of the patient-subject. Also, in context, it is natural to suppose that arguments about the rights of the physician and the duties of the patient-subject are to be resisted. The sort of duty which could be conceived and which the authors of the

Code want to resist is a duty on the part of the patient to society at large.[25,26,27,28] What the authors presumably want to resist here is not the idea that I may regard myself as owing a duty to my fellow citizens, or to my species, but that society may impose such a duty upon me, with attendant sanctions. A natural analogy might be drawn between the duties a soldier owes to his state and the duties a patient might be taken to owe; and, in particular, the duties a citizen owes to the state in the sense of an obligation to undergo military conscription. The core of the obligation to undergo conscription is the so-called 'free-rider' problem, where individuals enjoy the use of some social good (for instance civil liberty) without contributing to the social (and economic) costs necessary for the maintenance of that good. Conscription aims, among other things, to distribute fairly the chances of paying with injury or death the military costs of a state's liberty, in such a way as to avoid the free-rider problems that may be judged to arise if a war is fought with only voluntary enlistment. A similar argument concerns the development of new drugs. Drug development always involves testing for safety and efficacy on human beings. Since some people will be needed to be subjects for any given innovative treatment, is someone who persistently refuses to take part in drug testing as a subject, but who benefits from the outcomes of such testing, to be regarded as immoral? And if they are, what social sanctions might be merited? Related to this is the argument that convicted criminals might be regarded as owing some measure of participation in human experimentation as part of their 'debt to society', either because they have partially forfeited their right to refuse consent, or as a full or partial substitute for their penal servitude.[29,30,31,32]

ACTIVITY: Do you think we might have an obligation to participate in medical research? That argument has been put by the utilitarian bioethicist John Harris in his article 'Scientific research is a moral duty' (2005), in which he asserts that 'Biomedical research is so important that there is a positive duty to pursue it and to participate in it'. It might seem odd for a utilitarian like Harris to make assertions about 'duty', more usually associated with deontologists. A consequentialist or utilitarian, however, is likely to see the balance between social benefit and individual rights as needing to be weighted more towards social benefit.

The relevance of these arguments, which have an alarming sound to the liberal ear, is that many of them were tacitly or explicitly accepted in many states at the time the Nuremberg Code was being framed. And furthermore, the statist character of these arguments may be regarded as tendentious, but the moral arguments from analogy to what most liberal democracies (and perhaps all states) are prepared to accept are not trivial to refute. It is better to understand the refusal to press the analogy as founded not on self-vindicating moral principles, but on a stipulation that this is the set of moral standards in this limited area which the global community will now adopt and commit ourselves to abide by. The problem with this is that the principles of the Nuremberg Code were in part intended to be self-evident moral principles, against which the activities of figures such as Dr Josef Mengele could be judged. Later revelations about experiments carried out by Allied states following (tacitly or explicitly) the analogy between conscription and a 'duty' to participate in experimentation only underline the ironies of the Nuremberg stipulations; they do not, for all that, detract from the rightness of those stipulations.[33,34,35]

Duty and voluntary action   The gap that must be kept open is the gap between recognition that one may morally be under some partial obligation to take part in human experiments in the medical field and a statist position where this duty can be imposed upon citizens. One argument which may assist us is the argument that military and fiscal obligations are citizenship duties, rather than social duties, and the putative duty to participate in medical experiments is if anything, social, and not connected with citizenship. The analogy here that could be stressed is between the need for suitable subjects for medical experiments and the need for volunteer blood-donors. Another analogy may be with duties to charitable giving and to voluntary work in the community. Duties of this kind admit of a variety of interpretations, although most people will admit them, whatever their rationale for doing so. It might be that the religious tenets one adheres to stress charitable giving, for instance. A key feature of duties of this kind is that typically they are only regarded as meaningfully satisfied when the duty is voluntarily performed. There is a complication here: many states partially replace this duty with another kind of duty, the duty to pay progressive taxes as a redistributive measure, or as part of a welfare programme. This sort of enforceable duty is sometimes argued to be destructive of charitable virtues, and many resent doing under obligation what they would happily do out of charity. This type of argument is often made by communitarians.

So once again we return to voluntariness, as referred to in the Nuremberg Code, where we first met it as a barrier to coerced participation, and now we meet it as what makes participation morally significant.

'Inferring' consent

Paternalism
Patients, for a variety of reasons, linguistic, educational, psychological and social, frequently do not fully comprehend what they are being asked to consent to, or why, or in what their consent consists, or how far it extends.[36,37] And this is so on most tests – the most telling being the test of recollection: can they, after a decent short interval recall what they have consented to?[38,39] Whether one is entitled to conclude from this that the consent process is a waste of time, or dispensable at any rate, is a moot point, and one that has occupied much space in the medical and ethical journals. My opinion is that there is something suspicious about drawing absolute conclusions concerning the utility of patient consent from facts about the difficulty of achieving it. This is especially to be resisted when much of that difficulty may be regarded as founded upon imperfections in communication.

ACTIVITY: Ashcroft argues that the claim that subjects often or even sometimes find procedures difficult to understand cannot count as a justification for overriding their consent, particularly when this is because of difficulties of communication. List the kinds of factors that might make informed consent difficult in this way.

These imperfections may be regarded as being of three kinds. The first kind, the linguistic barrier, is contingent, where some individual or group of patients is unable to understand the information given, either because the information is insufficiently informative, or because the language used is obscure, or because, simply, the patient or doctor is not fully at home in the language being used (perhaps, as in a case reported in the *British Medical Journal*, they are first generation immigrants from Vietnam who have learnt English late in life).[40] Here all that is required is that efforts be made to ensure that these contingent imperfections in communication are removed.

The second kind of imperfection, cognitive barriers, might be regarded as necessary: simply, no non-medical professional can reasonably be expected to understand the details of the medical procedure, and so basing the requirement for consent upon a requirement that the patient understand those details would make consent almost impossible to obtain. Consequent upon that would be the necessity of abandoning the experiment. However, the number of experiments where the patient cannot be given a balanced and comprehensible description of the experiment, such that he understands and can make a decision about consent, must be vanishingly small.

The third kind of imperfection, social distortions, may be regarded as contingent but 'structural'; that is, the contingency relates not to any facts about the individual patient, doctor or treatment, but to social facts. The sort of social facts which are relevant are facts connected with social structure and what Habermas calls 'systematic distortions in communication', which are founded in power relations.[41] Examples of this include: patients not understanding that they are entitled not to give consent; patients not understanding the scientific purpose of the trial and supposing that the novel innovation is (a) more effective and (b) will be administered to them (when they may be randomized to the alternative arm); patients' interest in consent to being treated not being equivalent to the doctor's interest in consent to advance medical knowledge; differential attitudes in particular socio-cultural groups to the need for consensual decision-making and appropriate processes for making decisions; differential capacities and opportunities to exercise patients' rights.[42]

All of these 'distortions' to the process of giving voluntary consent can be related in part to social structural factors, and as such are properly the domain of social research rather than philosophy or medicine. But there are three main points to be noted here. The first is that the social context of the consent process (both the micro-context of the sick patient in the interview room in the surgery or hospital, and the wider social, political, cultural and economic contexts of the patient) is relevant to the quality and significance of consent. The second is that consent is obtained in a situation where power is involved in quite complex ways. And the third is that consent is a sort of action (technically, a speech act of a certain kind), such that there are conditions under which verbal consent fails to be consent in the relevant way.

The Nuremberg Code gives an explicit gloss to the meaning of 'voluntary consent' which indicates that the authors recognized that consent was an action involving understanding. The paragraph reads:

This voluntary consent] means that the person involved should have legal capacity to give consent; should be so situated as to be able to exercise free power of choice, without the

intervention of any element of force, fraud, deceit, duress, overreaching, or ulterior form of constraint or coercion; and should have sufficient knowledge and comprehension of the elements of the subject matter involved as to enable him to make an understanding and enlightened decision. The latter element requires that before the acceptance of an affirmative decision by the experimental subject there should be made known to him the nature, duration, and purpose of the experiment; the method and means by which it is to be conducted; all inconveniences and hazards reasonably to be expected; and the effects upon his health or person which may possibly come from his participation in the experiment.

This statement tells us quite a lot about the meaning of voluntariness. It tells us that consent is genuine only when free from intentional duress, and only when the giver is in a position to understand the significance and extent of what he is assenting to. In some ways this makes the consent requirement even more restrictive than the naked formulation, because it adds additional tests: notably the core of what later is known as 'informed consent'. Most of the literature on informed consent – and it is very extensive – concentrates on this question of what informed consent should be said to consist in. But it is also interesting that some tests we might set for assent to be consent are not mentioned, here or in any of the subsequent Codes. For instance, we might regard consent given under conditions of desperation as no more genuine than consent given under conditions of duress. And the ways in which desperation can be socially generated are numerous – not only the gravity and severity of an illness, but also economic need, for instance. And consent under desperation usually contains an intention that the novel treatment be received, and so (in the randomized controlled trial) does not intend randomized assignment.[43]

That this is so is illustrated by the subversion of randomization by AIDS sufferers in certain treatment trials in the late 1980s. This is a fine point. Arguably, these patients acted unethically in giving apparent consent to enrol under the treatment protocol, thus rendering the data in these trials almost useless (although usable to some extent under some interpretations), and perhaps necessitating further trials to retest the hypothesis. But on their part the argument that to be offered a choice between getting the drug, probability 0.5, and getting nothing was not a fair set of alternatives under the circumstances. That this is so has been recognized increasingly in AIDS trials, although multi-armed trials are considerably more expensive, require greater quantities of the probably rare, possibly dangerous experimental drug, and need the enrolment of proportionately more patients.[44]

Conclusion That the tests an experimental procedure should pass are more restrictive than those we place upon 'ordinary' treatment is not surprising. But what are these tests designed to achieve? As noted above, the tests on consent are meant to distinguish valid consent from invalid pseudo-consents, specifying relevant features of each; and consent itself is meant to ensure that patients are protected from undergoing risks and harms without their knowledge and agreement. Their force, in the Nuremberg Code at least, is to force doctors to seek consent, a matter which the code is quite explicit about, making it a duty upon doctors in the third paragraph of the first section of the Code:

> The duty and responsibility for ascertaining the quality of the consent rests upon each individual who initiates, directs or engages in the experiment. It is a personal duty and responsibility which may not be delegated to another with impunity.

A slightly curious feature of this formulation is that it makes of each doctor – in the first instance – his own gatekeeper. Later, both in Britain and in the USA, an additional institution was created, the Local Research Ethics Committee or Institutional Review Board, to oversee the implementation of this requirement and to assess all research for their ethical status (at least prima facie).[45,46,47] However, as yet no mechanism exists for ensuring that the researcher will actually do what he says he will in his proposal, and the 'with impunity' sentence in the Code is the weaker for this omission.[48,49] Certain mechanisms exist for enforcing this protective rule, notably the public sanction of the medical journals, which may refuse to publish studies conducted without valid consent processes, and the possibility of medical negligence torts in the case of experimental procedures carried out *sans* consent.[50,51,52] Out and out fraud with respect to consent is uncommon, so far as we know, and two doctors who forged signatures on consent forms were struck off by the General Medical Council's professional conduct committee.[53,54]

ACTIVITY: Thus far in this section we have investigated the concept of informed consent by means of a reading exercise using Richard Ashcroft's paper. It

seems clear, taking into account the limitations described by Ashcroft, that being informed constitutes at least part of what it means for consent to be valid. He has also pointed out some other requirements, notably that such consent should be competent and uncoerced. In the second part of this section we go on to investigate these requirements by means of a reading exercise on a paper by the Finnish medical lawyer Salla Lötjönen. Before you start reading the paper, we would like you to take a few minutes to consider the various ways in which obtaining valid consent might prove difficult in practice. If you were a member of a research ethics committee, what questions would you want to ask the researchers in order to ensure that the consent they would obtain would be valid? Then begin your reading of the paper.

Ethical and legal issues concerning the involvement of vulnerable groups in medical research

Salla Lötjönen

In the aftermath of the Second World War and during the trial of the doctors who took part in the inhuman experiments carried out during the Nazi era, the Nuremberg Code was drafted, in 1947. The first and foremost criterion of the Code was the voluntary consent of the human subject, which is also recognized in the United Nations Covenant on Civil and Political Rights (1966). Since then, the scope of the requirement for a free and uncoerced consent to experimentation has raised a considerable amount of discussion and it has been the basis for many additional international documents. Mostly, the discussion has concerned the voluntariness or the capacity of experimental subjects.

Voluntariness The voluntariness of the experimental subject comes into question most of all with regard to institutionalized persons, i.e. prisoners, soldiers, patients subject to involuntary treatment, and patients staying permanently in nursing homes, etc. There are some views which regard institutionalization as such as excluding voluntariness (e.g. *Kaimowitz* v *Michigan Department of Mental Health*). The fear has been that the institution's management or staff could unduly influence the self-determination of the subjects towards participation, or that potential research subjects in an institution would at least regard their choice as restricted even if that was not actually the case. It has also been proposed that subjects might participate in a research project in the hope of benefits such as early release, more attention, or simply a change in the daily routine, which have been thought to be inappropriate incentives for participation.

It is questionable whether such incentives really differ significantly from the incentives used at present outside of such settings, which include financial benefit, free or sometimes even better access to treatment or access to a better-monitored treatment. Additionally, the groups that are often involved in participating research projects are medical students and hospital staff. Until recently, only few guidelines or conventions have taken these groups to deserve special protection. For example, the Declaration of Helsinki or the Council of Europe Convention on Human Rights and Biomedicine (referred hereafter as the Biomedicine Convention) in their present form do not include provisions protecting these groups, even though the chance for at least indirect pressure from their superiors or colleagues can be obvious. Moreover, these groups often take part in research that is not likely to have any direct health benefit to them, which makes their use as experimental subjects even more problematic. Having said all this, the Additional Protocol to the Convention on Human Rights and Biomedicine, concerning Biomedical Research, which entered into force in December 2009, nevertheless does explicitly warn against undue influence, and instructs ethics committees to pay particular attention to vulnerable or dependent persons (Article 12). In addition, it insists that there be no discrimination against those who decline to participate in research (e.g. Article 14).

ACTIVITY: Stop here for a moment and consider the following case. In the light of the previous few paragraphs and using your checklist we would like you to analyse the case and to list the arguments in favour of the research being allowed to proceed and those against. In the end, after having considered both sets of arguments, what would you decide, and why?

A case of payment for research A research project focusing on specific CSF enzyme levels in neurological disease requires control measures. For this purpose, healthy participants are required who are willing to undergo lumbar puncture. Recruitment is slow. The researchers have funding and propose to pay each participant £800 in order to increase the recruitment rate. The participants are properly informed about the procedure and its risks and give valid consent to take part in the research. However, most would not have given consent were it not for the £800.

Now continue with your reading of the paper.

Competence Recently, the hottest debate in Europe has not been on the voluntariness but on the competence of research subjects. The two concerns can overlap, as in the case of a patient who receives involuntary psychiatric care for his or her mental illness. In the 1960s, a physician called Henry Beecher identified several research projects which had used children, often suffering from mental disability, as research subjects. Probably the best known of them, the Willowbrook study (Krugman *et al.*, 1960), concerned mentally retarded children in an institution, who were deliberately infected with hepatitis in order to examine the efficacy of the vaccine in preparation.

In the light of Willowbrook and several other studies, it is understandable that there are voices that would prefer to ban research on incompetent subjects. However, there is another side to the coin. If medical research on minors and other incompetents were to be banned altogether, gathering scientifically valid information on their development and diagnostics or finding suitable medication for childhood diseases or, e.g. Alzheimer's disease, would be seriously hindered. What is needed is a compromise that aims to protect the incompetent as well as to give science some space to explore.

ACTIVITY: What is it exactly that makes medical research on incompetent subjects different from research on those who are competent? And, if research on them should be allowed, under which conditions should it be allowed?

Self-determination What makes minors and incompetent adults special is, of course, their impaired ability to decide for themselves. Although in most countries the capacity to decide over one's own body does not strictly follow the age of majority, setting a clear line on whether a person is competent to make a health-related decision has proven to be very problematic. In some countries, strict age limits or tests of capacity have been imposed; in some others, more flexible formulations on the sufficient level of understanding have been set. The level of involvement of persons with impaired decision-making ability in research can be categorized in the following way: (a) independent consent (full capacity), (b) assent (both the consent of the subject and his or her proxy are required), (c) refusal (objection is valid despite incompetence and proxy consent).

One very interesting factor is the emphasis that is placed on the right of self-determination of the incompetent in medical research compared to medical treatment. Children can be taken as an example here. Whereas competence for deciding over minor, purely therapeutic measures can be achieved at quite an early age, competence for deciding independently on research procedures is considerably harder to achieve. A link can be made to the comparison of levels of competence required in consenting and refusing treatment. As the latter may bring some negative consequences to the incompetent person, his or her right to self-determination does not seem to stand on its own, but on a more consequentialist ground, on the outcome of the procedure (see, e.g. *Re W*).

The same may be said of the incompetent adult. In contrast to minors, adults enjoy a presumption of competence which seems to alter the situation in favour of the adult in terms of stronger involvement in decision-making. Additionally, adults who have been competent earlier, may have had the opportunity to state their opinion before becoming incompetent. In that case, their previous wishes should be given the same weight as advance directives. One could, however, think of a situation of an adult incompetent who has previously (e.g. at the early stages of dementia) stated his willingness to participate in research, but along with deteriorating mental capacity has become afraid of physicians and medical procedures. Should the previously stated will of the patient still be respected? That question will remain unanswered here. A lot will always stay within the discretion of the medical profession and depend on the circumstances of the individual case.

Nevertheless, as the outcome of the research procedure seems to weigh more than the autonomy of the patient in medical research, it leads to a situation where the refusal of the subject is his or her strongest means of self-determination. This right is very strongly protected, and the required level of competence is taken to be very low. When the Medical Research Act (No. 488 of Statutes, 9 April 1999) was drafted in Finland for example, a child as young as 5 was proposed to be given the right to refuse a research procedure. In the present Act, no definite age limits have remained, but the relevance of objection has been left to be determined by the age and maturity of the minor. In comparison, the refusal of an adult incompetent is always considered sufficient.

Proxy decision-making　If the subject is incompetent to decide for him or herself and he or she does not object, who can then decide on their behalf? In the case of a minor, the parents or the local authority have the power to make decisions over the child as his or her legal guardians. However, in the case of an adult, there are usually no provisions that make someone automatically his or her legal representative as in the case of a minor.

In the Finnish Medical Research Act, Section 7 of the Act states that incompetent adults may be research subjects in cases where written consent has been given by 'their close relative or other relative or legal representative'. The selection of people is thereby made quite extensive and may result in problems in a case of disagreement in the family. However, as the right to refuse is widely interpreted in medical research, it could follow that in the case of disagreement amongst the patient's relatives, one relative refusing to give consent would be sufficient to prevent the subject's participation.

ACTIVITY:　In England and Wales the Mental Capacity Act 2005 likewise sets a 'best interests' standard, but also allows for decisions to be made for, and on behalf of, incapacitated people. For treatment decisions, the Act creates the possibility of 'lasting powers of attorney', by which a donor, when competent, may confer on a proxy decision-maker the power to make decisions on his or her behalf in the event of losing capacity. In research, in addition to familiar safeguards such as the need for ethics committee approval, the Act requires the researcher to find someone close to the potential participant who is willing to be consulted about the appropriateness of their involvement or (if there is no such person) another person not otherwise involved in the research. If you were asked to make such a decision for a person lacking capacity, would you consider it right to allow that person to take part in research which might entail risks? How would you weigh up the countervailing argument that taking part in research is the altruistic action of an autonomous agent and should not be denied to people lacking mental capacity?

Scope of proxy decision-making　What then is the scope of proxy decision-making in medical research? Taking part in medical research is by definition not solely concerned with the patient's best interests. Here, a distinction between therapeutic and non-therapeutic research must be made. After all, with therapeutic research, the treatment given is at least connected to the patient's condition and may be of significant benefit to him or her. In fortunate cases, the experimental treatment may prove to be more beneficial to the patient than the standard treatment. Leaving aside the debate on so-called 'placebo-controlled' trials, very few objections towards incompetents taking part in therapeutic research have been made and proxy decision-making has been considered acceptable in therapeutic research at least in principle.

The problem then becomes clearly visible in non-therapeutic research. When the sole legal criterion in almost all of the European countries for proxy decision-making has followed the general rule of best interests of the incompetent person, how can an infringement of the incompetent person's bodily integrity be justified if there is no potential health benefit to be expected?

In England, prior to the Mental Capacity Act, the case of *Re F* followed the general principle of 'best interests', leaving it for the courts to decide whether the proposed procedure was in the best interests of the incompetent patient. Later, in the case of *Re Y*, the High Court gave more flesh to the interpretation of the 'best interests' criteria. It ruled that harvesting bone marrow from a severely mentally and physically disabled person to be used as a bone marrow transplant for her sister would be lawful. The court based its ruling on the grounds that preventing the death of Miss Y's sister would be for her 'emotional, psychological and social benefit' as the family was a particularly close one. It has been suggested that neither of the cases can be applied to solve the problem of proxy decision-making for medical research on adult incompetents because even a wide interpretation of the 'best interests' criterion would hardly ever be met in non-therapeutic medical research.

There seems to be a conflict here that cannot be solved using the traditional criteria. One suggestion to resolve the conflict is formulated in the Biomedicine Convention, which has been adopted e.g. into Finnish legislation. It provides a compromise that is needed to bridge the aim of protection and fear of exploitation into a constructive solution. Like the Helsinki Declaration, the Convention (and its recent Additional Protocol) make a distinction between whether the procedure has an expected therapeutic benefit to the patient or not. According to the Convention, in exceptional circumstances and under the protective provisions of national law, non-therapeutic research on the incompetent is also allowed. The provisions on non-therapeutic medical research on the incompetent in the Convention are based on two criteria: societal necessity and the principle of minimal risk. Both of them have to be simultaneously fulfilled.

Societal necessity   Societal necessity stems from the claim that if research on incapacitated persons were not permitted, this might in fact work against the interests of the group such a ban was designed to protect. If non-therapeutic research on the incompetent were prohibited altogether, existing medicines could not be tested on children before they reach the market and the physicians treating these patients would have to base their decision-making on estimating the right dosage using their own discretion instead of scientifically valid data. Mental illnesses could not be researched effectively, and certain illnesses of the ageing population would also be left without due regard.

The use of the term 'societal necessity' may be misleading in the sense that it may not be the society at large whose interests are at stake, but merely the group that the incompetent person belongs to. In order to ensure that the best interests of the subject are not interfered with for a purpose other than the original aim, provisions have been drafted so that if the prospect of benefit in taking part in the research is not directed to the subject him or herself, it should be directed 'to other persons in the same age category or afflicted with the same disease or disorder or having the same condition' (Article 17, para 2; see also Additional Protocol Article 15, para 2). Another illustration of the necessity argument is visible in the provision which states that if the research of comparable effectiveness can be carried out on individuals capable of giving consent, research on incompetent subjects may not be undertaken even in the case of therapeutic research (Article 17, para 1; see also Additional Protocol Article 15, para 1).

A third aspect to the notion of 'societal necessity' applies not only to vulnerable groups but addresses research ethics in general. It touches the general aims and the quality of the project. For example, if the design of the project is flawed, if it is merely duplicating what has already been scientifically proven or if the results are more directed to advance commercial rather than medical interests, the reason for conducting the project is medically speaking futile and therefore cannot fulfil the 'societal necessity' criteria (e.g. Additional Protocol Article 8).

Minimal risk   The other condition for conducting non-therapeutic research on incompetents is the criterion of minimal risk. The research must not entail more than a 'minimal risk and a minimal burden' to the subject (Article 17, para 2; see also Additional Protocol Article 15, para 2). This requirement resembles closely one of the interpretations given to the 'best interests' criterion, according to which the parental powers extend to cover also procedures which are not considered to be 'against the best interests' of the patient, e.g. taking a blood sample (*S v S, W v Official Solicitor*). In the explanatory report of the Biomedicine Convention some examples have been given as to what the term 'minimal risk' might mean. With regard to children, it lists 'ultrasonic scanning when replacing X-ray examinations or invasive diagnostic measures, incidental blood samples from newborns without respiratory problems in order to establish the necessary oxygen content for premature infants and discovering the causes and improving treatment of leukaemia in children for example by taking a blood sample'. The list is by no means complete. However, as can be seen from the list, a procedure is not considered acceptable or unacceptable merely on the basis of a consideration of the risk it poses; the risk is also evaluated in comparison to the aim of the research project.

Role of ethics committees   Ethical research on incompetent persons involves a lot of weighing and balancing of different aspects. Very often there is no legislation or clear guidelines for deciding on competence or making the risk–benefit calculations, which are of central importance in deciding about the ethics and legality of the research concerned. Fortunately, such decisions are not left solely for the researchers to decide: they can and must get approval for the proposed research project from the relevant ethics committees that are equipped to give a more objective opinion on the project. On the condition that the research ethics committees are provided with adequate resources and training to be able to efficiently supervise medical research involving vulnerable groups, some of the restrictions of medical research could be loosened, according to the example given by the Biomedicine Convention. As already said, this leaves a heavy responsibility for the ethics committees, and the need for ascertaining public confidence is apparent. As most of the documents processed by the committees are confidential, general trust should be maintained by paying special attention to the composition of the committees in order to ensure the objectivity of its decision-making.

ACTIVITY: At this point stop for a moment and, taking into account what you have read in the section so far, make a list of all the elements you consider to be required for consent to be valid. Next make a list of the various ways and circumstances in which these criteria are unlikely to have been met. Add these points to your checklist.

At the end of this section our checklist has added the following questions:

- Are the research subjects giving their informed consent?
- Are the research subjects competent to participate in the research?
- Are the research subjects subject to any form of coercion?

- Are the research subjects in a dependent relationship with the researcher?
- Is participation in the research in the subject's best interests?
- How big are the risks associated with the research?
- What are the likely benefits of the research?

Section 3: Researchers' responsibilities and developing countries

In this section we shall be expanding our discussion from individual research subjects to look at global issues about research methods, obligations and responsibilities. We will explore these questions in relation to a case of some research which was carried out on HIV infection and transmission in Africa, causing an international debate about whether or not it was ethical. In fact, the research caused so much dispute within the bioethics community that it led to demands for a revision of the Helsinki Declaration itself, the international declaration against which the ethical acceptability of research is usually evaluated. The debate turned on issues about Western researchers' responsiblities in Third World countries, particularly to subjects in the placebo arm of the trial. Now read through the outline of the case, think about the ethical questions it raises and put these on your checklist.

The case of HIV drug trials in developing countries

Between 1995 and 1997, a programme of 15 trials on maternal–fetal transmission of HIV, coordinated by UNAIDS, was carried out on 12 000 women in various parts of the developing world (Ethiopia, Ivory Coast, Uganda, Zimbabwe, Tanzania, South Africa, Malawi, Kenya and Burkina Faso). The research was conducted by researchers funded by the USA, France, Belgium, Denmark and South Africa. At that time it was estimated by the National Institutes of Health that there would soon be 6 million pregnant women in the developing world infected with HIV. Maternal–infant transmission of HIV occurred in approximately 15% of cases, with approximately 1000 HIV-positive babies born each day.

A particular regimen of the antiretroviral drug zidovudine had been shown by research in the USA and in France to reduce the risk of such transmission by up to 66%. The 'triple combination' regimen, involving three stages (oral doses whilst pregnant, intravenous doses during labour and further oral doses, for the child, up until six weeks after birth), was claimed to be too expensive for widespread use in the developing world [$800 per mother and infant according to Varmus and Satcher (1997). This was 600 times the annual per capita allocation for healthcare in Malawi]. Were it possible to develop an effective regimen of the drug which was less expensive than triple combination therapy and cheap enough for widespread use in the developing world, it would clearly have the potential to avoid the infection of a very large number of babies. In order to investigate the success of a lower dosage of the drug, researchers considered two alternative study designs. The first approach considered was to run a trial comparing a new cheaper regimen with placebo. The second approach considered was to compare the new regimen with triple combination therapy.

It was the first approach that was adopted in these trials. That meant that only half of the HIV-positive women actually received the drug regime, with the other half receiving a placebo. Had the trials been carried out in the developed world, they would have been considered unethical. The Declaration of Helsinki in its then-current (1989) version stated that 'The potential benefits, hazards and discomfort of a new method should be weighed against the advantages of the best current diagnostic and therapeutic methods'. However, given the absence of any such treatment locally, the researchers felt that the trials were justified because, without them, the women who received the reduced dose therapy and those who received the placebo would both have received nothing. The trial, it was claimed, would leave no one worse off than they would otherwise have been: some women would receive treatment they would not otherwise have had, and those who received placebos would be no worse off than they would otherwise have been. The researchers also argued that a placebo-controlled trial would produce results more quickly than a treatment-controlled approach.

ACTIVITY: Before you go on, stop here for a moment and consider whether this research project is an ethical one. Imagine that you are a member of the ethics committee that had to decide whether or not to approve this project. Make a list of arguments for and another of arguments against allowing the project to proceed.

In an influential article which originally appeared in the *New England Journal of Medicine*, two prominent critics, Peter Lurie and Sidney M. Wolfe, argued that these trials were indeed unethical, falling below the standard of the Declaration of Helsinki (Lurie and Wolfe, 1997). While they recognized that both critics and opponents of these trials agreed that perinatal HIV transmission was a grave international problem, that there was a role for research on this topic in developing countries, that finding cheaper interventions would benefit those countries hugely and that randomized trials were an effective way of identifying such interventions, they viewed the crucial ethical issue dividing them from proponents of the trials as the composition of the control or comparison group.

As Lurie and Wolfe wrote, 'The researchers conducting the placebo-controlled trials assert that such trials represent the only appropriate research design, implying that they answer the question, "Is the shorter regimen better than nothing?" We take the more optimistic view that, given the findings of ACTG 076 [the zidovudine regimen trials] and other clinical information, researchers are quite capable of designing a shorter antiretroviral regimen that is approximately as effective as the ACTG 076 regimen. We believe that such equivalency studies of alternative antiretroviral regimens will provide even more useful results than placebo-controlled trials, without the deaths of hundreds of newborns that are inevitable if placebo groups are used' (Lurie and Wolfe, 1997, p. 854). They continued, 'If the research can be satisfactorily conducted in more than one way, why not select the approach that minimizes loss of life?' (Lurie and Wolfe, 1997, p. 854).

According to Lurie and Wolfe, researchers working in the Third World are ethically obliged to provide treatment for control groups that corresponds with the standard of care in the sponsoring country, even if the standard of care in the country where the trials are being held is lower. (The only exception would be a trial that required massive infrastructure expenditure – say, building a new coronary care unit in a hospital.) Otherwise we risk enshrining double standards in research, Lurie and Wolfe asserted, with one standard for the rich world and another for the poor. They also pointed out that in any case, zidovudine was normally made available free of charge by the manufacturer for use in clinical trials. So to put the matter in terms of Aristotle's standard of justice, 'treating equals equally', there wasn't even a financial excuse for circumventing the ethical imperative of treating rich and poor alike.

Accepting that the control group in this case should receive a lower standard of care than they would in the First World – or in fact no care at all – gives researchers an incentive to choose subjects with minimal access to healthcare. Lurie and Wolfe pointed out some dangerous and exploitative implications of accepting such a double standard: 'Researchers might inject live malaria parasites into HIV-positive subjects in China in order to study the effect on the progression of HIV infection, even though the study protocol had been rejected in the United States and Mexico. Or researchers might randomly assign malnourished San (bushmen) to receive vitamin-fortified or standard bread. One might also justify trials of HIV vaccines in which the subjects were not provided with condoms or state-of-the-art counseling about safe sex by arguing that they are not customarily provided in the developing countries in question. These are not simply hypothetical worst-case scenarios; the first two studies have already been performed,[55,56] and the third has been proposed and criticized'[57] (Lurie and Wolfe, 1997, p. 855). Overall, Lurie and Wolfe explicitly agreed with the position taken in the same journal nine years earlier by Marcia Angell, who wrote that 'Human subjects in any part of the world should be protected by an irreducible set of ethical standards.'[58]

ACTIVITY: These seem strong and clear arguments, but what are the counter-arguments? We would now like you go on to read the next selection, in which the case for such trials was presented in a joint statement by two of the organizations funding the research, 'The Conduct of Clinical Trials of Maternal–Infant Transmission of HIV Supported by the United States Department of Health and Human Services in Developing Countries'.

A defence of HIV trials in the developing world

Based on the US National Institutes of Health and Centers for Disease Control and Prevention Statement[59]

In a joint statement (US National Institutes of Health and Centers for Disease Control and Prevention, 1997) the Directors of the two organizations funding the

research trials, the National Institutes for Health and the Centers for Disease Control and Prevention in the US [http://www.nih.gov/news/ mathiv/mathiv.htm, 1997], made the case for the research trials. The statement begins by reiterating the desperate need for the development of less expensive treatments for the developing world.

> One regimen of antiretroviral therapy has been shown to reduce substantially the likelihood of maternal–infant transmission of HIV. The identification of this successful regimen was the result of the National Institutes of Health's AIDS Clinical Trials Group protocol 076 (ACTG 076 or 076) in 1994. In spite of this knowledge, approximately 1000 HIV-infected infants are born each day, the vast majority of them in developing countries. This occurs, in part, because the regimen proven to be effective is simply not feasible as a standard of prevention in much of the developing world.
>
> There are two reasons for this lack of feasibility. Firstly, to follow the regimen that has proven efficacy requires that the women be reached early in prenatal care; be tested for and counseled concerning their HIV status; comply with a lengthy oral treatment regimen; receive intravenous administration of the antiretroviral zidovudine (ZDV or AZT) during labor and delivery; and refrain from breast-feeding. Additionally, the newborns must receive 6 weeks of oral AZT therapy. During and after the time the mother and infant are treated with AZT, both must be carefully monitored for adverse effects of exposure to this drug. In the developing world countries that are the sites of these studies, these requirements could seldom be achieved, even under the infrequent circumstance when women present early enough for the screening and care requirements of the 076 therapeutic regimen to be implemented. Secondly, the wholesale drug costs for the AZT in the 076 regimen are estimated to be in excess of $800, an amount far greater than these developing countries could afford as standard care. [...] Less complex and expensive alternatives are urgently needed to address the staggering impact of maternal–infant transmission of HIV in developing countries.

The authors go on to point out that this type of research trial was specifically called for by the World Health Organization's 'Recommendations from the Meeting on Prevention of Mother-to-Infant Transmission of HIV by Use of Antiretrovirals, Geneva 23–25 June 1994', on the grounds that it offered the best chance to get results quickly. The World Health Organization document argues that,

> Since the ZDV regimen studied in ACTG 076 is not applicable in those parts of the world where most MTI transmission of HIV occurs, placebo-controlled trials offer the best option for obtaining rapid and scientifically valid results.

In addition to their argument that placebo controlled trials would get results quicker than treatment-controlled trials the WHO also argued that,

> [Triple combination therapy] is not applicable [in the developing world] because of its cost and operational requirements. In those parts of the world, the choice of a placebo for the control group of a randomized trial would be appropriate as there is currently no effective alternative for HIV-infected pregnant women.

The WHO guidelines are taken by the NIH and CDC to:

> clearly indicate that the in-country healthcare capabilities of each country in which maternal–infant HIV transmission research is to be conducted must be used to define the type of research which is ethical and therefore permissible in that country ... [Many of the] arguments against the NIH and CDC supported studies appear to rest on the proposition that it is unethical to conduct a clinical trial unless it offers all participants a chance to receive an effective intervention if such is available anywhere in the world, even if it is not available at the site of the clinical trial. Ideally, this would be so for all clinical trials for all therapies. But the reality is that often it is not possible. The very purpose of the NIH and CDC supported studies of maternal–infant transmission of HIV in developing countries is to identify interventions other than those of 076 [triple combination] and we agree with the WHO Geneva panel's recommendation 2 that:

> it should be emphasized that the results of ACTG 076 are only directly applicable to a specific population. Moreover, the ZDV regimen employed in the ACTG 076 study has a number of features (cost, logistical issues, among others) which limit its general applicability. Therefore, no global recommendations regarding use of ZDV to prevent MTI transmission of HIV can be made.

The joint NIH and CDC statement argues that the 'primary consideration' when making decisions about

what constitutes an ethical research project in the developing world ought to be the extent to which, once the research has been completed, will the population represented by the study participants benefit from the results of the project? They go on to argue on the basis of this claim that to carry out research on the triple combination treatment would in fact actually itself have been unethical because it would have been testing a treatment which stands no chance of becoming standard treatment locally.

The International Ethical Guidelines for Biomedical Research Involving Human Subjects that were prepared by the Council for International Organisations of Medical Sciences (CIOMS) in collaboration with WHO are:

> intended to indicate how the ethical principles embodied in the Declaration [of Helsinki] could be effectively applied in developing countries.

To evaluate interventions that they could not implement realistically would be exploitative of those in the participant country since there would be no likelihood of meeting requirement 15 of the Guidelines that obliges:

> any product developed [through] such research will be made reasonably available to the inhabitants of the host community or country at the completion of successful testing

Therefore, we have determined that the more compelling ethical argument is against using a regimen that if found to be superior in the study could not possibly be used in the prevention of maternal–infant transmission of HIV in the host country. Turning once again to Malawi for example, health officials there refused to permit the conduct of a study involving a full course regimen of AZT (such as that used in ACTG 076) because they believed it would be unethical to undertake such a study in Malawi given that its very limited resources and poor health infrastructure make the introduction of AZT as standard treatment for HIV-infected pregnant women unfeasible. Instead, the health officials wanted research on alternative treatment approaches that might reduce maternal–infant transmission of HIV. The justification and ethical foundation for the NIH- and CDC-supported studies incorporate the reality that the clinical trials are examining other alternatives that could actually be used for the majority of HIV-infected pregnant women and mothers in the countries in which the clinical trials are being carried out.

ACTIVITY: Now, having read these two sets of arguments, return to the activity with which you began this section. Imagine you were a member of an ethics committee which had been asked to approve these trials. Compare the arguments. Which do you find the most persuasive? What are your reasons?

At the end of this section we had added the following questions to our research ethics check list:

- Are the risks posed by the research so great that even if subjects consented the research would still be unethical?
- What inducements and benefits are ethical to offer to research subjects where the local standard of care is comparatively low?
- Are there risks to others than those who are being asked for their consent?
- What are the responsibilities of researchers to nationals of other countries than their own?

The bioethicist Ruth Macklin has offered another set of questions relating to 'double standards' in Third World research trials, including specific consideration of the ongoing benefits which researchers may owe to the countries in which the research was conducted. (This question of benefit-sharing has been extensively debated in recent years, with the introduction of guidelines in 2000 by the United Nations HUGO group suggesting that 2% of profits should return to the country hosting the research.)

(1) How can biomedical research be designed and conducted so as to contribute to the health needs of developing countries and at the same time contain adequate protections for the rights and welfare of the human subjects recruited for these studies?
(2) If a particular study may not be conducted in the sponsoring country for ethical reasons, is it acceptable to carry out an identical study in a developing country, and if so, with what justification?
(3) When completed research yields successful products or other beneficial interventions, what obligations, if any, do the sponsors have to the community or country where the research was conducted?
(4) Should the provisions of international ethical guidelines for research, such as the Declaration of Helsinki, be interpreted and applied in the same way in resource-poor counties as they are in wealthier countries? (Macklin, 2004, p. 12)

Macklin later concludes that 'Since research in today's world is a global enterprise, justice in international research calls for treating subjects equally whether they live in Boston or Botswana, Utah or Uganda' (Macklin, 2004, p. 254). This is a tall order, but it seems an appropriately stirring note on which to end this chapter on research ethics.

We began the chapter by examining the reactions and dilemmas of an individual research subject, Jan. The Nuremberg Code was understandably concerned to reinstate the rights of the individual against the collective after the abuses of the Nazi period. However, much modern research, for example in population genomics (Mitchell and Happe, 2005) concerns entire families or collectives. An individualist approach to informed consent may be insufficient to cover those instances, particularly among Third World populations whose cultures are based on lineage rights and duties rather than individual entitlements. For example, a research proposal to study the genome of the people of Tonga was rejected by local people because it failed to take into account the importance of family and lineage in protocols for consent (Dickenson, 2007). The controversy surrounding HIV trials in developing countries has illustrated another 'global' aspect of research ethics: the justice or injustice of 'double standards' pertaining to Western and non-Western populations.

ACTIVITY: As the final key points activity in this chapter, we would now like you to return to the research ethics checklist you have been constructing as you have worked your way through this chapter. Below is a summary of some of the questions we noted as we worked through the various activities, including issues about benefit-sharing and other questions of justice which arise in this final section. Have a look at it in the light of your own list and critically assess it. Remember that the list is meant to take the form of a series of questions one might ask a researcher or ask oneself about a research project.

An incomplete research ethics checklist

- What is the balance of harms and risks likely to occur as a result of the research? Is the proposed research going to offer some benefit?
- Is the study going to answer the proposed question?
- Is it necessary for this research to be carried out on human participants? Could the answers be

gained in the laboratory, or by animal studies? Or might animal studies also be ethically problematic?

- Are the participants going to be asked to give their consent? Is there a consent form? Is it clear and understandable? Who will be asking the potential participants for their consent? Are there risks to others than those who are being asked for their consent?
- Are the research participants giving their informed consent? Will participants have sufficient information to be able to consent?
- Is there a Patient Information Sheet?
- Is this information presented clearly and in a way participants will be able to understand?
- Are the research participants competent to participate in the research?
- Are the research participants subject to any form of coercion?
- Are the research participants in a dependent relationship with the researcher?
- Is participation in the research in the participant's best interests?
- Is it clear to the participants that they can withdraw from the study at any time and that this will not affect the quality of their treatment?
- Is it made clear that the participant can refuse to participate and that this too will not affect the treatment received?
- How big are the risks associated with the research?
- Does the study put participants at unacceptable risk?
- Might the validity of the research participants' consent be questioned as a result of their distress or vulnerability?
- Why is the research to be carried out on incompetent and vulnerable patients?
- Could such groups lose out as a result of not being researched? Does the research involve deceit or covert methods?
- Is the research question worth investigating?
- Has it been done before? Does the methodology offer the likelihood of achieving aims?
- Is the confidentiality of the research subjects protected?
- Are the risks posed by the research so great that even if subjects consented the research would still be unethical? What inducements and benefits are ethical to offer to research subjects where the local standard of care is comparatively low?

- What involvement do commercial biotechnology firms have in funding the research or in extracting benefits from it?
- Is there any conflict of interest with the researcher's right to publish and with researchers' scientific obligations?
- Have researchers and their university or institute declared all financial interests?
- If patents or other intellectual property are likely to result from the research, who will own them?
- Is there an ongoing right for participants to share in financial benefits or to share information from the research?

Appendix: The Nuremberg Code

From 'Trials of War Criminals Before the Nuremberg Military Tribunals Under Control Council Law No. 10', Volume 2, Nuremberg, October 1946 – April 1949 (Washington, DC: US Government Printing Office, 1949, pp. 181–2).

The great weight of the evidence before us is to the effect that certain types of medical experiments on human beings, when kept within reasonably well-defined bounds, conform to the ethics of the medical profession generally. The protagonists of the practice of human experimentation justify their views on the basis that such experiments yield results for the good of society that are unprocurable by other methods or means of study. All agree, however, that certain basic principles must be observed in order to satisfy moral, ethical and legal concepts.

(a) The voluntary consent of the human subject is absolutely essential. This means that the person involved should have legal capacity to give consent; should be so situated as to be able to exercise free power of choice, without the intervention of any element of force, fraud, deceit, duress, overreaching, or other ulterior form of constraint or coercion; and should have sufficient knowledge and comprehension of the elements of the subject matter involved as to enable him to make an understanding and enlightened decision. This later element requires that before the acceptance of an affirmative decision by the experimental subject there should be made known to him the nature, duration and purpose of the experiment; the method and means by which it is to be conducted; all inconveniences and hazards reasonably to be expected; and the effects upon his health or person which may possibly come from his participation in the experiment. The duty and responsibility for ascertaining the quality of the consent rests upon each individual who initiates, directs or engages in the experiment. It is a personal duty and responsibility which may not be delegated to another with impunity.

(b) The experiment should be such as to yield fruitful results for the good of society, unprocurable by other methods or means of study, and not random and unnecessary in nature.

(c) The experiment should be so designed and based on the results of animal experimentation and a knowledge of the natural history of the disease or other problems under study that the anticipated results will justify the performance of the experiment.

(d) The experiment should be so conducted as to avoid all unnecessary physical and mental suffering and injury.

(e) No experiment should be conducted where there is an a priori reason to believe that death or disabling injury will occur; except perhaps, in those experiments where the experimental physicians also serve as subjects.

(f) The degree of risk to be taken should never exceed that determined by the humanitarian importance of the problem to be solved by the experiment.

(g) Proper preparation should be made and adequate facilities provided to protect the experimental subject against even remote possibilities of injury, disability or death.

(h) The experiment should be conducted only by scientifically qualified persons. The highest degree of skill and care should be required through all stages of the experiment of those who conduct or engage in the experiment.

(i) During the course of the experiment the human subject should be at liberty to bring the experiment to an end if he has reached the physical or mental state where continuation of the experiment seems to him to be impossible.

(j) During the course of the experiment, the scientist in charge must be prepared to terminate the experiment at any stage, if he has probable cause to believe in the exercise of good faith, superior skill and careful judgement required of him that a continuation of the experiment is likely to result in injury, disability, or death to the experimental subject.

References and notes

* The four principles were first described in Fulford and Howse (1993).

** Adapted with permission from Richard Ashcroft, 'Autonomy and informed consent in the ethics of the randomized controlled trial: philosophical perspectives'. In Ashcroft, R. E., Chadwick, D. W., Clark, S. R. L. *et al.* (1997). Implications of socio-cultural contexts for ethics of clinical trials. *Health Technology Assessment*, 1(9), 1–67.

1. Annas, G. J. and Grodin, M. A. (ed.) (1992). *The Nazi Doctors and the Nuremberg Code: Human Rights in Human Experimentation*. Oxford: Oxford University Press.

2. Advisory Commission on Human Radiation Experiments Research Ethics and the Medical Profession (1996). *Journal of the American Medical Association*, **276**, 403–9.

3. Caplan, A. L. (1992). Is there a duty to serve as a subject in biomedical research? In *If I were a Rich Man Could I Buy a Pancreas? And Other Essays on the Ethics of Healthcare*, ed. A. L. Caplan, Chapter 6. Bloomington, IN: Indiana University Press.

4. Emson, H. E. (1992). Rights, duties and responsibilities in healthcare. *Journal of Applied Philosophy*, **9**, 3–11.

5. Rothman, D. J. (1987). Ethics and human experimentation: Henry Beecher revisited. *New England Journal of Medicine*, **317**, 1195–9.

6. Jones, J. H. (1993). *Bad Blood: The Tuskegee Syphilis Experiment*. Glencoe, IL: Free Press.

7. Annas, G. J. (1992). The Nuremberg Code in US courts: ethics versus expediency. In *The Nazi Doctors and the Nuremberg Code: Human Rights in Human Experimentation*, ed. G. J. Annas and M. A. Grodin. Oxford: Oxford University Press.

8. Bush, J. K. (1994). The industry perspective on the inclusion of women in clinical trials. *Academic Medicine*, **69**, 708–15; Dresser, R. (1992). Wanted: single, white male for medical research. *Hastings Center Report 22 (Jan/Feb)*, 24–9; McCarthy, C. R. (1994). Historical background of clinical trials involving women and minorities. *Academic Medicine*, **69**, 695–8; Mastroianni, A. C., Faden, R. and Federman, D. (1994). Women and health research: a report from the Institute of Medicine. *Kennedy Institute of Ethics Journal*, **4**, 55–61; Merton, V. (1993). The exclusion of the pregnant, pregnable and once-pregnable people (a.k.a. women)

from biomedical research. *American Journal of Law and Medicine*, **XIX**, 369–451; Merkatz, R. B. and Junod, S. W. (1994). Historical background of changes in FDA policy on the study and evaluation of drugs in women. *Academic Medicine*, **69**, 703–7.

9. Warren, C. A. B. and Karner, T. X. (1990). Permissions and the social context. *American Sociologist*, Summer, 116–35.

10. Lesser, H. (1989). Obligation and consent. *Journal of Medical Ethics*, **15**, 195–6.

11. Freedman, B., Fuks, A. and Weijer, C. (1992). Demarcating research and treatment: a systematic approach for the analysis of the ethics of clinical research. *Clinical Research*, **40**, 653–60.

12. Reiser, S. J. (1978). Human experimentation and the convergence of medical research and patient care. *Annals of the AAPSS*, **437**, 8–18.

13. Reiser, S. J. (1994). Criteria for standard versus experimental therapy. *Health Affairs*, **13**, 127–36.

14. *Op. cit.* Note 3.

15. Allmark, P. (1994). An argument against the use of the concept of 'persons' in health care ethics. *Journal of Advanced Nursing*, **19**, 29–35.

16. Gillon, R. (1993). Autonomy, respect for autonomy and weakness of the will. *Journal of Medical Ethics*, **19**, 195–6.

17. Pellegrino, E. D. (1990). The relationship of autonomy and integrity in medical ethics. *Bulletin of the Pan-American Health Organization*, **24**, 361–71.

18. Karlawish, J. H. T. and Hall, J. B. (1996). The controversy over emergency research: a review of the issues and suggestions for a resolution. *American Journal of Respiratory Critical Care Medicine*, **153**, 499–506.

19. Sheldon, T. (1995). Consent is not always essential, say Dutch experts. *British Medical Journal*, **310**, 1355–6.

20. Jonas, C. and Soutoul, J. H. (1993). Biomedical research in incapacitated people according to French law. *Medical Law*, **12**, 567–72.

21. Hodgkinson, D. W., Gray, A. J., Dala, B. *et al.* (1995). Doctor's legal position in treating temporarily incompetent patients, *British Medical Journal*, **311**, 115–18.

22. Gifford, F. (1986). The conflict between randomized clinical trials and the therapeutic obligation. *Journal of Medicine and Philosophy*, **11**, 347–66.

23. Shumm, D. S. and Speece, R. G. (1993). Ethical issues and clinical trials. *Drugs*, **46**, 579–84.

24. Perry, C. B. (1994). Conflicts of interest and the physician's duty to inform. *American Journal of Medicine*, **96**, 375–80.

25. *Op. cit.* Note 3.

26. Emson, H. E. (1992). Rights, duties and responsibilities in healthcare. *Journal of Applied Philosophy*, **9**, 3–11.

27. Jonas, H. (1969). Philosophical reflections on experimenting with human subjects. *Daedalus*, **98**, 219–47.

28. Fethe, C. (1993). Beyond voluntary consent: Hans Jonas on the moral requirements of human experimentation. *Journal of Medical Ethics*, 19–103.

29. Rothman, D. J. (1987). Ethics and human experimentation: Henry Beecher revisited. *New England Journal of Medicine*, **317**, 1195–9.

30. Beecher, H. K. (1970). *Research and the Individual.* London: J. and A. Churchill.

31. Beecher, H. K. (1966). Ethics and clinical research. *New England Journal of Medicine*, **274**, 1354–60.

32. Popper, S. E. and McCloskey, K. (1995). Ethics in human experimentation: historical perspectives. *Military Medicine*, **160**, 7–11.

33. Buchanan, A. (1996). Judging the past: the case of the human radiation experiments. *Hastings Center Report*, **26** (May/June); 25–30.

34. Burchell, H. B. (1992). Vicissitudes in clinical trial research: subjects, participants, patients. *Controlled Clinical Trials*, **13**, 185–9.

35. Evered, D. C. and Halnan, K. E. (1995). Deadly experiments. *British Medical Journal*, **311**, 192.

36. Silverman, W. A. and Altman, D. G. (1996). Patients' preferences and randomized trials. *Lancet*, **347**, 171–4.

37. Rosenzweig, S. (1933). The experimental situation as a psychological problem. *Psychological Review*, **40**, 337–54.

38. Daugherty, C., Ratain, M. J., Grochowski, E. *et al.* (1995). Perceptions of cancer patients and their physicians involved in Phase trials. *Journal of Clinical Oncology*, **13**, 1062–72.

39. Susman, E. J., Dorn, L. D. and Fletcher J. C. (1992). Participation in biomedical research: the consent process as viewed by children, adolescents, young adults and physicians. *Journal of Pediatrics*, **121**, 547–52.

40. Nguyen-Van-Tam, J. S. and Madeley, R. J. (1996). Vietnamese people in study may have had language difficulties. *British Medical Journal*, **313**, 48.

41. Habermas, J. (1979). *Communication and the Evolution of Society.* London: Heinemann Educational.

42. Alderson, P. (1995). Consent, and the social context. *Nursing Ethics*, **2**, 347–50; Alderson, P. (1988). Trust in informed consent. *IME Bulletin* (July) 17–19; Andreasson, S., Parmander, M. and Allebeck, P. A. (1990). A trial that failed, and the reasons why:

comparing the Minnesota model with outpatient treatment and non-treatment for alcohol disorders. *Scandinavian Journal of Social Medicine*, **18**, 221–4; Angell, M. (1984). Patients' preferences in randomised clinical trials. *New England Journal of Medicine*, **310**, 1385–7; Beech, C. L. (1995). Compliance in clinical trials. *AIDS*, **9**, 1–10; Brownlea, A. (1987). Participation: myths, realities and prognosis. *Social Science and Medicine*, **25**, 605–14; Daugherty, C. K., Ratain, M. J. and Siegler, M. (1995). Pushing the envelope: informed consent in Phase I trials. *Annals of Oncology*, **6**, 321–3; DeLuca, S. A., Korcuska, L. A., Oberstar, B. H. *et al.* (1995). Are we providing true informed consent in cardiovascular clinical trials? *Journal of Cardiovascular Nursing*, **9** (3), 54–61; Fox, R. (1996). What do patients want from medical research. *Journal of the Royal Society of Medicine*, **89**, 301–2; Gostin, L. O. (1995). Informed consent, cultural sensitivity and respect for persons. *Journal of the American Medical Association*, **274**, 844–5; Grimshaw, J. M. (1990). Clinical trials: patient perspectives. *AIDS*, **4**, Suppl. **1**, S207–8; Joseph, R. R. (1994). Viewpoints and concerns of a clinical trial participant. *Cancer*, **74**, 2692–3; Kotwall, C. A., Mahoneym L. J., Myers, R. E. and Decoste, L. (1992). Reasons for non-entry in randomised clinical trials for breast cancer: a single institutional study. *Journal of Surgical Oncology*, **50**, 125–9; Lilleyman, J. S. (1995). Informed consent: how informed and consent to what? *Pediatric Hematology and Oncology*, **12** (6), xiii–xvi; Llewellyn-Thomas, H. A., McGreal, M. J., Thiel, E. C., Fine, S. and Erlichman, C. (1991). Patients' willingness to enter clinical trials: measuring the association with perceived benefit and preference for decision participation. *Social Science and Medicine*, **32**, 35–42; McGrath, P. (1995). It's OK to say no! A discussion of ethical issues arising from informed consent to chemotherapy. *Cancer Nursing*, **18**, 97–103; Winn, R. J. (1994). Obstacles to the accrual of patients to clinical trials in the community setting. *Seminars in Oncology*, **21** (4, Suppl. 7), 112–17.

43. Logue, G. and Wear, S. (1995). A desperate solution: individual autonomy and the double-blind controlled experiment. *Journal of Medicine and Philosophy*, **20**, 57–64.

44. Epstein, S. (1991). Democratic science? AIDS activism and the contested construction of knowledge. *Socialist Review*, **21**, 35–64.

45. Benson, P. R. (1989). The social control of human biomedical research: an overview and review of the literature. *Social Science and Medicine*, **29**, 1–12.

46. McKay, C. R. (1995). The evolution of the institutional review board: a brief overview of its history. *Clinical Research and Regulatory Affairs*, **12**, 65–94.

47. McNeill, P. M. (1993). *The Ethics and Politics of Human Experimentation*. Cambridge: Cambridge University Press.

48. Byrne, P. (1988). Medical research and the human subject: problems of consent and control in the UK experience. *Annals of the New York Academy of Sciences*, **530**, 144–53.

49. Reiser, S. J. and Knudsen, P. (1993). Protecting research subjects after consent: the case for the 'Research Intermediary' *IRB: A Review of Human Subjects Research*, **15**, 10–11.

50. DeBakey, L. (1974). Ethically questionable data: publish or reject? *Clinical Research*, **22**, 113–21.

51. Rosner, F., Bennet, A. J., Cassell, E. J. *et al.* (1991). The ethics of using scientific data obtained by immoral means. *New York State Journal of Medicine*, **91**, 54–9.

52. Smith, R. (1996). Commentary: the importance of patients' consent for publication. *British Medical Journal*, 313, 6.

53. Carnall, D. (1996). Doctor struck off for scientific fraud. *British Medical Journal*, **312**, 44.

54. Dyer, O. (1996). GP struck off for fraud in drug trials. *British Medical Journal*, **312**, 798.

55. Heimlich H. J., Chen X. P., Xiao B. Q. *et al.* (1996). CD4 response in HIV-positive patients treated with malariatherapy. Presented at the 11th International Conference on AIDS, Vancouver, B. C., July 7–12, 1996.

56. Bishop W. B., Lauscher I., Labrodarios D. *et al.* (1996). Effect of vitamin-enriched bread on the vitamin status of an isolated rural community – a controlled clinical trial. *South Africa Medical Journal*, **86**, Suppl. 458–62.

57. Lurie, P., Bishaw, M., Chesney, M. A. *et al.* (1994). Ethical, behavioral and social aspects of HIV vaccine trials in developing countries. *Journal of the American Medical Association*, **271**, 295–301.

58. Angell, M. (1998) Ethical imperialism? Ethics in international collaborative clinical research. *New England Journal of Medicine*, **319**, 1081–3.

59. With permission from US National Institutes of Health and Centers for Disease Control and Prevention. 'A defence of HIV trials in the developing world and Prevention' (1997), from 'The Conduct of Clinical Trials of Maternal–Infant Transmission of HIV Supported by the United States Department of Health and Human Services in Developing Countries.' Available at http://www.nih.gov/%20news/mathiv/mathiv.htm

5 Mental health: consent, competence and caring

We begin this chapter with the case of Mr AB from Italy, because it raises not only important ethical issues in itself, but also ethical questions about mental health more widely. Are there morally significant differences between psychiatric medicine and medicine of other kinds? Are there also morally significant differences between various psychiatric conditions? If so, what are the implications of these differences for the practice of psychiatric medicine?

Central to Mr AB's case are questions about autonomy and mental competence, which we will further explore by returning to the case of Mr C, whom we encountered in the first chapter, on decisions at the end of life. The autonomy of the psychiatric patient is a core theme in the ethics of mental healthcare. As such, in the second section of this chapter, we move to examine ideas associated with autonomy, like the freedom or liberty of a psychiatric patient and the limits (if any) that can be placed on his or her freedom (such as through involuntary treatment or hospitalization). The boundaries of autonomy also feature in the third section, which focuses upon the mental health of children and young people. In that section, as in the previous one, we will explore the tensions that can arise between protecting the patient's autonomy and protecting their welfare. You will see, at many points, that there appears to be conflict between an approach premised on patients' rights and more paternalistic approaches to psychiatric treatment and care. However, in the final section of this chapter, we will investigate a different way of thinking about mental health ethics, which seeks to resolve the tension through consideration of the ethics of care.

We would like you to start by reading the case of Mr AB. As you do so, we would like you to consider the extent to which you feel that the difficulties which arise in the case are morally significant or 'ethical' and the extent to which they are simply a practical or clinical matter. To what extent do you think it is possible to make such a distinction? Do clinical decisions such as those concerning Mr AB always have an ethical dimension?

Section 1: Autonomy, competence and mental health

The case of Mr AB

Mr AB was a 90-year-old man who suffered from dementia. After several years of being cared for at home by his wife, Mr AB was finally admitted to a special care unit in northern Italy because his wife no longer felt able to bear the demands which caring for her husband placed upon her.

On admission to the unit, a clinical and multidimensional evaluation of Mr AB's condition revealed him to be severely cognitively impaired and to be extremely frail as a result of malnutrition. Mr AB was capable to some limited extent of walking and also of eating but was dependent upon others in virtually every other respect. Although he was able to walk, Mr AB found balance very difficult and needed the support of a carer. The doctors who saw him also recorded that he had severe 'behaviour disorders' associated with dementia, such as anxiety and agitation.

The physician responsible for Mr AB's care designed a walking rehabilitation programme for him and the nurses in the unit tried to improve his nutritional status by means of personal care and attention during meal times and by the use of nutritional supplements. It was also decided to reduce the levels of psychotropic drugs with which Mr AB had been treated while he was living at home.

After 20 days of treatment at the special care unit, Mr AB's cognitive and functional status had improved dramatically and he was now able to walk alone, without help. His behaviour disorders were also less severe and disturbing (especially his anxiety and agitation) despite the fact that his treatment with psychotropic drugs had been reduced.

After 35 days at the unit, however, Mr AB developed a fever and cough which became progressively worse. This was diagnosed as pneumonia. As a result of the pneumonia, Mr AB became much more confused again and was no longer able to walk. He also lost the ability to feed himself. All this resulted in a dramatic and serious decline in Mr AB's health. It was felt that Mr AB's life would be at risk unless his pneumonia was treated and he received some nutrition.

After discussing the patient's condition with his wife, the physician started treating Mr AB intravenously with fluids and also with antibiotics. However, during attempts to administer intravenous drugs Mr AB became very irritable and agitated. He also refused food during assisted meals.

After further consultation with Mr AB's wife, short-term physical restraints were adopted by the hospital staff, both during the administration of drugs and during assisted meals. After 2 weeks Mr AB recovered from pneumonia and returned to his previous daily nourishment and drug therapy.

ACTIVITY: Make a list of the distinctively ethical (as opposed to clinical) questions presented by this case. Next to each of these, note down your reasons for your decision. How easy is it to identify a distinction between a clinical and an ethical problem? What is it which marks the difference, if there is any? If you think no difference can be found, then what are the implications of this for ethics and practice?

At first sight the case of Mr AB might be considered an everyday one involving a series of relatively straightforward clinical decisions. He entered the unit in a very poor condition and was given a course of treatment which increased his quality of life greatly. This course of treatment was interrupted by his pneumonia which was itself then treated, thereby allowing Mr AB to return to his earlier much-improved condition. From a utilitarian or consequentialist perspective, that is if we judge the morality of actions and choices in terms of their consequences, the treatment seems to have been justified, at least on first inspection. The patient's quality of life was improved greatly both by his admission to the unit and his consequent treatment, including the use of restraints. Nevertheless, the use of restraints and compulsory treatment on a patient clearly raises ethical questions of great

importance independently of their short-term consequences. Whilst it is not clear that the patient was actually refusing treatment, its administration was obviously making him extremely anxious and agitated. Under what conditions is it right to override someone's wishes and in fact to physically force treatment upon them on the grounds of an assessment of their 'best interests'?

John Stuart Mill once famously argued that the moral thing to do, from a utilitarian point of view, was to respect and uphold the liberty of individuals insofar as such liberty is compatible with the liberty of others (Mill, 1993). We therefore have to think very carefully indeed before we use utility/best interests as a justification for overriding the freedom and wishes of patients.

The main ethical consideration which we felt to be a feature of the case on first sight was this tension between the healthcare professional's duty to respect the choices and wishes of the patients in their care and the complementary duty to act for the patient's benefit. Sometimes, perhaps mostly, these two duties pull in the same direction: i.e. the patient wants to have the treatment which will most obviously benefit them. However, in this example the carers felt that this was not the case and that their responsibility to act for the patient's benefit was more important than to respect the patient's 'wishes'. To what extent do you agree with this?

One of the features of work with at least some psychiatric patients, of course, is that it is often unclear just what the patient's wishes are, and this throws a different light on the tension between wishes and welfare. Assuming for a moment that the patient was indeed attempting to refuse the treatment, there is clearly a sense in which he is a danger to himself and putting himself at risk by refusing both nutrition and treatment for his pneumonia. To what extent do we have the right and perhaps the duty to physically restrain another person from doing what they want to do (assuming we know what this is), even where we consider it to be harmful to them or to be against their best interests? Such a conflict might often be interpreted in terms of paternalism (doing something against the patient's wishes, for their own good) versus the patient's right to choose. However, the right to choose will hinge on the extent to which the patient is *competent* to make the choice in question. The argument here, put simply, would be that Mr AB by virtue of his confusion, his dementia and his anxiety was incapable of having sufficient understanding of his condition or of the proposed treatment to enable him to make an informed choice, either to refuse or to accept his treatment, thereby 'justifying' the healthcare professionals' attempts to act in his best interests despite his protests.

Stefano Boffelli, an Italian old-age psychiatrist, comments on the case as follows.

> The patient, after admission, was judged to be incompetent in taking decisions about himself: cognitive status testing showed a severe decline, [which was] also worsened by the heavy psycho-pharmacological treatment administered at home. The patient was also frail: malnutrition, frequently found in nursing home patients, was the main risk factor for developing pneumonia. However, the patient was not in the end stage of the disease, as was shown by the clinical improvement after rehabilitation. The patient had never written an advance directive about medical treatment before the onset of dementia. So decisions about rehabilitation and the pharmacological treatment of his pneumonia were discussed with his wife, as a substitute decision-maker.
>
> The decision to use physical restraint (for a short time only) was taken with the caregiver. Both in the doctor's and in the caregiver's view, restraining the patient was judged to be an acceptable process to administer drugs and nourishment. Mr AB's wife said of the outcome that ensuring his recovery from pneumonia was worthwhile, even if obtained through short-term discomfort. The patient's reactions against the nurses (agitation and irritability) were interpreted as the effects of dementia, not as an attempt to refuse treatment.
>
> (Boffelli, 1999, personal communication)

ACTIVITY: To what extent do you agree with the doctor and the patient's wife that restraining the patient was an acceptable process in order to administer drugs and nutrition? What arguments can you think of against this view? What do you think about the wife's view that the restraint was simply a 'short-term discomfort' for her husband? To what extent (if any) should we be willing to override the patient's wishes and freedom in favour of what we consider to be their best interests?

In the UK the Mental Capacity Act 2005 sets out the conditions that must be satisfied if restraint is to be used, which are helpfully summarized in guidance issued by the Royal College of Nursing, stating:

> Restraint is defined in the Act as action that uses, or threatens to use, force to secure the doing of an act which the client resists, or restricts the client's liberty of movement, whether or not the client resists. This legal authority to restrain a client is allowed only if the following three conditions are satisfied:
>
> - The client lacks capacity in relation to the matter in question.
> - The nurse reasonably believes that it is necessary to do the act in order to prevent harm to the client.
> - The act is a proportionate response to (a) the likelihood of the client's suffering harm and (b) the seriousness of that harm.
>
> (Royal College of Nursing, 2008, p. 9)

As the title of the Act implies, 'capacity' is a central concern here. In the case of the treatment of a fully competent patient we would surely consider it unacceptable to restrain a patient in this way in order to forcefully treat them. It is only in cases where we consider the patient incapable of making an informed choice that we even contemplate such things. Thus it would seem that the physician and the patient's wife are basing their claims upon the argument that there is a morally relevant difference between the practice of psychiatric medicine with patients who are not fully competent and that with those who are.

It is important to remind ourselves at this point that for most psychiatric patients there is no doubt about their competence. Most are fully competent. Most psychiatric patients are seen as outpatients for a wide variety of psychological problems. For this reason and as a result of the variety of types of mental illness, it is important to remind ourselves that psychiatric illness is not a homogeneous category. Indeed, as we shall see in the next section, the question of competence is still a matter of considerable debate even in the treatment of long-term inpatients.

The autonomy of psychiatric patients

As Mr AB's case illustrated, psychiatric medicine can give rise to a conflict between healthcare professionals' duty to respect the wishes of their patients and the duty to work in their best interests. The problem is particularly acute in situations where the patient's competence to make informed choices appears to be compromised. Were it legitimate to claim that psychiatric patients such as these are simply incapable of making informed choices about their treatment as a result of the incompetence associated with their illness, we might be justified in arguing that it is the duty of those who take care of them to make decisions on such patients' behalf, in their best interests. But to what extent is it true to say that patients are either competent or incompetent in any general sense, and to what extent are psychiatric patients actually capable at least sometimes of making such autonomous choices?

One way of answering this question would be to ask those who work most closely with psychiatric patients, such as psychiatric nurses. Maritta Välimäki and Hans Helenius did just this, by means of a questionnaire submitted to 127 professional nurses working on long-term wards in four hospitals in Finland, of whom 117 replied (Välimäki and Helenius, 1996). Over half of the nurses (53%) considered self-determination 'very important' to psychiatric patients, with an additional 33% rating it as 'rather important'. A mere 1% thought autonomy was not at all important for their patients. Those who did consider self-determination important often phrased their response in terms of the patient's self-esteem and human rights, regardless of any mental illness. Along with these rights-based views, however, 40% of nurses expressed an outlook which could be regarded as consequentialist: that affording self-determination to patients would also improve their clinical outcome. Patients involved in planning their own treatment, for example, would be better motivated to follow through with the treatment regime.

> When someone is admitted to psychiatric hospital, especially for a long period of time, that person may be deprived to a lesser or greater extent of humanity. Every possible means is important in this situation (to avoid this). We cannot expect good results in treatment if patients are not allowed to look after themselves in hospital.
>
> (Välimäki and Helenius, 1996, p. 365)

However, the minority of nurses who felt that self-determination was *not* an important consideration argued that the patients they worked with were typically not competent to make decisions about their own lives. These nurses felt that in this kind of situation it was the duty of the carer to protect the patient.

> Realistically speaking, most long-term patients are unable to evaluate their own treatment or to get over their illness. Therefore the only way they can cope in their everyday life is if they are told what to do.
>
> (Välimäki and Helenius, 1996, p. 366)

Certainly it is difficult to see how allowing Mr AB to continue to refuse treatment would have enhanced his quality of life but, as the majority of the nurses claimed, not all cases are like this one. As Välimäki and Helenius argue at the end of their paper,

> The important thing to recognise is that even though a patient is unable to make independent decisions in certain areas of life, that does not have to mean that all freedom and independence in all areas has to be closed down. It is extremely important for patients' self-determination and moral dignity that they are allowed to make at least some decisions, however trivial. It is quite clear that no one can have an unlimited or absolute right to self-determination, let alone the right to harm other people or put them in jeopardy. When principles of health care are in conflict, the important thing is to try and strike a sensible, and sensitive, balance.
>
> (Välimäki and Helenius, 1996, p. 370)

This strikes us as a humane and practical approach, which enables due regard to be had for the patient's self-determination. But what do patients themselves think about this issue? As a follow-up to their research into the attitudes of psychiatric nurses, Välimäki and Helenius, along with Helena Leino-Kilpi, carried out some further research into the attitudes of psychiatric patients themselves about the importance of self-determination (Välimäki *et al.*, 1996). They found that many patients were actually ambivalent about whether they had a right to take part in making decisions about their own care, with 75% in favour of such a right but 10% opposed. However, a majority of patients had actually taken part in decision-making (65%). The most contentious issue was the right to refuse treatment: only 39% of patients thought they had such a formal right, although a slightly higher percentage (42%) had actually refused treatment at some point.

The competence of psychiatric patients

In their later study, Välimäki, Leino-Kilpi and Helenius found that psychiatric patients themselves had difficulty in determining whether or not, or to what extent, patients have a right to refuse treatment. We think that this difficulty stems, at least in part, from the complex questions that arise when considering the competence of psychiatric patients. What are the criteria for competence? Are they universal – or do we need to be alert to the risk of multicultural misunderstandings? Even if we can establish competence, what is a competent psychiatric patient able to refuse?

These questions all arise in the case of Mr C, which will be familiar from the first chapter. Here, in addition to reiterating our earlier point that competence is decision-specific for all patients, we will reveal some further facts of the case and consider additional questions more specific to psychiatric practice.

The case of Mr C

Mr C, a 68-year-old patient suffering from paranoid schizophrenia, developed gangrene in a foot during his confinement in a secure hospital. He was removed to a general hospital, where the consultant surgeon diagnosed that he was likely to die imminently if the leg was not amputated below the knee. The prognosis was that he had a 15% chance of survival without amputation. Mr C refused to consider amputation. The hospital authorities considered whether the operation could be performed without Mr C's consent and made arrangements for a solicitor to see him concerning his competence to give a reasoned decision. In the meantime, treatment with antibiotics and conservative surgery averted the immediate threat of imminent death, but the hospital refused to give an understanding to the solicitor that in recognition of his repeated refusals it would not amputate in any future circumstances. There was a possibility that Mr C would develop gangrene again. An application was made on Mr C's behalf to the court for an injunction restraining the hospital from carrying out an amputation without his express written consent. On behalf of the hospital it was contended that Mr C's capacity to give a definitive decision had been impaired by his mental illness and that he had failed to appreciate the risk of death if the operation was not performed. (*Re C* (Adult: Refusal of Treatment) [1994] 1 All ER 819.)

Now consider the following additional facts. Which, if any, is relevant?

- Mr C had emigrated from Jamaica in 1956, with his passage paid by the woman with whom he had lived since 1949. He stabbed her after she left him in 1961.
- Since that time Mr C had been confined either in prison or in a secure hospital.
- For the past six years he had been accommodated in an open ward and was described as having 'mellowed', having become more sociable and even-tempered.

- Mr C was very adept with finances; he had saved all of his earnings during his 30 years' time in the secure hospital.
- However, when his solicitor asked him to whom he intended to leave his savings, he replied 'I'll leave it for myself, for when I come back'.
- Mr C's delusions included the belief that he was a world-famous vascular surgeon who had never lost a patient.
- Mr C also believed that his doctors were torturers.
- Mr C's refusal of amputation reflected his religious convictions, although it was not part of a formal creed.

Let's begin with the question of Mr C's Jamaican origins. The high percentage of psychiatric patients of West Indian ancestry has often been remarked on, but opinion is divided on the extent to which their comparatively high rate of psychiatric diagnosis reflects actual pathology, or simply an ethnocentric tendency in psychiatrists to 'pathologize' behaviour which is quite normal in another culture. Unwitting discrimination is a potential risk here (Reich, 1998), but so too is 'psychological relativism': 'the abandonment of universal principles of mental disorder ... [with the result that] cure of mentally ill ethnic minority patients [becomes] impossible except within a totally culture-specific model of therapy ... This approach makes every human being a mere reflection of his community, an individual without identity or uniqueness, completely subordinated to his ethnicity' (Benhabib, 1997). In a similar vein, we might well ask whether it is right to take a relativistic, 'hands-off' approach because of Mr C's religious beliefs?

Ultimately, neither multicultural nor religious factors seem particularly relevant to the assessment of Mr C's competence. (Indeed, he had been sentenced to prison, and then transferred to a secure psychiatric hospital, because of a serious assault, which would be a crime in any culture.) Mr C's psychotic delusions seem to have a greater bearing on his competence. Nigel Eastman, a consultant psychiatrist, thought that these delusions affected Mr C's belief in the doctors' prediction that he had only a 15% chance of cure without amputation. This seems plausible: if Mr C thought his 'rivals' were jealous of his 'medical reputation', he probably would have discounted their opinion, particularly if he also believed that they were inflicting another form of torture on him by proposing to cut off his leg. His delusions might even be seen as the cause of the crisis: because he thought the doctors were torturers, he did not report his leg infection until it was dangerous. If so, there would be an argument that Mr C should not be allowed to refuse the amputation – even though that was treatment for a physical rather than a mental disorder. In the UK a distinction between refusing psychiatric treatments and other interventions is made by section 63 of the Mental Health Act: as we have seen, a compulsorily detained psychiatric patient may not refuse treatment intended to improve his or her mental condition, but retains the right to reject treament for physical disorder. One could certainly argue that Mr C's physical disorder was related to his mental disorder in its origins, although was is less clear the amputation would actually have a beneficial impact on his mental disorder.

Furthermore, despite his delusions, Mr C was competent in other areas, such as finances. Does this extend to competence to refuse medical treatment? It is important to remember that *there is a presumption of competence in adults*, and that *a finding of mental disorder does not automatically undermine that presumption*. Although English law governing competence has moved on since Mr C's case (with the Mental Capacity Act 2005), these principles remain firm. In the court hearings, expert witnesses testified that Mr C's preferences were shared by many other people with vascular disease, whose competence was not in doubt. Refusing to get on the treadmill of possible repeated amputations is common in such patients. Mr C had strong views that he would prefer to die with two legs than survive with one. These, too, have been expressed by other people facing or experiencing amputation, and have nothing necessarily to do with psychotic delusions.

We should recognize also that chronic vascular disease and the possibility of renewed gangrene meant that there was no guarantee that Mr C would necessarily survive in the long run even if he accepted the procedure. Indeed, the consultant vascular surgeon, Dr Rutter, did testify that below-the-knee amputation carries a 15% mortality risk. This raises questions about rationality and risk preferences. It is always tempting for clinicians to reject patients' treatment decisions which do not correspond to the doctors' own evaluation for the best chance of success. But patients are entitled to their own risk preferences; refusing a procedure which the doctor thinks likely to succeed is not in itself proof of irrationality or incompetence. Indeed, the courts have agreed that:

> Prima facie, every adult had the right and capacity to decide whether or not he will accept medical intervention, even if a refusal may risk permanent injury to his health, or even lead to premature death. Furthermore, it matters not whether the reasons for the refusal were rational or irrational, unknown or even non-existent.
>
> (*Re T* [1992], p. 664)

The criteria for competence, as enunciated in Mr C's case, are functional; they concern the ability to make this particular decision, not 'rationality' in the abstract. The touchstone is whether mental disorder had reduced the patient's understanding of the *nature, purpose and effects* of the proposed intervention to such an extent that he or she is incapable of making this particular decision. To repeat an important point from Chapter 1, even a patient whose delusions are plainly irrational may be competent to make a treatment decision if he or she fulfils the following criteria:

(1) Comprehending and retaining information relating to the decision
(2) Believing the information
(3) Weighing it in the balance when making a choice.

This is a *functional* test of competence, which is in essence retained by the Mental Capacity Act 2005. According to that Act in section 3(1), professionals in England and Wales might have reason to judge a patient incompetent if that patient is unable:

(a) to understand the information relevant to the decision,
(b) to retain that information,
(c) to use or weigh that information as part of the process of making the decision, or
(d) to communicate his decision (whether by talking, using sign language or any other means).

The new test, like the test adopted in the case of Mr C, focuses upon competence to make *this particular* decision. Mr C was found competent to refuse the proposed amputation, despite the doubts that had been expressed by his principal consultant psychiatrist, Dr Ghosh, and even Dr Eastman, who thought that Mr C failed the second test, i.e. he did not believe what the doctors told him. (You will notice that this requirement is no longer present in the 2005 Act.)

What was important, according to Mr Justice Thorpe, was Dr Eastman's testimony that Mr C did not believe the doctors had actively caused his condition, even though he believed that they were torturers.

'Plainly, C's capacity is reduced by his mental illness. But for him [Dr Eastman] the decision as to whether it is sufficiently reduced remains marginal in the absence of any direct link between the persecutory delusions and his present condition.' That Mr C was able to meet the third criterion, weighing the information, was shown by his acceptance of the possibility that he might yet die as a result of refusing amputation, although he expressed faith that God and good medical/nursing care would see him through. Overall, Mr Justice Thorpe wrote in his opinion, 'His answers to questions seemed measured and generally sensible. He was not always easy to understand and the grandiose delusions were manifest, but there was no sign of inappropriate emotional expression. His rejection of amputation seemed to result from sincerely held conviction. He had a certain dignity of manner that I respect' (*Re C*, 823).

> ACTIVITY: Are these the sorts of factors you would include in assessing a patient's competence. Are there any other factors? Drawing on the cases of AB and C, plus any other cases you may have encountered, draw up a list of the factors which you would want to use in measuring competence.

One point which we must always remember is that competence and incompetence are not clear polar opposites. As Välimäki and Helenius earlier suggested, there may be *degrees of competence* and people's competence may be *fragmented*, such that they are highly competent in some respects whilst being incompetent in others. This is an important insight, which suggests that the assessment of a patient's competence ought to be carried out on a case-by-case basis and that a patient may be competent in some matters to a greater degree than she is in others. The claim that competence is often a matter of degree also implies that whilst patients may not be able to make an informed choice alone, they may well be able to participate in decision-making with some assistance.

The (UK) General Medical Council and most doctors now recognize this:

> A patient's ability to make decisions may depend on the nature and severity of their condition, or the difficulty or complexity of the decision. Some patients will always be able to make simple decisions, but may have difficulty if the decision is complex or involves a number of options. Other patients may be able to make decisions at certain times but not others, because fluctuations in their condition impair their ability to understand, retain or weigh up information, or communicate their wishes.
>
> (General Medical Council, 2008, para 66)

The General Medical Council instructs doctors to ensure that they 'share information in a way that the patient can understand and, whenever possible, in a place and at a time when they are best able to understand and retain it' (2008, para 18). Through such (simple) efforts the doctor can best ensure that their patient possesses the capacity to take a particular decision.

There are two additional points worth noting in relation to the case of Mr C. First, the case established that the hospital could not operate without Mr C's express written permission even if he became incompetent in the future, for example, if he became comatose in the event of a serious relapse. This is the principle of the living will or, more properly, *advance directive*, which states in advance what treatments a patient would want to accept or (usually) refuse. The Mr C case established that advance refusals are broadly valid in law and, as we saw in the first chapter, they have since been granted statutory recognition in the Mental Capacity Act 2005. (In the event, Mr C did not actually become incompetent, so there was no need to activate an advance directive, nor did he die: he survived, with the 'dry' form of gangrene in a useable but 'mummified' leg.)

Although the Mr C case did not go so far, it leads to interesting speculation on whether a mentally ill person who is still competent should be allowed to formulate wishes in advance regarding involuntary hospitalization (Berghmans 1992, 1994; Brock, 1993; Savulescu and Dickenson, 1998). Notably, this sort of psychiatric advance directive is now allowed for in the Dutch system:

> In November 2005 and November 2006 respectively, the Dutch House of Representatives and the Dutch Senate consented to a proposal, first made in March 2002 by the then Dutch cabinet, to legally support the introduction of Ulysses arrangements in psychiatry ... A Ulysses arrangement [which takes its name from the story of the Sirens and Ulysses, the Latin name for the Greek hero Odysseus, in Homer's epic *The Odyssey*] is an arrangement between a patient suffering from a chronic relapsing serious psychiatric illness and professional care providers, at a time when the patient is competent, about the use of involuntary

admission and/or treatment during a future epi-
sode of relapse when the patient will not be competent. A Ulysses arrangement can be considered
a special type of advance directive. It concerns
patients who consider it desirable that others
intervene during episodes of relapse, but who, at
the same time, have experienced that when in
crisis they resist these very interventions.

(Gremmen *et al.*, 2008)

Second, the case illustrates how active advocacy
can improve a patient's functional competence to
make healthcare decisions. The involvement of a
strongly patients' rights-minded solicitor, Lucy Scott-
Montcrieff, allowed Mr C to make his convictions felt.
The judge, Mr Justice Thorpe, can also be seen as a
kind of patient advocate in that he interviewed
Mr C in hospital, actively soliciting his testimony.
More frequently, the role of patient advocate falls
to nurses and sometimes to doctors. Alternatively,
there may be governmental ombudsmen charged
with this duty – particularly in Scandinavia. In the
Netherlands, legislation requires all mental hospitals
to have a patient advocate, whose tasks are to advise
and inform patients, and to act as intermediary
between the patient and healthcare professionals.

Through such measures as the appointment of an
advocate, it is therefore possible to protect and promote the autonomy of the patient. Of course, as we
have seen throughout this introductory section, the
fact that in some cases the patient's autonomy, identity
and rationality are in question adds a particularly
interesting and difficult ethical dimension to work
in psychiatry, not least if the patient's choice looks
likely to cause them harm. The tension between an
approach premised on respect for autonomy and an
approach premised on paternalism is often central to
dilemmas arising in mental health ethics. We will
continue to explore this tension throughout this chapter, starting – in the next section – with the liberty of
the patient.

Section 2: Liberty, consent and compulsion

In this section, we will continue to explore the
autonomy of psychiatric patients, but we will shift
our focus from the basis for autonomy in competence:
towards autonomy in the sense of freedom or liberty,
and so to patients' rights to be free to live where they
choose, to receive only that treatment to which they

consent, and to behave in ways that might even be
harmful to them.

We begin this section with a paper by Ron
Berghmans, which outlines the rights of psychiatric
patients in the Netherlands, and which we then
compare with Italian legislation that goes so far as to
outlaw psychiatric long-term hospitalization altogether.
However, the patients'-rights position runs into problems, Berghmans argues, when it allows psychiatric
patients to reject treatment aimed at alleviating their
mental illness. By way of contrast, in England patients
have had their rights limited, at least in relation to
informal admission to hospital. The distinct legal models in operation in the Netherlands, Italy and England
therefore provide us with different ways of thinking
about autonomy, competence, vulnerability and risk
to self, which, as we have seen elsewhere in this chapter,
raise particularly difficult ethical issues in psychiatry.
We close this section with an especially vivid illustration
of the ethical tensions, in Kerry Gutridge's paper
exploring the extent to which we might consider psychiatric patients free to injure themselves.

We start our consideration of these themes with
Berghmans's article.

Protection of the rights of the mentally ill in the Netherlands

Ron Berghmans[1]

Introduction

In my article I will address a number of issues with
regard to autonomy and patients' rights in Dutch mental health care. First, I will describe a number of developments that were aimed at strengthening and
protecting patient rights and autonomy. These developments have led to a reform of the law as well as to
the creation of special facilities for the protection of the
rights of committed mentally ill patients.

An issue of central importance in this debate concerns the morality and legality of the use of coercion
towards the mentally ill, and the limits of the mentally
ill patient's right to refuse supervision and treatment.

Protecting the rights of the mentally ill In the
Netherlands, a strong movement for the protection
of patients' rights has significantly contributed to a
process of law reform, taking place from the start of
the 1970s up until the enactment of a law on compulsory admission in 1994.

This law (officially: the Act on Formal Admissions
to Psychiatric Hospitals) can be seen as a political
compromise between two competing views with

regard to the morality of coercive treatment of the mentally ill. Firstly: the view, based primarily on the moral principle of beneficence, that considers mental health care exclusively as a benevolent service to alleviate the suffering of mentally ill people. Central to this view is the idea that the mentally ill are suffering from a mental disease, that their freedom is more or less compromised, and that their capacity to make choices in some or all domains of decision-making is defective.

This traditional emphasis on beneficence is contested by those who adopt a civil rights-based view and focus on the corresponding moral principle of respect for the autonomy of persons. This second view regards persons principally as bearers of rights that deserve respect and, first and foremost considers persons as free and responsible agents. This assumption also applies to the mentally ill, who are considered to have the same civil rights as any other citizen.

Within the first view, that of beneficence, a paternalistic outlook dominates, and the use of coercion and of compulsory treatment in the care of the mentally ill is seen as a necessary element in the provision of mental healthcare. The civil rights view by contrast takes a strong anti-paternalistic position, and considers uninvited beneficence as an intrusion upon the ultimate freedom of persons to live their own way of life (Berghmans, 1996).

ACTIVITY: Stop here for a moment and make a chart of the conflicting concepts and premises associated with the two views Berghmans identifies. The two contrasting views can be characterized in different ways, but we have headed them 'paternalism' and 'civil rights'. Our chart begins like this:

Paternalism	Civil rights
Key concept: Beneficence	Key concept: Autonomy
Mentally ill are different	Mentally ill have the same rights
Patient's autonomy is compromised	Autonomy should be respected
Coercion may be necessary	Coercion is intrusive and wrong

Now continue with Berghmans's paper.

The law In the Netherlands, a distinction can be made between the informal and formal admission of patients to mental hospitals. The informal or 'voluntary' admission to a mental hospital before 1994 – the

year when the revised law came into force – was reserved for all cases in which the patient *did not object* to hospitalization. If the patient objected, a court order was needed (formal admission). Generally, about 85% of patients residing in mental hospitals had the status of informal patient, and 15% the status of formal patient.

The reformed law has changed this state of affairs dramatically. Under the changed law, a formal procedure is necessary if a person 'does not exhibit the necessary willingness to be hospitalized'. This implies that it is not only persons who object to hospitalization, but also persons who do not object and at the same time do not exhibit a willingness to be hospitalized (i.e. certain mentally handicapped persons and psychogeriatric patients) who are subject to formal procedures. Formerly, these groups (the 'non-objecting and non-consenting') were considered to be informal, 'voluntary' patients.

ACTIVITY: In the Netherlands some 85% of patients in mental hospitals were formerly admitted as 'informal' patients, so long as they did not actively object. What are the implications of this fact for (a) psychiatric practice and (b) the definition of consent to treatment?

Our answer to (a) is that abolition of the 'informal' admission procedure will have massive resource implications for practice in any system where informal patients are in such a vast majority. Formal admission procedures or appeals will entail enormous amounts of time. There is also a risk that some patients may fall through the net – not meeting the criteria for formal admission, because they do not have a treatable mental disorder, but still needing help. In other words, beneficence, the obligation to confer benefit, could justify retaining a general policy of 'informal' admission.

But, perhaps surprisingly, we could also argue *in favour* of informal admission from the viewpoint of the *patient's rights*. This would be a more sophisticated version of the argument from autonomy, running something like this: Does requiring active consent to treatment enhance or *threaten* the autonomy and dignity of patients with (for example) dementia, learning disability and autism? If such patients are incapable of giving meaningful consent, they cannot be admitted informally, even if they would benefit. Is this a formalistic interpretation of patients' rights which does nothing for the dignity and welfare of vulnerable people without real capacity to consent? Would their autonomy actually be enhanced by treatment that made them better able to live a more normal life?

Our answer to (b) is that consent to treatment must be active in other areas of medicine; it is simply not good enough to read the absence of *dissent* as consent. Surgeons who did that would rapidly find themselves the subject of legal actions for battery or negligence. Consent serves two functions: first, it provides the legal justification for what would otherwise be trespass to the person and a violation of the patient's bodily integrity. In clinical practice, second, it creates the basis of trust and relationship between doctor and patient. (*Re W* [1992]) So consent is not to be taken lightly; but the practical implications of taking consent seriously in relation to the demented, autistic or learning-disabled patient are tremendous, as our answer to (a) suggested. This is the essential conflict.

Now go on to read the next section of Berghmans's paper.

Under the law, a person can be involuntarily committed if the following conditions are met:

(1) he suffers from a mental illness;
(2) he is dangerous to himself or others;
(3) this dangerousness is a result of the mental illness;
(4) he does not exhibit the necessary willingness to be hospitalized; and
(5) there is no alternative way to prevent the dangerousness.

After a patient has been coercively committed to a psychiatric hospital, the psychiatrist has the legal duty to negotiate a so-called treatment plan with the patient. The treatment plan aims at the amelioration of the disorder that has led to the danger that the patient posed to himself or others before he was committed. After being informed about the proposed treatment plan, the patient can consent to or refuse treatment. If the patient is considered to be incompetent or decisionally incapacitated, the physician has the duty to discuss the treatment plan with a proxy of the patient. This representative of the incompetent patient also can consent to or refuse treatment.

This implies that a compulsorily (formally) admitted mentally ill patient has the legal right to refuse treatment. The fact that a patient is involuntarily committed in the mental hospital is a necessary, but not a sufficient, ground to overrule a treatment refusal. In other words: the decision regarding compulsory treatment is a separate decision based on grounds other than the decision regarding compulsory admission to the mental hospital.

Compulsory psychiatric treatment implies that a treatment plan is executed in the case where disagreement exists over this treatment plan between the psychiatrist and the patient (or his representative), or in the case where the patient (or – for an incompetent patient – his legal representative) refuses treatment. Compulsory psychiatric treatment aims at averting the danger to himself or others resulting from his mental illness.

Compulsory psychiatric treatment can only be legally justified

– insofar as it is plausible that without this treatment the danger which was the reason for the compulsory commitment cannot be eliminated within a reasonable timeframe;

or

– insofar as this treatment is absolutely necessary to avert the danger to the patient or others in the mental hospital.

As far as the right to refuse treatment is concerned, the Dutch law makes no distinction between the refusal of treatment by a competent patient, and treatment refusal by an incompetent patient.

A refusal of treatment by an incompetent patient may raise serious ethical problems in the practice of mental healthcare. The patient can be formally detained, but unless he becomes a serious danger to him or herself or others, treatment aiming at improvement of the mental condition of the patient cannot take place if he or she opposes such treatment.

ACTIVITY: Berghmans has moved on from the question of informal admission to the patient's equal right to refuse treatment even if he or she satisfies the criteria for compulsory admission. Here too, the paternalistic approach has been rejected in favour of an autonomy-centred strategy. How far do you think the right to refuse treatment should extend? Should it apply equally to a refusal of psychiatric treatment and to a refusal of general medical treatment? As we saw earlier in relation to Mr C, in the UK this last distinction is made clear by section 63 of the Mental Health Act: broadly speaking, a compulsorily detained psychiatric patient may not refuse treatment intended to improve his or her mental condition, but retains the right to reject treatment for physical illness. However, if the physical disorder is caused by the mental disorder, or if physical treatment is part of a plan of care designed to help the mental disorder – for example, in forcible feeding of patients with anorexia nervosa or compulsion to self-harm by refusing food – the distinction is not so clear (*R (B)* v *Ashworth Hospital Authority* [2005] UKHL 20).

Although the Netherlands is well known for its libertarian approach to social policy, the Italian legislation is surprisingly even more far-reaching. While the Italian system relies heavily on implicit consent in other contexts, spurning the language of rights (Calzone, 1996; Calzone and D'Andrea, 1996) nonetheless long-term psychiatric hospitalization has been banned entirely in Italy.

> The trend in recent years has been to admit patients into psychiatric units in general hospitals only when absolutely necessary, treat them aggressively, and then discharge them to the next appropriate level of treatment (day centres, therapeutic communities, supervision in the community, day hospitals, halfway houses).
>
> (Mordini, 1997)

As possible rationales for long-term hospitalization, Italian law accepts neither the notion of preventative detention, on the basis of risk to the community, nor of forcible treatment in the patient's best interest, on the grounds of necessity. The former is unacceptable because it constitutes a form of discrimination: no one else can be detained on the basis of crimes which they might commit in the future, but only after the offence. The latter is thought surplus to requirements: sophisticated pharmacology can keep florid symptoms under control, it is felt, without the need for long-term hospitalization. However, compulsory short-term hospitalization is allowed under three strict conditions:

- The patient refuses treatment after all attempts to negotiate have been exhausted.
- No other solutions are available (community care, hostels, or self-help communities).
- The degree of mental illness is so severe as to require immediate intervention. Although the law does not define this term, there is broad agreement that 'severe' means either that the patient's life is at risk or that his compelling interests are at risk.

It is worth noting – in the absence of these risks – that it is doubtful whether mere evidence that the patient's mental health will deteriorate consitutes sufficient reason for compulsory hospitalisation.

(Mordini, 1997)

The autonomy rights of psychiatric patients appear central to the Italian model – although, as Berghmans explains in the conclusion to his paper, they can come at a cost.

> **In conclusion** Coercive treatment and the protection of patients' rights in psychiatry is a complex issue raising a number of medical, legal, ethical and policy questions. Societal developments have led to a strong emphasis on the moral principle of respect for the autonomy of persons. The mentally ill have been given liberty rights which they had traditionally lacked under the guise of paternalistic psychiatric beneficence. In a number of jurisdictions this has led to a right of mentally ill people to refuse treatment. In the Dutch context, a major emphasis was given to the negative right of the mentally ill to be left alone. Respecting the autonomy of the patient first and foremost is interpreted as a duty not to interfere with the affairs of the mentally ill person.
>
> Recognizing a 'right to be left alone' may be devalued to a 'right to rot' if communities and mental health professionals use this liberal principle to legitimate indifference and lack of compassion. On the other hand, psychiatric coercion, although generally motivated by good intentions, involves prima facie a morally offensive action. In particular in mental healthcare, interventions may deeply intrude into the physical and mental integrity of the subject. In these cases moral reasons reaching beyond the presumed best interest or benefit of the patient are needed to provide an ethical justification of coercive treatment.

The 'right to be left alone' to which Berghmans refers is, as he notes, a 'liberal principle'; in other words, it rests on the idea of *liberty*, a concept which has arisen a number of times in this chapter. The right Berghmans mentions is sometimes described as 'negative liberty': freedom *from* arbitrary power. Political philosophers will often distinguish this from positive or welfare rights: the freedom *to* act, enjoy certain benefits and to be accorded entitlements (Berlin, 1969). Should we think of psychiatric patients as having not just the negative right to be free from compulsory hospitalization, but also the positive right to treatment which

111

will benefit them? If so, then the distinction between the paternalistic model and the patients' rights view begins to look less firm.

The right to liberty is actually one of the rights protected by the European Convention of Human Rights, under article 5. Its application to 'informal' admission in the UK was tested in a case known as 'Bournewood' (HL v UK 45508/99 [2004] ECHR 471):

The Bournewood case

Mr L was a severely autistic man, with profound learning disability and complex needs, requiring 24-hour care. After spending many years in a psychiatric hospital, Mr L lived with foster carers for three years. Whilst attending a day centre, he became extremely agitated. Staff were unable to contact his carers, and Mr L was informally admitted to hospital. Mr L was unable to speak, so that he had no ability to communicate consent or dissent to hospital admission, but his consultant concluded that Mr L's apparent compliance rendered formal admission unnecessary. Whilst he was being assessed, Mr L was denied access to his foster carers, on the grounds that he might attempt to leave with them before he was fit for discharge.

The European Court of Human Rights decided that this amounted to a deprivation of Mr L's liberty. The judges noted that Mr L had no recourse to the protections offered by the Mental Health Act 1983, such as the ability to challenge his detention and the restrictions on treatment. The lack of procedural safeguards and access to the court amounted to a breach of article 5.

Since this ruling, the Mental Capacity Act 2005 has been enacted for England and Wales, an amendment to which provides a set of safeguards that must be in place where an individual is deprived of their liberty. The amendment, which came into effect in 2009, allows for the detention of an incapacitated patient, provided that the decision made is the least restrictive of the available options, and is in the patient's best interests. The guidance emphasizes the importance of following available procedures, appropriate documentation, and taking care to ensure, as far as possible, that the patient remains in contact with those close to him or her.

Central to this legislative scheme is a concern with the best interests of the patient, albeit twinned with a need to respect the patient's autonomy wherever possible. Of course, sometimes there will be conflicts between the two, as we see in our next reading. The central question is: to what extent should we be willing to allow a psychiatric patient freedom to act, when their actions might cause them harm?

Free to self-injure?

Kerry Gutridge

Allowing a psychiatric patient the freedom to injure themselves is controversial, particularly when you know the injury is virtually certain to occur. Intuitively, allowing injury appears to be in opposition to a professional's duty of care. As such, it seems a case can be made for restricting a psychiatric patient (or service user) in their freedom to act in such a way. However, the professional's duty of care needs to be balanced against respect for autonomy, properly understood. If a service user wants to self-injure, should their decision be respected or is this an example of an aberrant understanding of autonomy?

In mental healthcare practice, the decision to allow self-injury is complicated, because prohibiting the behaviour could have a detrimental effect on the therapeutic relationship between a service user and their psychiatric team. The service user may resent the frustration of their choice and the imposition of searches and perhaps even physical restraint. Moreover, if someone who regularly self-injures is determined to act, then any efforts to enforce restrictions on choice may lead to worse physical consequences overall. Acting covertly and quickly to avoid detection, a patient may impulsively use dangerous means to injure themselves. Concealing or suppressing their self-injury may increase their distress and make them want to injure more urgently and more seriously.

Further complication arises when one considers the reasons why an individual self-injures. It is widely accepted that self-injury is used as a means of coping with distressing emotions; however, these emotions may be precipitated by various experiences (e.g. different types and degrees of abuse or neglect). Moreover, the injury can be associated with fluctuating, varied and complex feelings (e.g. overwhelming emotional pain, self-hatred, or 'unreality': Bristol Crisis Service for Women, 1995).

If a service user wants to self-injure, then a professional is faced with a difficult choice: do they prohibit self-injury by restricting a patient's liberty, which may in fact cause an escalation of the undesirable behaviour, or do they allow self-injury, which risks

---

potentially misinterpreting respect for autonomy and thereby allowing the patient to undertake an unjustifiable (and harmful) action? If a professional allows injury to occur, are they colluding in a patient's self-punishment or allowing the patient the freedom to use a rehearsed and familiar coping strategy?

To address this dilemma one needs to consider whether allowing self-injury is legal and ethical, with particular reference to the concept of autonomy. I will argue that allowing self-injury is not unlawful but that current unregulated practice poses risks for the professional. I will suggest that allowing self-injury can be defended using an account of individual autonomy if one accepts that psychiatric professionals have a positive obligation to increase a patient's autonomy.

In recent years, some mental health units and voluntary services have advocated allowing particular patients to continue to self-injure whilst they are residents in mental healthcare facilities. Proposed or implemented management strategies are not always documented, so it can be difficult to specify the exact nature of the approach. Moreover, when made public, specific strategies have been misunderstood, partly as a result of sensational and misleading reporting. For example, seemingly inaccurate claims have been made about the provision of 'cutting rooms' and clean blades for service users on demand. Partly in response to this media attention, and in the interest of transparent practice, one unit decided to document how they manage allowing self-injury. They specified their preference for harm-minimization, rather than prohibition of self-injury in certain, defined, circumstances. For harm-minimization to be considered by the team, a patient needs to use self-injury to cope with distressing emotions, have mental capacity to consent to the approach and not have suicidal intent. If this is the case, and the patient expresses a wish to self-injure, a harm-minimization care plan can be completed.

The legal position and professional guidelines   If the members of such a unit examine legal cases and professional guidelines they will find it difficult to determine whether they can, and should, allow self-injury to occur within their inpatient facility.

The issue has not come directly before the courts and the approach is not standard practice (Hewitt, 2004, p. 148). One possibility is that the practice might be considered negligent, in other words contrary to what responsible health professionals would do. Such a finding could lead to liability in civil law, for which compensation might be due. For a negligence claim to be refuted, the unit's lawyer would need to justify the existence of the approach as well as the

appropriateness of the practice for the patient in question (Hewitt, 2004, p. 156). It is an interesting question whether consensus within one team is sufficient to prevent a civil negligence claim from succeeding.

Healthcare professionals also have a duty to prevent patients detained in mental health care facilities from committing suicide. Article 2 of the Human Rights Act 1998 places the unit under a duty to protect the right to life, and there is also the possibility that allowing self-injury which leads to death might amount to assistance in suicide, contrary to section 2 of the Suicide Act 1961. Epidemiological research indicates that there is an association between self-injuring and suicide (Hawton et al., 2003), although there are problems with interpretation of these studies. It is often difficult to determine whether a patient's death is accidental or intentional. According to Allen, service users can regularly distinguish between behaviour that is suicidal in nature and self-injury that is not (Allen, 1995) – but it is less certain whether this distinction is always obvious to their professional carer. In any case, the question still remains whether accidental death is likely to occur. If a service user dies accidentally, the professional needs to demonstrate they have shown reasonable care in their provision of advice and treatment or, again, they risk an allegation of negligence. Are the harm-minimization strategies used, such as sterilization of implements and observation for behavioural changes, sufficient to defend against such a claim?

Allowing self-injury is not unlawful per se, but the prospect of a finding of negligence is more likely whilst the practice is unregulated. Guidelines developed by the National Institute for Clinical Excellence to address the physical, psychological and social assessment and treatment of individuals in the first 48 hours after self-harming (NICE, 2004) suggest that wound care and safer cutting techniques can be discussed with people who repeatedly self-injure. However, the guidelines are silent on the appropriateness of allowing self-harm to occur in healthcare facilities. The Codes of Practice for the Mental Health Act 1983 stated that individuals should be protected from self-injury if the drive to self-harm is the result of a mental disorder for which they are receiving care or treatment, but this statement has been removed from the 2007 Codes of Practice (Department of Health, 1999, para. 19.30). Without national guidelines on appropriate harm-minimization strategies, teams who allow self-injury are operating in legal uncertainty.

Ethical practice: examining liberty   Beauchamp and Childress see self-governance as being afforded a substantial degree of freedom from the controlling influence of others (Beauchamp and Childress, 2009, p. 99); that is, they understand 'acting autonomously' as being allowed to act with a sufficient degree of negative liberty. Negative freedom to act is permitted when certain other conditions for autonomy obtain. One of these conditions is the possession of particular mental capacities, such as the ability to act on the basis of one's own, self-chosen, desires or plans: that is, having 'the capacity for intentional action' (Beauchamp and Childress, 2009, pp. 99–100). This definition is functional, since autonomy is judged in relation to a specific act, with the act itself being seen as either intentional or nonintentional (Beauchamp and Childress, 2009, p. 101).

The effect of a disorder on intentional decision-making raises deep philosophical questions about determinism. For current purposes it is worth considering whether any diagnosis, for example of depression or personality disorder, would mean that self-injuring is necessarily non-voluntary. According to Harris, with service users, 'there is no [moral] ground at all for paternalistic interference with their decisions unless it is clear in their individual case, and in the case of the particular decision in question, that they are not maximally autonomous with respect to their decision' (Harris, 1985, p. 217). This clarity is not provided by the presence or absence of a diagnostic label.

Although a patient has legal capacity, internal cognitive inconsistencies or damaging emotional states may be present which challenge whether their choice is maximally autonomous. It is important to note that assessment of whether a service user is maximally autonomous is not a measurement against an objective ideal. One is considering how the patient might feel if she is able to reflect sufficiently on her reasons and motivations to self-injure. Christman believes that internal consistency is sufficient for positive liberty (the freedom to act); however, he concedes that potentially (though not necessarily) beliefs can be subject to an epistemic, not moral, external requirement (Christman, 1991, p. 355). Using this external condition, an individual who has access to reliable factual evidence can interfere with the unwitting choices of others to increase another's self-mastery.

An example of a possible cognitive inconsistency is a conflict between desires to injure and not to injure, of a degree that prevents the patient from forming volitions about self-injury – in other words, that prevent her from reaching conscious choices or decisions. Inconsistency may be indicated if the service user says she wishes she did not self-injure but she

believes she is compelled to do so against her better judgement. Emotional states that may compromise autonomy include low self-worth. According to Benson, 'free agents must have a certain sense of their own worthiness to act, or of their status as agents' (Benson, 1994, p. 650). If an individual ceases to trust themselves to govern their actions competently, then this can affect their ability to act autonomously (Benson, 1994, p. 657). Abuse and neglect may have damaged a service user's opinion of herself to such an extent that she holds attitudes towards herself which preclude the necessary sense of worth to be optimally autonomous. If she does have low self-worth, her self-injury may *in part* be associated with self-hatred and could act as a form of punishment.

ACTIVITY: In a study questionnaire, adolescents were asked to describe why they self-injured. A significantly higher number of females than males said they used self-injury as a form of self-punishment (Rodham *et al.*, 2004), although an earlier study did suggest that, while girls are more likely to self-injure, a substantially increased proportion of deliberate self-harm is undertaken by males (Hawton *et al.*, 1997). This raises questions about gender and self-injury. In light of these wider social questions, do you think that a policy permitting self-harm can be considered ethical?

If a patient is not maximally autonomous, the question then becomes whether, and how, action should be taken to improve her autonomy in relation to her choice to self-injure. If it is accepted that there is a positive obligation to improve autonomous functioning in psychiatric practice in general, then it is logically possible that this obligation applies to this specific action (Campbell *et al.*, 1997, p. 169). What needs to be established then is whether prohibition of self-harm or toleration of harm acts as a means to increased autonomy. Establishing the answer rests in part on empirical findings, but it also relies on one's understanding of human development and psychological change. If one follows Harris' reasoning and accepts that 'self-determination improves not with time but with practice' (Harris, 1985, p. 199) one may choose a therapeutic approach that enables the individual to rehearse and develop new alternative coping strategies. This approach may depend on an initial acceptance of self-injuring as a means of coping, which gradually leads to encouragement to change. This acceptance will, in part, provide a therapeutic space where the motives and reasons for self-injury can be explored.

Dworkin claimed that 'our self-esteem and sense of worth are bound up with the right to determine what shall be done to and with our bodies and minds' (Dworkin, 1988, p. 95). If this is the case, a patient may benefit from retaining a significant amount of control and choice within the therapeutic relationship, to mitigate against other factors that have reduced their self-worth and in turn their autonomy.

Given these claims, allowing self-injury may be ethically permissible if it acts as a means to improving autonomy, for example, because it improves engagement with psychotherapy. This argument for allowing self-injury does not stand alone. To help a patient *and* to minimize collusion in self-punishment, a healthcare professional should try to understand the meaning of the injury for the individual: e.g. is the behaviour a habitual coping strategy or self-abuse? This assessment is unlikely to be straightforward – both factors may motivate the action or there may be other reasons and complications.

It seems reasonable to suggest that the level of self-understanding necessary to determine what motivates one's self-injury might only be reached after detailed self-exploration. If prohibiting self-injury prevents this exploration, it could prevent (or at least reduce the probability of) a patient's recovery. In sum, although allowing self-injury poses some difficult dilemmas for professionals (and, of course, for service users themselves), a (cautious) case can be made for permitting the practice with *some* patients, as an autonomy-enhancing step on the road to its reduction and, ideally, removal.

Although Gutridge's ultimate goal is to improve the patient's welfare, she nevertheless defends the idea that we might allow a patient to continue harming herself while we pursue that goal. You may feel that this takes respect for autonomy too far and that it places too little weight on the need to protect patients – particularly vulnerable patients in our care. Gutridge wants to resolve the tension in a way that promotes the patient's autonomy and welfare in the longer term. This sort of thinking can sometimes also be detected in relation to younger people, particularly young children, who will need to be afforded a degree of freedom in order to develop, but not so much freedom that they risk seriously damaging their current and future interests (and, indeed, freedom). It seems we need to proceed cautiously – but we should also be wary of

presuming an *absence* of autonomy on the part of the young person, even when that person is enduring psychiatric difficulty. It is to this issue we turn in our next section.

Section 3: Children and young people: presumed incompetent?

One might suppose that the freedom due to an individual will depend, at least to some degree, on the age of that individual. However, we have also seen throughout this book how important it is to respect an individual's autonomy – and, we might reasonably argue, one's autonomy does not wholly depend on one's age. Instead, the key concept must be competence, which we earlier examined in relation to Mr C, where we saw how fundamental the presumption of competence is in relation to adults. Even Mr C, with profound psychotic delusions arguably related to his physical disorder, was found competent to make decisions relating to that illness, although the result might have been his death. In this section we will begin with an example which illustrates how the opposite applies to children and young people. The case involves a 16-year-old girl with anorexia nervosa, a life-threatening condition – like Mr C's – and again on the borderline between the purely physical and the purely mental.

The Case of 'W'

'W', aged 16, was orphaned at the age of eight, when her mother died of cancer. Three years earlier, her father had died of a brain tumour. Together with her brother and sister, W was taken into the care of the local authority; her aunt, who had been named as testamentary guardian, was unable to care for the children. After a foster placement broke down, she was moved to a second family, but her new foster mother developed breast cancer. Her grandfather, to whom she was very attached, died shortly thereafter, when W was 13. A few months later W began losing weight; she had been suffering from depression and a nervous tic for some time before, and she was referred for her eating disorder to the same clinic which had been treating her other conditions. But sessions with a clinical psychologist at the clinic did not really resolve the problems, and shortly before her 15th birthday W was admitted on an inpatient basis to a specialist London residential unit for children and adolescents. Here she began injuring herself by picking at her skin and other forms of self-harm. A few months later her condition had deteriorated to the point where she had to be fed by nasogastric tube, to which she consented; her arms were encased in plaster to prevent her picking at her skin.

The local authority decided to move W to another treatment unit, to which W was opposed. She had developed a good relationship with staff at the first centre, she argued – although it was also true that she had occasionally been violent towards staff there. However, the original treatment centre wanted to continue working with W and opposed the move. Her weight was now stable at about seven stone. In March 1992 W reached the age of 16 and exercised her right to be represented by a solicitor of her own choice. Under the provisions of the Family Law Reform Act 1969, which treats the treatment choices of 16- and 17-year-olds as equally valid to an adult's, it appeared that W would have the right to refuse the transfer. The authority made a formal application to the High Court to test whether this was so, requesting leave to move W to a named treatment centre without her consent, and to give her whatever treatment the new centre deemed necessary, also without her consent.

The High Court ruled that W was competent, with Mr Justice Thorpe – also the judge in the C case – stating: 'There is no doubt at all that [W] is a child of sufficient understanding to make an informed decision.' This was consistent with the evidence of Dr G, a consultant psychiatrist specializing in anorexia nervosa, who noted: 'I am convinced that she has a good intelligence, and understands what is proposed as treatment'. It might seem, therefore, that because W was competent, she would be allowed to refuse both transfer to the second centre and the 'blank cheque' which the authority was seeking for her treatment there.

One could certainly argue that the treatment at issue in W's case, the possibility of further artificial or even forcible feeding, is medical treatment rather than psychiatric treatment, and that she should have been allowed to refuse it, in the same way that Mr C was allowed to refuse amputation. But because there is a presumption of incompetence for minors under 18, this was not the case. W had no right to say no, it was held in both the High Court and the Court of Appeal.

The effect of the W case is that young people under 18, even if found competent, are not allowed to refuse consent to treatment so long as someone with parental responsibility consents. (In W's case the local authority had parental responsibility.) The case of W went beyond an earlier judgement, that of 'R',

which held that a young person of fluctuating mental condition was not competent to refuse treatment (in R's case, antipsychotic drugs). W was found competent but denied the right to refuse treatment none the less.

Whereas in the case of Mr C the court was impressed by his dignity of manner and self-control, in W's case her attempts to control her environment, carers and body itself were viewed as pernicious. Lord Donaldson called W's desire for control a pathological symptom of her condition: 'One of the symptoms of anorexia nervosa is a desire by the sufferer to "be in control", and such a refusal [of treatment] would be an obvious way of demonstrating this' (Re W, p. 631). This looks particularly odd compared with the C case (although the W judgement pre-dates C). It seems quite likely that Mr C's refusal was a manifestation of his schizophrenic delusions – giving rise to his pathological distrust of the clinicians – even if it was also a desire held by other sufferers from vascular disease. Lord Donaldson argued that W's anorexia undermined her 'Gillick competence', the formulation laid down in an earlier case establishing that the test is the ability to understand the nature and purpose of the proposed treatment. The test in the Gillick case (1985) was whether the child had 'sufficient understanding and intelligence to enable him or her to understand fully what is proposed' (Gillick, p. 423). None the less, Lord Donaldson, in the Court of Appeal, declared that this was not enough in W's case:

> What distinguishes W . . . is that it is a feature of anorexia nervosa that it is capable of destroying the ability to make an informed choice. It creates a compulsion to refuse treatment or to accept only treatment which is likely to be ineffective. This attitude is part and parcel of the disease and the more advanced the illness, the more compelling it may become. Where the wishes of the minor are themselves something which the doctors reasonably consider to be treated in the minor's best interests, those wishes clearly have a much reduced influence
>
> (Re W, p. 637).

W had broken unit rules at her current treatment centre with impunity, it was noted. A judgement in her favour would merely be another form of capitulation, reinforcing her sense that she, not the clinicians, was in control. Throughout the judgement the language of discipline, control and hierarchy is evident. Whereas the judge in C seems to regard Mr C as his equal, the judgements in W are given from a paternalistic position. Thus the W case reinforced the important principle in UK law that children and young people are presumed incompetent to refuse treatment, although they may give consent. This is the limit to which their competence can extend.

ACTIVITY: Do you agree with the judgement in the W case? What would you have decided had you been a judge?

Your answers to these questions may well have rested on the perceived competence (or incompetence) of W. Of relevance here is a recent study by Jacinta Tan, a consultant child and adolescent psychiatrist, and colleagues, which found that 'In terms of intellectual measures such as understanding and reasoning, even severe anorexia nervosa patients may be judged to be competent to make treatment decisions. However, this study shows that with respect to thinking processes and values, the participants report difficulties that are relevant to competence' (Tan *et al.*, 2006, p. 279). The authors therefore suggest that competence to refuse treatment may indeed be compromised in patients with anorexia nervosa – but not necessarily in ways captured by conventional legal approaches to 'competence'.

Although the source of the difficulty may not be that to which Lord Donaldson referred, Tan's research arguably leads us to the conclusion he reached: W is not competent. It may well be that in the particularly pressing circumstances of W's case you would also have erred on the side of paternalism. This is an understandable interpretation of professional responsibility in the context of a life-threatening emergency: W's weight was just over five stone at the time the judgement was given – although it is also worth pointing out that her weight only began to drop so radically when the court proceedings began, having been stable at seven stone before that.

You may also feel that it is perfectly reasonable to require a higher 'tariff' for refusal of consent than for acceptance of treatment. The consequences of treatment refusal, some argue, are generally more severe, because treatment would not be suggested unless it was of benefit (Buchanan and Brock, 1989). On the other hand, one might argue that this wrongly assumes the doctor's opinion about the probability

of treatment succeeding is always correct (Devereux *et al.*, 1993).

Your decision may also depend on whether the proposed treatment is life-saving. What happens when forcible treatment cannot be justified on the basis that it could save the patient's life? – as the court accepted in the W case. One such difficult example is electro-convulsive therapy, which is sometimes used with younger people (Zaw, 2006). Another – more common – example involves the use of pharmacological means of dealing with a young person's psychiatric difficulty.

ACTIVITY: In which circumstances, if any, do you judge it appropriate to administer psychoactive drugs to young people? Consider the legal case of *Re W*: do you think that the judges' reasoning in that case can be applied to psychopharmacology? In particular, would you require the young person's consent to such treatment? In the following paper, Carlo Calzone, an Italian child psychiatrist, explores some of the issues.

Drug treatment in child psychiatry

Carlo Calzone[2]

Psychopharmacotherapy in childhood and adolescence raises three types of ethical issue:

(1) The lack of certainty about the outcome of treatment as concerning risks and benefits;
(2) The relationship between psychoactive drugs and personal freedom;
(3) The rights of non-autonomous patients.

1. The lack of certainty about the outcome of treatment is related to the following aspects:
(a) We cannot transfer onto children the results of experiments on adults because of the uncertain response to drugs of an immature central nervous system. The paradoxical effects of many drugs on this age group, e.g. stimulants and benzodiazepine, are well known.
(b) With under-age subjects, experimental protocols need to be more stringent. In Italy, for example, drugs and placebos cannot be compared and this obviously limits research.
(c) Individual variance, a well-known phenomenon in pharmacology, is much higher in children and adolescents because of interfering development processes and of the social–psychic context in which they take place.

(d) In developing subjects, untoward effects, also long-term ones, can be especially unpredictable and serious (e.g. late dyskinesia caused by antipsychotic drugs).

2. The use of psychoactive drugs can be seen as a limitation to personal freedom because:
(a) Some drugs, such as benzodiazepine or SSRIs, can induce addiction.
(b) Pharmacotherapy actually changes the patient's personality. Think, for example, of the changes that can be induced by drugs in manic-depressive or schizophrenic patients.
(c) The elimination of symptoms, albeit accepted as socially useful, can be felt by the patient as a loss. In this sense, I would like to mention the case described by Oliver Sacks (Sacks, 1992) of the patient with Tourette's syndrome, who discontinued his therapy with haloperidol on non-working days, because he wanted to revert to his own 'Tourette personality'.

3. The lack of autonomy in under-age patients can be ascribed to various factors, such as:
(a) Physical and cognitive limits.
(b) Emotional dependence on adult figures.
(c) Economic dependence.
(d) Legal limitations, varying from one country to the other, such as the age of majority or the concept of liability of adolescents.

These three factors are not independent and start a vicious circle that discourages many clinicians from prescribing psychoactive drugs in childhood and adolescence. A careful work-methodology and an ethical evaluation of each case can help child psychiatrists in the choice of using drugs according to the principle of benefits accruing to the young patient.

The judges' reasoning in *Re W* would appear to justify treating a young person against his or her will, on the *sole* consent of someone with parental responsibility. This may be particularly questionable in the area of psychopharmacology, not only because of the obvious affront to respect for patient autonomy, but also because our assumptions about serving the patient's welfare may not be entirely safe in this context. As Calzone appreciates, we cannot always be certain about the effects a particular drug will have on a younger patient – indeed, sometimes the effects can be very grave (McGoey and Jackson, 2009).

Yet there will also be circumstances in which some such treatment is indicated. Calzone advocates robust psychiatric evaluation, coupled with careful diagnosis, close observation and cautious increases in dose. He also recommends that the prescription should only be issued once a treatment plan has been agreed and approved, specifically by the patient's parents. He also writes: 'Always obtain the parents' informed consent, to be kept with other records, since very often authorised therapeutic indications do not allow many drugs to be used on children'.

Whether this goes far enough is open to question: certainly, a case can still be made for (better) protecting the autonomy of the young person – although its advocates will still have to navigate difficult issues pertaining to the child's welfare. However, as we will explore in the final section of this chapter, this needn't mean that we are stuck with a stark dichotomy, in which we either protect autonomy or promote paternalism.

Section 4: Caring in the therapeutic relationship

Until now in this chapter, we have contrasted two approaches to psychiatric ethics: the *rights-based* view and the *paternalistic* model. The analysis has tended to be critical of medical paternalism and more supportive of the patients'-rights approach, although we have also focused on the limitations of that approach, for example in Berghmans's critique. However, you may still be left with the feeling that although analysing the differences between the models helps to clarify your thinking, the two approaches impose an artificial straitjacket on actual clinical practice. Is there room for another approach?

In this final section we provide a more extended, exploratory discussion of ethical theory, in an article written by a practising clinician, a forensic psychiatrist with a particular interest in medical ethics and ethical theory: Dr Gwen Adshead, consultant psychiatrist at Broadmoor Hospital in the UK. In the article, Adshead argues for what has come to be known as an ethics of care approach. (Alternative models of autonomy are considered at greater length in the 'Autonomy' chapter.)

The idea that it is possible to build an approach to biomedical ethics around the concept of care is one which has become increasingly popular, particularly among nurses and theorists of nursing (e.g. Bradshaw, 2009), as well as among some feminist bioethicists, although others are sceptical about its tendency to reinforce gender stereotypes about women as 'naturally' caring (Sherwin, 2002) But just what is meant by the ethics of care? Before you go on to read the paper by Gwen Adshead, we would like you to read the following extract from a paper by Peter Allmark (1995) in which he provides an outline of this approach.

Amongst nurse theorists the idea of an ethics of caring is especially popular. Nursing has long sought to gain an identity separate from medicine and some writers hope that care may be the key to finding this identity. Caring has roots in the work of Carol Gilligan (Gilligan, 1982). The key idea is that the detached, impartial observer ideal of morality, characteristic of ethics since the Enlightenment, is flawed and inappropriate, particularly for women. In its place is recommended an approach stressing involvement in the situation, with an attitude of care for others also involved. As such, the importance of relations between people in their practical reasoning is highlighted rather than the more common approach stressing abstract principles ...

Blum (1988) lists what he sees as some of the differences between 'impartialism' and the ethics of care. (I) The care approach is particularised. It does not abstract from the particular situation and attempt to see, for example, which principles are operative, or what is the ethical framework. Gilligan and Noddings (Noddings, 1984) have both criticised Gandhi for his 'blind willingness to sacrifice people to truth', that is, some form of abstract truth. (II) The care approach is involved. It does not see the person making moral decisions as a radically autonomous self-legislating individual. Rather she is tied to others. Autonomy is not seen as some kind of ideal. Involvement with the person on whom one acts draws on capacities of love, care, empathy, comparison and sensitivity. This dimension of moral understanding is ignored by the 'impartialist' approach. (III) For the care approach, moral reasoning does not involve rationality alone but an intertwining of emotion, cognition and action. Noddings quotes Hume with approval. It seems that for both, 'Reason is, and ought only to be, the slave of the passions'. (IV) The care approach is not concerned with universalistic right action. Gilligan talked instead of situationally based responses based on the 'cognisance of interdependence'.

ACTIVITY: Bearing this description in mind, we would now like you to go on and read the paper by Adshead, listing as you do so the features of this approach which you consider its strengths and those which you judge its weaknesses.

A different voice in psychiatric ethics

Gwen Adshead[3]

Introduction

In this section, I will argue that the perspective of an ethic of care is of particular relevance to psychiatric treatment, where therapeutic relationships are themselves the vehicle of treatment. The limitations of a rights-based, or justice-based vision alone, will also be discussed.

Different voices in bioethics There are multiple theories of ethical reasoning in healthcare, including those based on interpersonal relating (Beauchamp and Childress, 1994). In relation to psychiatry, the dominant discourse has been one of an ethic of justice/rights, with considerable debate about the rights of vulnerable people to treatment, to be protected from coercion, and competing rights of public safety and personal freedom (Fulford and Hope, 1994).

Within psychiatric ethics, concern for rights and justice must be important because patients are made vulnerable by their mental illness, and are also vulnerable to abuse by others. I will suggest that ethical debates in psychiatry which focus solely on conflicts between two principles, and set up ethical dichotomies (e.g. respect for beneficence or respect for autonomy), cannot address the complexity of the lives of individuals and the relationships in which they are embedded, both in the past and in the present. A rights/principles account that does not consider the patient within a matrix of relationships runs a risk of over-simplifying the patient's autonomy, and thus not doing justice (an appropriate word) to the complexity of the dilemma for this person.

The case of Miss A

Miss A suffered from borderline personality disorder. In childhood, she had experienced prolonged and extensive sexual abuse by her father. As a result, she suffered from depression, and intermittent feelings of loathing towards her own body, which resulted in acts of deliberate self-harm and episodes of self-starvation. She was admitted to a psychiatric hospital and over

119

a long period of time developed a reasonable relationship with her male psychiatrist, who was concerned for her welfare.

During one admission (after a period of years), Miss A's weight began to drop so dramatically that her doctor threatened to force-feed her in order to save her life. She went to court to get an injunction to prevent him from doing so. The dilemma here for both the patient and the doctor is obvious. Respecting her autonomy may result in her acting so riskily to herself that she suffers harm, and dies.

It may be relevant when contemplating this dilemma to consider how force-feeding is a symbolic re-enactment of the original abuse (she was subjected to forced fellatio over a period of time). The experience of child abuse frequently leaves individuals with real concerns about the extent to which they are in control of their own bodies even if retaining control incurs risk.

A relevant issue is that of Miss A's self concept, i.e. her attitudes of herself towards herself (Attanucci, 1988). Her own ambivalence about herself ('I don't matter ... I do matter') was mirrored in the attitudes of staff, who alternatively saw her as incompetent to care for herself and needing to be force-fed; or as manipulative and trying to bully them. This mirroring also replicated the relationship between herself and her parents. Legal argument focused on her competence to make decisions and refuse help (but that will not be examined here).

On a rights/principles perspective, or even a utilitarian analysis, there is a tension between Miss A's view of what was right for her, and the staff's view. A broader view of her welfare, which included thinking about her past, and present relationships with caretakers, might understand the dilemma as part of the concern that abused adults have about their control over their own bodies. By supporting her at these times when she was at her most self-destructive, it might be more possible to understand her self-destruction (and thus her ethical conflict with staff) as a response to her own previous experiences of abuse. Time could also be offered to staff to explore their feelings about Miss A, which might help to reduce the tension between them, and help them to feel less threatened by Miss A's expression of autonomy.

Autonomy and relationship   One of the limitations of a rights-based or a principles approach rests on the definition of autonomy. Rights-based accounts of autonomy provide a rather static atomistic picture of autonomy which allows little flexibility and disallows the importance of connections between persons (Christman, 1988). What is needed is a more complex notion of autonomy within a relationship: a synthesis and dynamic of independence in in-dependence. The reality is that most of us, but especially those who are made vulnerable by physical or mental disability, actually need connections with others in order to act freely. The case of Mr T demonstrates the impact of physical disability on psychological autonomy, and also the importance of family relationships when making assessments of harms and benefits.

> **The case of Mr T**
>
> A 21-year-old young man was maimed by a truck at the age of 10, leaving him disabled. His persisting disability provides a caring role for his mother. He allows his mother to do things for him that he is capable of doing; he is also ambivalent about going out, expressing concerns about others' response to his disability. His mother supports him in his reluctance, and suggests that it is too difficult for him to go out. Attempts to increase his opportunities for socialization (money for taxis, identification of peer groups) are met with verbal aggression by his mother, and benign sabotage on the part of the patient. The young man's family appears to be connected together by his disability so that attempts to rehabilitate him out of the house, which would indeed do him 'some good', seem to cause distress within the family system. Active interventions to motivate him may actually do him harm, in the sense that they disarrange a complex family dynamic.
>
> Changing that family dynamic requires a subtle assessment of harms and benefits, and an understanding of the relationships between all members of the family. A less subtle analysis of harms and benefits, which focused on only the young man's physical context and not his emotional one, may lead to difficulties, and clinical failure. Such failures are not uncommon, particularly in the area of psychiatric care in the community, and may reflect the lack of training which clinicians receive, both about the scope and nature of their ethical duties and the nature of relationships between people (Carse, 1991).

Discussion: Psychiatry and relationships There are many types of healthcare relationships within medicine, and not all are equivalent in terms of time, mutuality and complexity. Relationships characterized by brief discrete episodes, where the patient's independence or self-esteem are not threatened, are arguably different from those where the condition is life-long, wide-ranging in terms of effects and causes substantial disability. In this situation, the patient forms a complex system of relationships with all his carers, including healthcare professionals (Agich, 1990). Feelings arise on both sides of these relationships, which affect the perceptions of responsibilities and are an important aspect of any empathic connection between carers and patients.

Such a broader contextual vision of psychiatric illness addresses the impact of the illness on a patient's relationship, both towards himself and with his carers. The patient's self is understood as construed in terms of relationships with others, with knock-on effects for understanding his capacity for agency and the exercise of autonomy. Sutton (1997) describes the ethical difficulties presented by adolescent patients with mental health problems, whose autonomy is not only interconnected but also developing. Understanding the self in the context of dependent relationships allows for a dimensional understanding of the capacity for agency in psychiatric patients, from those whose capacity is more limited by psychotic or dementing illnesses, to those whose capacity is less limited by neurotic disorders.

It is perhaps in the field of neurotic disorders that the issue of relationships becomes more prominent. Healthy relationships appear to be important for normal adult mental health, insofar as they may protect against mental illness (Mullen, 1990). People suffering from neurotic depression or anxiety frequently describe failures in relationships as their presenting problem. Both depression and anxiety encourage people to withdraw from relationships, which increases a sense of isolation and anxiety.

The importance of relationships is even clearer in relation to the so-called 'personality disorders' (such as Miss A's). The conceptual status of these disorders has long been debated, particularly whether they can be considered 'illnesses'. What is clear is that their essential feature lies in an inability to make and sustain relationships. For example, a significant feature of antisocial personality disorder is an increased capacity to be detached from other people and the lack of empathy in connection with others (American Psychiatric Association, 1994). One of the defining criteria of 'borderline personality disorder' is

instability of relationships, which are characterized by intense positive attachments followed by quick rejections and fluctuating attachments (American Psychiatric Association, 1994).

Therefore therapeutic relationships within psychiatry have a number of significant features. First, the patient and their psychiatrist (and/or GP) are likely to be involved in a developing relationship over time, where the psychiatrist has to manage the patient's dependence, while facilitating his independence. Second, the illness itself may have profound influence on the relationships that the patient forms: with his doctor, and with his other carers, and those important to him. Third, the ability to make relationships may be affected by the illness.

Lastly, the contribution of the psychiatrist is just as important to the relationship, as any other aspect of treatment. This is particularly true in the context of those specifically psychotherapeutic relationships where there is a high degree of dependence on the therapist, which is developed by a regular consistent meeting over a long period of time. The psychiatrist contributes either by a direct impact on the patient, so that changes in the psychiatrist given can actually have an effect upon mental health of the patients (Persaud & Meus, 1994), or indirectly by the effect of her feelings on therapeutic decision-making.

The inequality which is a traditional feature of the doctor–patient relationship may be in some circumstances analogous to the inequality of power and knowledge in parent–child relationships. The therapeutic relationship can also be said to echo two aspects of effective parenting: namely care and containment of distress. A supportive approach by psychiatrists to decision-making by the dependent patient will (hopefully) be different from usurpation of judgement or strong paternalism. Present-day ethical dilemmas may reflect difficulties in past relationships with parents, who may not have been able to let the patient be themselves. A failure to appreciate this may mean that important emotional influences are left out of the ethical reasoning process.

Conclusion: Four principles and psychiatric relationships The two cases outlined above (drawn from real cases, but not based on any individual patient) show the complexity of relationships that have to be considered in the management of ethical dilemmas that affect psychiatric patients. Miss A's case highlights how an ethical dilemma may be understood in terms of the relationships between a patient and the multidisciplinary team. Mr T's case demonstrates how difficult it can be to delineate harms and benefits in the case of patients who are chronically dependent on others, and where their interests may have a direct bearing on the interests of the patient.

ACTIVITY: Here is a comment about this paper by one of our critical readers, Win Tadd. As you read it think about whether you agree with the point being made and about how Adshead might respond.

> I'm not sure what Adshead is claiming in the case of T. I assume her to be arguing that simply to focus on T's 'dependence' or his 'lack of autonomy' when considering his case, as she claims the principlist approach requires of us, would be to overlook many other important ethical considerations. In relation to this case I think that Gerald Dworkin's (1988) account of autonomy would avoid many of her concerns. He argues for example that any theory of autonomy should not 'imply a logical incompatibility with other significant values' and therefore, 'the autonomous person [should] not be ruled out on conceptual grounds, from manifesting other virtues or acting justly'. In T's case it might be the case that he truly values and understands his mother's need to feel 'needed' and therefore, as a consequence, 'autonomously' decides to allow himself to be dependent upon her.
> (Tadd, 1999, personal communication)

Now continue with your reading of Adshead's paper.

'Bare' principlism, which addresses ethical dilemmas in psychiatry only in terms of competing principles (such as beneficence versus autonomy) may not do justice to the complexity of the relationships and feelings that may be involved between the psychiatrist and the patient, and between the patient and his family. Too strong an emphasis on competing principles may cause clinicians caught up in ethical dilemmas to ignore important relationships in the patient's life, which are ethically significant (Jinnet-Sack, 1993).

The issue of respect for justice also needs careful consideration in relation to psychiatric patients. Real concerns about the abuse of psychiatric patients led to an undoubtedly valuable trend towards de-institutionalization and an emphasis on individual human rights. Nevertheless, the lack of services, care and the presence of stigma in the community has meant that patients could sometimes be abandoned with their autonomy respected: 'dying with their

rights on'. Such outcomes seem to suggest an understanding of justice as having an 'all or nothing' quality. It also seeks justice in an adversarial form, where A is pitted against B. In cases where A is a dependent member of the same society as B and where A and B are not as different as they may seem, then a more complex analysis is needed.

Principles theory needs to be supplemented, developed and enriched by other perspectives, including the ethic of care (Pellegrino, 1994; Robertson, 1996). This would appear to be particularly true in the practice of psychiatry and psychotherapy. This approach is also likely to have some value in other settings where patients suffer from long-term disabilities, and where relationships with others are both a significant part of their problem and part of the approach to treatment.

ACTIVITY: What do you consider to be the strengths and weaknesses of an approach based on the ethics of care? Peter Allmark (1995) argues that the concept of care used in this context is hopelessly vague because it lacks either normative or descriptive content. By this he means that it does not enable us to make a distinction between times when we are caring for the right things or the wrong things, and it cannot tell us whether we are expressing our care in the right way. In short, he argues that 'care' is used by ethics of care theorists as if it is always and inevitably a good thing. This, he argues, is to leave the concept seriously under-examined. Do you agree with this? If so, why? How does this criticism bear on Adshead's article?

In order to consider this question and the relative strengths of this and the other approaches we have discussed in this chapter, we would now like you to look at an extract of a report on this issue by the Danish Council of Ethics. As you read through it we would like you to consider just how far this rights-based approach is compatible with the ethics of care.

Rights and care in psychiatry: The Danish situation

In 1998, the Danish Council of Ethics produced a report on *Conditions for Psychiatric Patients*. In it they proposed, after much discussion, a set of rights for psychiatric patients. In summary the rights they proposed were as follows:

(1) The right to good hospital standards

The Council of Ethics feels, in principle, that anyone admitted to a psychiatric ward should have the possibility of staying on a private ward. There should be no compulsion to place mentally disordered admissions on multiple-bed wards unless it reflects the patient's wishes or is in some other way deemed appropriate for the sake of the person concerned. The Council then, does not feel that the right to a private ward (as argued by the Kallehauge Committee below) ... should be confined to cases where it can be said to be medically indicated.

In their report, the Council refer to the Kallehauge Committee who argued for five rights relating to good hospital conditions: (I) the right to stay on a private ward, where medically indicated; (II) the right to stay in modern structural conditions; (III) the right to a suitable offer of employment and teaching; (IV) the right to at least one hour in the fresh air daily and (V) the right to go out accompanied, as and when desired.

(2) The right to differentiated offers of treatment

In principle the Council of Ethics considers it essential for safeguarding psychiatric patients' personal integrity and achieving the best possible relationship of trust between the psychiatric patient and the treatment system that the Psychiatry Act provide clarification and assurance that in as far as possible treatment will consider the patient's own perceptions of his or her own symptoms, paying the greatest possible heed to the patient's own wishes with regard to choice of treatment forms. Only a tiny minority of patients are totally incapable of relating to their own condition and to what is happening to them.

(3) The right to a continued stay on a psychiatric ward.

As a working basis, the Council of Ethics feels that the hospital authority assumes special responsibility for the health and wellbeing of a mentally disordered person the instant that person is subjected to coercive measures. In the Council of Ethics' opinion, therefore, there is also a concomitant obligation to ensure that patients who have been subjected to coercion in connection with admission are not discharged until there is a reasonable likelihood of their being able to cope outside of the psychiatric ward. The Council of Ethics therefore feels that, for such patients, introducing a right of continued stay on the psychiatric ward should be considered until such time as they are deemed fit for discharge and the requisite extra-mural measures are in place.

(4) Limits on the use of coercion

There is scarcely any way of avoiding the use of coercion on the mentally disordered in some cases. However, it must be maintained that using force is a serious intervention and every effort should therefore be made to try and restrict such measures wherever possible ... The Council of Ethics therefore feels that restricting the use of coercion in as far as possible must be upheld as a central and vitally important objective in organizing mental health treatment.

(5) The right to a patient counsellor in cases of involuntary treatment

The Council of Ethics holds the view that for the sake of patients' civil rights a provision should be introduced whereby involuntary measures must be added to the ward's coercion records and trigger the right to a patient counsellor. Doing so would also enable these patients to complain about certain measures.

(6) The right to complain and to appeal

The Council of Ethics feels that the right of appeal should be organized in such a way as to make it as easy and manageable as possible.

> **ACTIVITY:** For your final activity of this chapter we would like you to apply the Danish rights to the two cases described by Adshead. Do you get different outcomes? What does this mean for Win Tadd's claim that the rights-based approach and the ethic of care are not necessarily incompatible?

We have seen throughout this chapter how the tension between respecting autonomy and protecting and promoting welfare can give rise to intense dilemmas in mental healthcare. As the Danish Council of Ethics observed, psychiatric care and treatment will sometimes involve practices that go against the patient's wishes (and maybe even their rights) – but its recommendations also show that there are ways of ensuring that we can maintain respect for the patient. One way of doing this, which Adshead suggested, is by supplementing our approach to respecting autonomy with the adoption of a caring attitude, which is alert to the patient's individual situation and their relationships with others. Indeed, a more nuanced understanding of autonomy also requires us not to assume automatically that a patient's choice must always be respected – for example, if it seems to conflict with other deeper values, as Dworkin suggests. Equally, respecting autonomy in a self-injuring patient with a history of abuse appeared potentially problematic if it ignored or colluded with that history. The patient's individual situation, highlighted by the ethics of care, is also foremost in anything but the barest, most simplistic notions of autonomy, which will rarely be helpful in the clinical situation. Conversely, whilst we may not be able to eradicate the dilemmas of autonomy and competence entirely, there will be ways of steering an appropriate course towards respecting the patient's rights and serving their welfare.

Notes

1. Reproduced with permission from Ron Berghmans, 'Protection of the rights of the mentally ill in the Netherlands'. Paper presented at the Tenth EBEPE Conference, Turku, Finland.

2. Reproduced with permission from Carlo Calzone, 'Drug treatment in child psychiatry'.

3. Adapted with permission from Gwen Adshead, 'A different voice in psychiatric ethics'. Paper presented at the Tenth EBEPE Conference, Turku, Finland.

Long-term care: autonomy, ageing and dependence

Introduction

Open any book on medical ethics and look at the contents page. Look at the front page of any national newspaper. In nearly all cases the focus will be on dramatic cases, crises situations or situations in which clinicians and families are faced with what are often called 'ethical dilemmas'. Yet the day-to-day practice of medicine and healthcare more generally is not like this. One danger of this concentration on crises is that it creates the impression that medicine and healthcare are otherwise ethically unproblematic. Nurses, doctors and other healthcare professionals know that this is not the case. Many of the most difficult and, indeed the most interesting, ethical aspects of healthcare are those that arise in daily and long-term care. In this chapter we investigate ethical issues relating to long-term care, such as truth-telling and deception, confidentiality, the ethics of mealtimes and feeding, of mobility, the ethical difficulties raised by work with patients suffering from dementia, and dealing with intimate relationships between patients.

Section 1: Truth-telling

The Case of Mr D

Sixty-eight-year-old Mr D, who has moderate dementia of the Alzheimer's type, lives at home with his wife. He is active and fit, which makes him quite demanding for Mrs D to nurse, given that he is also prone to wander and to forget where he lives. She welcomes the respite given by his attendance at a day-care centre, which he enjoys: he is very sociable.

Lately, however, Mr D has become worried about going to the day-care centre because he thinks he is losing time off work. He has never really stopped believing that he is still employed, although his increasing dementia forced him to retire six years ago. Now he insists that he cannot afford time to 'relax' because his deadlines at work are too pressing.

There have been unseemly tussles with the staff of the day-care centre van when it comes to collect Mr D, and Mrs D is embarrassed by the scenes in front of the house. She is also increasingly exhausted because she is no longer getting the respite she needs.

Missing the company of the day-care centre has made Mr D morose and irritable, increasing the tensions at home. He has also become increasingly obsessive, muttering that 'he never has any time any more' and complaining that his work burdens seem to grow and grow. He desperately needs more time at the office, he says angrily, and blames his wife for being unable to drive, so that she cannot take him to work.

The ambulance staff have suggested to Mrs D that she could tell her husband that the van is a taxi, calling to take him to work. They are sure that the staff at the centre will go along with the fiction that this is Mr D's new office. These little deceptions happen all the time with patients like Mr D, they reassure her: sometimes patients are given medications in secret at the day-care centre, for example. Somehow Mrs D doesn't actually find this terribly reassuring.

(Based on a case in Hope and Oppenheimer, 1996)

ACTIVITY: Stop here for a moment and ask yourself what should be done in the case of Mr D. What ethical issues are involved? Make a list of the arguments for and against telling him that the day-care centre van is his taxi to work.

What arguments for and against the deception did you come up with? Here are some of the arguments that we identified:

Arguments for:
- The burden on Mrs D will be greatly reduced if she is spared the scenes and given time to recuperate from her heavy burdens in providing long-term care for Mr D.
- It is unlikely that Mr D will find out the truth; the day-care centre staff can be trusted to keep up the fiction.

- Long-term care arrangements for Mr D are otherwise satisfactory, and he can be maintained at home, with respite care, for a longer period. Alternative nursing home arrangements may be difficult to set up, and costly.
- No one is harmed and everyone benefits: Mr D benefits from and enjoys his day-care centre; his obsession will be reduced; Mrs D will get the rest she needs.

Arguments against:

- Mrs D is not happy about the deception.
- Mr D may be very angry if he finds out he has been lied to, and may refuse to attend the centre ever again.
- This 'little' lie may lead to others; already the staff suggest that deception is routine, extending even to administration of medicines in secret. Although there is evidence that such practices do sometimes occur (e.g. Kirkevold and Engedal, 2005; Whitty and Devitt, 2005), they raise considerable ethical issues, not least in psychiatry (e.g. Hope, 1996; Wong et al., 2005). A climate of deception is easily created but not so easily undone.
- There is a shift from 'reality orientation' towards the 'validation' of Mr D's delusions if we accept that he should be lied to rather than being confronted with them *as* delusions. Arguably, this breaches the clinical duty of care.

(Widdershoven, 1996)

You may have noticed that virtually all of these arguments are concerned with the likely consequences (harmful or beneficial) of deception of this kind; they are therefore consequentialist arguments. Perhaps the strongest arguments against deception, however, are those which are sometimes called deontological or 'duty-based'. From a deontological perspective we might say that we have a duty to tell the truth and that:

- Deceiving Mr D in this way is simply dishonest. Lying is morally wrong. It diminishes the status of the person being lied to, denying him or her the opportunity to act as a free agent on the basis of correct information. It manipulates and uses people in an unacceptable way. This is inconsistent with respect for Mr D's dignity and integrity.

But is this last argument necessarily true? Many practitioners would find it very moralistic. Some might argue that ethical absolutes like this have no place in clinical practice, that pragmatic considerations should win the day (and probably that Mr D should be deceived for his own good). But if you look at some of the arguments *for* the deception, you'll find that they, too, have an ethical component. Look, for example, at the argument that 'no one is harmed and everyone benefits'. This eminently pragmatic argument actually rests on moral principles: the conception that we have an ethical obligation to maximize benefit and minimize harm. If the first principle of clinical practice is 'first do no harm' (*primum non nocere*), we would have to be certain that no clinical harm will come to Mr D from the deception. We might want to distinguish clinical harm from social harm, such as marital stress, which seems less obviously the concern of the practitioner. However, if staying at home all the time increases the risk that Mr D will become more anxious or that his dementia will worsen, we might argue that avoiding the deception does in fact impose a risk of clinical harm. Conversely, if Mr D discovers that he has been lied to and then refuses to co-operate with his caregivers, clinical harm could also result.

Similarly, the argument that everyone benefits rests on a slightly different conception of the practitioner's duties: to benefit patients positively, not just to avoid harming them. Conceivably that might extend to a view that their long-term benefit outweighs any short-term harm, so that 'first do no harm' could be overridden. For example, even if it is admitted that there is a risk of short-term harm in deceiving Mr D, one might argue that the chance of successful long-term care management is increased if we take the small risks entailed in lying to him. On the other hand, someone who was committed to benefiting patients first and foremost might equally well argue that the benefits of lying to Mr D are by no means clear. Perhaps there is some other, less obvious treatment strategy which might achieve comparable benefit and avoid the wrong of lying?

So the principles of doing no harm (sometimes called *non-maleficence*) or maximizing benefit (sometimes called *beneficence*) don't actually tell us which way to proceed in the case of Mr D. At this early stage of the chapter, it's not as crucial to find a solution as to suggest that the comparatively 'ordinary' and 'everyday' kind of case which Mr D represents does raise ethical dilemmas which need careful analysis.

ACTIVITY: Your final activity in this section forms a bridge to later parts of the chapter. We would like you to begin reading an article by the Dutch philosopher and medical ethicist Guy Widdershoven. The first section of the article appears here, but your reading of it will be resumed later in the chapter. As you read this part of Widdershoven's article, ask yourself what the implications are (1) for the case of Mr D, and (2) for long-term care of the elderly more generally.

Truth and truth-telling

Guy Widdershoven[1]

Truth is an important value in our lives. We do not want to be deceived, and we usually find it difficult to deceive others. Yet truth-telling is not a simple matter. Often we are not sure whether we should tell somebody else what we know, or how we ought to tell it. In every long-term relationship, a lot goes on which could be told, but actually is not. One might decide not to say what one actually thinks because it would take too much trouble to explain. One might refrain from correcting another person's views, because doing so would not be productive. In such cases it seems better to remain silent than to tell the truth. But how exactly can we justify such actions (or maybe better: omissions)?

In healthcare, several approaches to the issue of truth-telling can be found. The first is developed by defenders of *principlism* in biomedical ethics. They hold that the decision whether or not to tell the truth can be made by applying various principles, especially the principle of respect for autonomy and the principle of beneficence, to the case at hand. The second set of approaches is based upon a *therapeutic* perspective. This approach can be applied in various ways. Within the therapeutic perspective, some, the proponents of Reality Orientation Therapy (ROT), claim that truth-telling is crucial because it helps the patient (especially the demented patient) to orient himself in the world. Telling the truth is helpful because it keeps patients in touch with reality. Others, whilst also starting from a therapeutic perspective, deny that truth-telling is of itself therapeutically helpful and argue for a process of *validation*, claiming that one should not confront patients with reality, but attune to their way of meaning-making.

ACTIVITY: Stop reading here for a moment and think about what these different approaches might say about Mr D. Has our discussion so far left any of these perspectives out?

We would say that so far we have discussed Mr D's case mainly in terms of principlism and Reality Orientation Therapy. We looked at the force of doing no harm and

the hope of benefit, drawing on the principles of non-maleficence and beneficence. We also mentioned an argument against lying to Mr D which turns out to be derived from Reality Orientation Therapy: that there is a shift from confronting Mr D with reality to validating his delusions if we tell him the ambulance is a taxi to work. But we have not looked explicitly at the rightness or wrongness of validation: we merely assumed that it was a bad thing.

Now continue with your reading of Widdershoven's article.

The case of the forgetful mourner

In 1995, the *Hastings Center Report* published a case-study, titled 'The forgetful mourner'. In it an 86-year-old woman has been admitted to a nursing home following the heart attack of her son, with whom she lived. After two years, her son dies. She attends the funeral. Yet afterwards she continues to ask for her son, as though he were still alive. When she is told that he is dead, she shows much distress. Each time the staff try to explain the situation to her, she reacts as though she is hearing the news for the first time.

The staff do not know what to do. Should they keep trying to tell her the truth, or should they remain silent about her son's death? In the latter case, she might become convinced that her son is neglecting her, which might cause her a great deal of emotional pain. The doctors think that it is necessary to try and convince her that her son is dead. After 15 attempts without success a nurse proposes to dress her in the clothes which she wore at the funeral. The dress seems to remind her of her son. She speaks gently of him. After the ritual, she no longer asks for him. Yet she continues to mention his name every now and then.

In medical ethics, the issue of truth-telling is seen as an instance of medical ethical problems in general. Medical ethical problems are characterized by a conflict of principles (Beauchamp & Childress, 1994). The principles which are relevant to medical ethics are: respect for autonomy, beneficence, non-maleficence and justice. Ethical problems arise when these principles call for different kinds of actions. Respect for autonomy might mean that one executes the conscious wishes of a patient even if these are not in his own interest. In such a case, respect for autonomy conflicts with beneficence. According to principlism, the doctor should weigh the principles, and follow the principle which is the most important in the case at hand.

The issue of truth-telling can easily be integrated into this approach. On the one hand, the principle of respect for autonomy urges us to tell the truth to a patient. In hiding the truth, we do not take him seriously. On the other hand, the principle of beneficence might entail that we care for the patient's wellbeing by not telling him what we know. He might become upset by the news, and his condition may get worse. The care-giver has to become aware of such conflicts, and judge what is best in the concrete situation. By balancing the principles, the care-giver can decide what to do in a justified way.

Applying the principlist approach to the case described above (the 'forgetful mourner'), the first significant thing is the evident tension between respect for the patient and acting in the patient's best interest. Respecting the patient would mean continuing to tell her the truth. But since this results in distress, the patient's wellbeing is seriously harmed by this procedure. Therefore, one should consider ending the attempt to make her see the truth. In this case, one might argue that the policy of the doctors should have been ended long before they actually stopped. The harm done seems to be much larger than any possible gain. After ending the attempts to tell her the truth, one might try and look for means to make her more at ease. The intervention of the nurse can be regarded as aimed to comfort the patient. This intervention is not inspired by respect for autonomy, it is motivated by the wish to enhance the patient's wellbeing. Both in theory and in practice, beneficence appears to be stronger than respect for autonomy. The principlist approach to the problem of truth-telling emphasizes tensions experienced by the care-giver. The care-giver feels the need to respect the patient, or to enhance his wellbeing. Within the dominant principlist approach it might be said that the patient's feelings are not relevant to medical ethics.

In therapeutic approaches to care for the elderly, in contrast to those which are principlist, especially in relation to care for people with dementia, the perspective is radically different. The emphasis is not on the moral considerations of the care-giver, but on the experiences of the care-receiver. Reality Orientation Therapy and validation are two, mutually conflicting, approaches in this field; yet they have in common the claim that interventions should focus upon the condition of the care-receiver.

According to ROT one should stimulate and actively help elderly people to keep in contact with reality, or to regain contact with it. The idea is, that by giving the right information about the environment and about the things that are going on around the patient, one can help him to orient himself better. Care-givers applying ROT constantly comment upon their actions ('now we are going to wash, and next you will get dressed; would you like to put on your red dress? Here it is . . . ', etc.). They ask the patient about his life, using aids such as photographs to help the patient remember important people, such as parents or children. They will correct the patient if he is mistaken, and help him if he is not able to use the right words or perform the right actions all by himself.

Telling the truth is a fundamental aspect of ROT. One should not keep silent about what is happening, even if the patient has trouble in understanding it. One should not refrain from correcting the patients' mistakes, albeit in a gentle way. The aim of ROT is not to confront people with their mistakes, but to help to correct them. Applying principles of ROT to the case described above, one should not focus upon feelings of obligation or guilt on the part of the care-giver, but on the experience of the patient. One should try to make the patient aware of the fact that her son is dead, in such a way that she can accept it. One might use a photograph of the son, or another memory of him, to explain about his death. Actually, the intervention of the nurse functioned in this way: it somehow reminded the woman of the funeral, and thus made her son's death real for her. From a therapeutic perspective, it is important that the patient feels safe and comfortable. In this respect, the attempts of the staff to tell her the truth right away were not adequate. They did not help her accept the facts, but made her afraid. Telling the truth is not a virtue in itself: it has to be told in a way that is conducive to helping the patient to orient herself better, and to regain access to reality. The nurse's ritual appears to be a good way to convey the truth to the woman. It brings her in contact with reality in a productive way.

A second therapeutic intervention which focuses upon the patient's experiences is *validation*. Instead of telling the patient what is actually the case, as in ROT, one focuses upon the patient's feelings. The idea is not to enhance the patient's view of reality, but to show interest, and to accept the patient as he is. Strange or objectively wrong utterances may have a meaning for the patient. It is important to grasp this meaning, and help the patient to formulate it. The crux of validation is to make contact with the patient.

A good way of doing this is to respond in a bodily way, by hugging, for example.

Truth-telling plays hardly any role in validation. The objective situation is not important; the emphasis is on the patient's feelings. Telling the truth might easily lead to frustration. Focusing upon truth or falseness might also obscure why a person or event is meaningful for the patient. Instead of correcting the patient's views, one should find out what his utterances mean.

Applying the technique of validation to the case of the forgetful mourner, one would try to understand the patient's feelings about her son. From this perspective one should not try to tell her that he is dead, but focus on the fact that he obviously is important to her, and elaborate upon this. If the patient mentions her son, one might react by commenting that she obviously misses him very much. In this way, the patient is invited to express her feelings about her son. In this process, a mixture of feelings, both positive and negative, may come up. Thereby, the patient may be induced to rework her past, and to develop a new sense of self. From this perspective, the attempts of the staff to 'break the news to her' are clearly incompetent. She becomes so upset that she is not able to experience any feelings about her son. The intervention of the nurse is much more helpful; it evidently enables the woman to give her son a new place in her life. The nurse's intervention is not a matter of truth-telling at all; afterwards the woman still does not really know that her son is dead, but she has developed a new relationship towards him.

ACTIVITY: What do you think about this suggestion? Does it resonate with your own experience?

We will end our reading of Widdershoven there for now, but we shall be returning to the article in Section 3. Let's end this section by relating what you have just read back to the case of Mr D with which we began the chapter.

In long-term care, where relationships with patients can be established and where patients' values and preferences may come to be known more deeply than in acute care, the question of truth-telling is linked to how the patient construes reality. Although Mr D is moderately demented, his construction of reality is still important. (This relates back to whether carers should validate or challenge how the patient sees the world.)

A *principlist approach* to the case of Mr D might analyse it in terms of the concepts of autonomy,

beneficence and non-maleficence and in terms of the conflicts between them. For example, Mr D's autonomous right to be told the truth might be seen to be in conflict with the view that 'everyone benefits and no one is harmed' by telling him a little white lie.

A *therapeutic perspective* might focus instead on how Mr D construes reality. Telling him that the ambulance is his taxi to work risks confirming his delusional construction of reality. Telling him the truth, according to Reality Orientation Therapy, might arguably keep him in better touch with reality. But so far that strategy does not appear to be working; it only results in painful scenes – just as staff attempts to tell 'the forgetful mourner' that her son was dead only succeeded in upsetting her.

Perhaps an alternative validation-based approach which respects Mr D's view of the world might be to ask what work represents to Mr D. Why is it so important? – or more accurately, why is the loss of it so important? Is there any way in which he could be made to recognize the truth – that he is no longer working – in a similarly inventive manner to that which the nurse devised for bringing the reality of the son's death home to the 'forgetful mourner'?

We will leave you with this question for now. Truth-telling, as illustrated by the everyday cases of Mr D and of the 'forgetful mourner', raises issues about how we approach practical and ethical dilemmas in long-term care, but it does not exhaust the list of those dilemmas – far from it. In Sections 2 and 3 we will discuss a range of other common ethical quandaries in long-term care, analysing them in some of the terms to which Section 1 has introduced you but extending our analysis into new areas as well.

In each of those sections, we will follow the plan of Section 1, beginning with an everyday case in long-term care and drawing out the implications. This may seem odd: medical ethics is more often conceived of in terms of 'big' issues such as euthanasia. But as the Swedish nursing lecturers Anne-Cathrine Matthiasson and Maja Hemberg have perceptively written,

Ethics is concerned with how we ought to act toward one another. What is good and bad, what is right and wrong when acting toward another individual? Within the study of medical ethics, these questions are often equated with dramatic decisions about life and death, or consequences of the latest advances within medical technology and research. Ethics, however, is not only concerned with the spectacular or with questions of life and death. In general wards of hospitals or in nursing homes, particularly in the daily care of the elderly, lies a type of everyday ethics with countless small down-to-earth decisions concerning the various aspects of care. These actions are not subject to analysis every time they are performed. Rather, they reflect consciously or unconsciously the fundamental attitudes which carers express in their everyday actions. In seeking assistance in concrete situations, it is therefore imperative that we are aware of the values upon which we base our reflection.

(Matthiasson and Hemberg, 1997, p. 1)

Section 2: Autonomy, competence and confidentiality

Restraint, wandering and mobility

We begin this section with another everyday sort of case in long-term care of the elderly, provided by Tony Hope, an English medical ethicist and old-age psychiatrist.

The case of Mrs B

Mrs B, who suffers from moderate to severe Alzheimer's disease, frequently wanders from the nursing home where she is living. She has poor traffic sense. Not long ago, she wandered out into the road. A car swerved to avoid her and crashed into a tree. The driver suffered mild bruising and was very shaken, but was not seriously hurt.

ACTIVITY: Consider how you would act in this case if you were responsible for Mrs B's care? Jot down some possible options and the arguments for and against them.

You probably found yourself balancing Mrs B's 'right' to wander freely, without restraint, against the risk of harm to herself and the public. The usual analysis of Mrs B's case would pit her 'right to wander', based on a claim that her autonomy should be protected for as long as possible, against the harm to others and *to* herself which might result from her wandering. In her own best interests, should she be prevented from wandering? There are also the interests of others to consider. Whether or not the motorist was seriously hurt this time, a fatal accident could occur next time. So perhaps you found yourself considering whether she should be restrained from wandering; alternatively,

you might have considered tracking or tagging, depending on the legitimacy of those strategies in the legal and professional codes of your country.

Compared with Mr D, Mrs B seems much less able to decide for herself, although walking around freely still seems important to her view of the world. She may well be incompetent to judge the risk to both herself and to others from her wandering, whereas Mr D's understanding of his situation has fluctuated. Competence is a crucial concept in law, dictating different treatment strategies for competent and incompetent patients. If the patient is competent, he or she has the right to refuse treatment, even if this treatment would be life-saving; to treat in the face of a competent refusal would be to assault or trespass against the patient. However, if the patient is not competent, it may well be appropriate to restrain them, provided that such restraint can be justified in their best interests.

Truth-telling, the issue in the case of Mr D, is premised on the assumption that the patient is to some degree competent to understand the truth and act on it. In the case of Mr D, what the carers actually hoped was that he would act on a lie – that the day-care centre van was a taxi to his office – but they still treated him as able to act on information that was given to him, as competent in that sense. In English law, we are first to presume that the patient *is* competent, but we are entitled to conclude that he or she is not competent if they are not able to understand the relevant information, retain it, use or weigh it to reach a decision, or communicate their decision (Mental Capacity Act 2005, section 3(1)).

But although truth-telling and negotiation are not so much the issue here as in the previous example, autonomy is still relevant. English law is nowadays particularly alert to the need to justify any interference with autonomy, in the sense of a 'deprivation of liberty', and the law includes safeguards for protecting the interests of incompetent patients (e.g. Gunn, 2009). Yet, even if we might *legally* be entitled to restrain Mrs B, this does not mean that we can easily do away with the *ethical* issues (e.g. Nuffield Council on Bioethics, 2009, pp. 105–9). Barring Mrs B from walking around the grounds is likely to feel like imprisoning her to her carers, whether it is done by means of a locked door, sedation or tracking devices. It feels like a significant invasion of her rights, even though she is almost certainly not competent (Gastmans and Milisen, 2006; Sammet, 2007). There are risks of elder abuse if such strategies are followed too frequently, and most professionals are sensitive to this – indeed, it is notable that the American Psychiatric Association *et al.* (2003) have issued a special publication aimed at reducing restraint and seclusion. However, as Tony Hope's analysis below demonstrates, they may not feel they can let their sensitivity be the only consideration.

> In balancing best interests, the degrees of risk and harm need to be weighed against the distress caused by restraint and the loss of pleasure due to the loss of freedom. In my view, arguments against the use of restraints either on the grounds of loss of dignity or on the grounds that it is important for people with dementia to be given the same freedom as normal people should not be given much weight. It could be argued that restraining Mrs B constitutes an abuse. Alternatively, it could be argued that allowing her to wander, risking grave harm, is also a form of abuse – an example of neglect.
>
> (Hope, 1997)

But what about cases in which the patient is less obviously incompetent, although the risks of harm are just as serious? Take the case of Mr A, summarized below.

The case of Mr A

Mr A is a 72-year-old retired railway conductor who lives with his wife in the house of their 43-year-old daughter and her family. Still active on the family smallholding, he is increasingly frustrated by difficulties in operating machinery and in finding his way about the house. Accompanied by his wife and daughter, he visited Dr B's clinic for memory disturbance, where he was diagnosed with hypertension, arteriosclerotic occlusive disease, and multiple subcortical perivascular lesions on a computer scan of his brain. The overall diagnosis was subcortical vascular dementia with a moderate degree of impairment. It emerged that Mr A also had considerable impairment of his short-term memory (e.g. telephone numbers) and long-term recall (e.g. names of old friends). However, he denied strenuously that his mental powers were in any way impaired.

In the course of the consultation, Dr B asked Mr A whether he drove a car. Mr A replied that he did, and Dr B warned him that he should stop, from a medical point of view – because of his memory impairment. Mr A absolutely refused to consider stopping: he was in perfectly good health, he insisted, and still very fit.

'I'm a lot better driver than all those young lunatics!' Mr A's daughter interrupted at this point to describe two small car accidents which her father had recently caused. Mr A then announced, out of the blue, that he had just decided to buy a new car. If there was any problem, it lay in the old car, not in his driving. And there the matter rested, at least in the doctor's consultation.

Privately Mr A's wife and daughter agreed between themselves that the only possible solution was to hide the car keys. But Mr A managed to locate them, and drove off to a reunion of his railway colleagues without any incident. When he returned, it was with a new copy of the car keys, and a bad mood that lasted for days at home. Mr A's wife has now lost any will to prevent her husband from driving: she can't bear his anger, she says, and in any case he was perfectly all right last time he drove. Perhaps he doesn't have dementia after all, she remarked to the doctor on her own next visit to his surgery.

ACTIVITY: How would you analyse this case? Think in terms of (a) the possible decisions which Dr B could take and (b) the reasoning behind those decisions.

Dr B's options range from doing nothing to full-scale psychiatric interventions. In between lies the option of reporting Mr B to the driver licensing authorities, on the grounds that he is a danger to others. However, that would raise issues about *confidentiality* in the doctor–patient relationship. This is one element in the reasoning which might enter into Dr B's decision: that information obtained in the course of doctor–patient consultation is normally private, and that it would be wrong to reveal it to the licensing authorities.

In most countries, however, the obligation of confidentiality is not absolute. Where public interest in disclosure outweighs the public interest in ensuring confidentiality, health professionals are permitted – though normally not obliged – to breach confidentiality (Herring, 2008, p. 210). 'Most countries have legislation which gives to the doctor the right to be freed from the obligation of confidentiality, when there is a danger to the health or life of other people' (Dalla Vorgia, 1997). The exact scope of the obligation varies from country to country, as do guidelines issued to practitioners by their professional bodies. In the UK, General Medical Council guidelines (2009) allow disclosure to prevent a risk of death or serious harm to others, and do require doctors to inform the Driver and Vehicle Licensing Authority of any patient who is unfit to drive but cannot be persuaded to stop.

Other limitations on absolute confidentiality may occur in cases of child abuse or of dangerous psychiatric patients being discharged into the community: here again, disclosure of confidential information may be permitted. (See, for example, an English case involving a patient in a secure hospital who challenged disclosure of a confidential psychiatric report on his dangerousness to the medical director of the hospital and to the Home Office: W v. *Egdell*, 1990.) UK case law holds that professionals may disclose confidences in order to protect the public, provided that these conditions are satisfied:

- There must be a real and serious danger to the public.
- The risk must be an ongoing one.
- Disclosure must be to a person or body with a legitimate interest in receiving the information.
- Disclosure must be strictly limited to the information about risk, not all the patient's details.

(Herring, 2008, pp. 211–12)

What lies behind the general duty of confidentiality? (Even if Dr B can legally breach that duty – after further attempts to persuade Mr A to stop driving voluntarily – it is not a duty lightly to be broken.) We might seem to be back with the principles of autonomy versus beneficence again, as we were in one possible interpretation of the case of Mr D in the previous section. That is, Mr A's autonomy, his right to judge his own competence to drive and the freedom which driving brings, would have to be balanced against enhancing public safety by reporting him. This is certainly one set of considerations that Dr B might be considering. But we saw in the previous section that there are alternative ways of thinking, too: in that case, involving truth-telling, in terms of validation versus Reality Orientation Therapy. Whereas in the principlist approach tensions experienced by the caregiver were to the fore, both validation and ROT focus on the condition of the care-receiver, according to Widdershoven. For example, in the case of Mr A, trying to understand his condition on a personal level might involve asking why mobility is so important to him. Does he miss the daily travel which his job as a railway conductor used to give him, for example?

ACTIVITY: Now read the following analysis of the case of Mr A by Tony Hope. As you read, ask yourself whether Hope is offering an alternative to a principlist analysis, or a more sophisticated version of it. How does he construe autonomy?

Commentary on the case of Mr A

Tony Hope[2]

At first sight this case may appear to be a conflict between respecting Mr A's autonomous desire to drive, and the risk he poses to others. However, it is not as straightforward as that. Consider first autonomy. What would it be to respect his autonomy, to allow him to do what he now wants (i.e. to drive); or to do what he might have said about this situation prior to his dementia?

It is normally only considered possible to 'respect someone's autonomy' if that person is competent with regard to the decision to be made. Is this man competent to make a decision about whether he should drive? Two important considerations in making a decision are the risk to others and the risk to oneself. Since Mr A is not aware that he is suffering from dementia and does not appear to understand these two risks, I do not think that he is competent to make a decision about his driving.

In these circumstances, respecting autonomy is more a question of respecting the view he would have had before the onset of dementia than respecting his current desire to drive. Therefore, from the point of view of autonomy, the key issue is what he might have said about the situation had he been asked about it prior to the dementia. I suspect that most people would say that they would prefer to be prevented from driving in these circumstances rather than risk seriously harming another person. However, I have no good evidence for this belief, and in any case the issue here is what would Mr A have wanted.

Thus, I see the conflict in this vignette as being between the value and pleasure which Mr A gets from continuing driving (this might include the value of retaining some independence, over and above simply the pleasure from driving) against the risks he poses to other people and himself. Most countries have laws to prevent some people from driving, principally because of the risk which they pose to other people. Such laws typically prevent people with certain illnesses such as epilepsy from driving (under certain conditions) as well as preventing those who have been found guilty of certain criminal offences from driving. Society deems it right to prevent people from driving if they pose an excessive risk to others, even if this overrides their own autonomous views.

Of course, all driving poses a risk to others, so that as a society we clearly have judged that some risk can be taken in the interests of individuals and society from allowing most adults to drive. Thus the issue seems to be that at some point the risk to others outweighs the benefit to the individual. In England, at any rate, an assessment of how much a person wants to drive, or even how valuable it is to a person to drive, is not considered relevant. For example, the criteria as to what frequency of epileptic fits should prevent a person from driving do not differ depending on how much pleasure a person gets from driving, or whether driving is a necessary part of his job. In the UK the criterion for epilepsy is that you can only drive if you have been free from fits for one year (or have only had fits whilst asleep for the last three years).

Thus it would seem that the issue of whether a person ought to be prevented from driving should essentially be a question of whether the risk that person poses to others is greater than some threshold. What risk does Mr A pose? Presumably he poses a greater risk than he did before the dementia. But that by itself would not justify stopping him driving on the grounds of risk to other people. Does he pose a greater risk than many normal 18-year-old men? Let us suppose that the figures suggest that people with the degree of dementia of Mr A actually pose less risk of harm than do young adult males, who have a relatively high accident rate. Is there any justification for allowing the 18-year-old to drive, but not Mr A? Here are some possible justifications:

(1) The fact that Mr A poses a greater risk than previously. However, this does not justify banning Mr A whilst allowing the 18-year-old to drive.

(2) The combination of increased risk *plus* the fact that he is no longer fully competent. Suppose an 18-year-old man drives dangerously and causes an accident. He would be held fully responsible for what he had done. However, were Mr A to cause an accident, he is likely not to be considered responsible. Although the question of whether or not the driver could be held responsible does not help the victim of the accident, it does provide the victim with the potential for some kind of redress, either civil or criminal. But this argument does not seem to me a convincing reason for treating Mr A differently from the young man.

(3) If Mr A were to cause an accident, his insurance company might well not pay compensation to the victim, on the grounds that the company was not aware that Mr A suffered from dementia. Thus, unlike the victim of the 18-year-old driver, whose age is a known risk factor to the insurance company (and who pays a higher premium accordingly), Mr A's victim would

receive no compensation. This seems to me to provide a powerful reason why either the doctor or Mr A's family should inform the insurance company of Mr A's condition. However, if the company were still willing to insure Mr A (perhaps at higher cost), it does not seem to me to provide a reason to prevent Mr A from driving.

(4) The most powerful argument for preventing Mr A from driving is that this is what Mr A would have wanted had he been asked when competent. My view is based on an empirical belief (which might be false) that most people would be concerned not to cause an accident through having dementia but no insight into it.

At the end of his analysis Tony Hope returns to the interesting re-interpretation of autonomy which he offered at the beginning. In this view, autonomy is not simply doing what you please, but acting in a responsible, competent manner. Really respecting Mr A's autonomy doesn't mean giving in to his current desires, a lack of insight into his condition or concern for the risks he imposes on others. It means treating him as a rational moral agent, and holding him to the standards of responsibility that a rational agent would accept. Respect for persons in this view means treating others as 'citizens of the kingdom of ends' (in the words of the eighteenth-century philosopher Immanuel Kant): as moral agents, not objects of care. It has been argued by other modern medical ethicists that autonomy in this sense means honouring the patient's ability to behave unselfishly, rather than giving him everything he wants (Lindemann Nelson and Lindemann Nelson, 1995).

To return to the question which we asked you to consider while you were doing this activity, Hope can thus be seen as using both a principlist and a non-principlist approach to analysing the case of Mr A. Whilst he concentrates first on the principles of autonomy and beneficence, he notes immediately that they are too simplistic as usually presented. His elaboration of autonomy turns out to be rather more like the approach suggested by Widdershoven, in fact. Rather than simply accepting Mr A's desire to drive at face value, as an expression of his autonomy, Hope asks whether it is a competent and responsible wish. If not, it needs questioning in much the same way that Reality Orientation Therapy suggested in the previous case examples.

Autonomy and its critics

Emerging from our analysis so far are different ways of understanding the concept of autonomy. In the next paper, Ruud ter Meulen, a Dutch psychologist and medical ethicist, proposes a broad view of autonomy which, he suggests, has particular relevance in caring for older people.

ACTIVITY: As you read this article, ask yourself what the implications are for practice of the broader view of autonomy which ter Meulen proposes. How would it affect the case of Mr A? (We will return to some of the concepts to which ter Meulen refers in Chapter 9, in which we consider in depth the various meanings – and relative weightings – autonomy can have.)

Care for dependent elderly persons and respect for autonomy

Ruud ter Meulen[3]

The safeguarding of autonomy is an important principle in care for the chronically ill. This is particularly true in the care of the dependent elderly. Policies in most European countries are aimed at allowing elderly dependent people to live in their own homes for as long as possible. Even once they have left their own homes, autonomy continues to be an important consideration in care management. In many nursing homes, elderly patients are given maximum opportunity for independent living and for shared decision-making. As an example, I refer to a 1993 policy paper of the Dutch Association of Nursing Home Care (NVVZ), which states that nursing home care should be about more than mere physical management. Instead, it should be aimed at making itself superfluous: at reducing, stabilizing or even removing the requirement for care. In communication with the client, caregivers should respect individuals' choices as much as possible, in order to enable clients to live their lives according to their own values.

In this context autonomy is defined as participation and the right to self-determination. Autonomy is commonly defined in various ways: as 'self-rule', 'making your own choices' or 'being able to live independently'. The right to self-determination is a necessary condition for realizing one's autonomy. However, the question is whether it is a *sufficient* condition for autonomy.

In this paper I will argue for a broad concept of autonomy in which aspects of identity and identification play an important role. This broadening of the concept of autonomy will be preceded by a philosophical and sociological critique of the way autonomy is usually conceived in healthcare ethics. This broad concept of autonomy will be illustrated in long-term care management for chronically ill and dependent elderly persons.

In healthcare and healthcare ethics, the concept of autonomy is for the most part exclusively described as the freedom to make choices and to follow one's own preferences. 'Freedom' is often defined negatively, that is 'not hindered by others'. The right to information, the principle of free and informed consent and the safeguarding of privacy are important and enduring moral principles in our healthcare system, and they apply to the care of dependent elderly persons as well. Nevertheless, the relations between individuals would be impoverished if they were exclusively defined in these terms. Such relationships will have a predominantly formal and procedural character, but would lack sufficient moral, psychological or emotional content.

Agich (1993) directs our attention to discussions in American psychiatry, where, in his view, the right to self-determination has degenerated into 'a right to rot'. In that context, the ideal of freedom is radically explained as the right of individuals 'to be left alone'. Legal procedures have increasingly disrupted the relationship between physicians and other care professionals on the one hand, and patients on the other. However, in European healthcare systems, one can observe the same tendencies. In the Netherlands, for example, physicians are increasingly afraid of a lawsuit for 'malpractice'. As a consequence, they tend to adopt a defensive attitude and limit their services to necessary care, on the condition that patients have given their explicit consent.

The relationship between individuals, particularly that between patients and healthcare professionals, will turn then into a predominantly contractual relationship. This is a relationship which is defined in terms of rights and allows no room for personal virtues like solidarity and personal involvement. The change into a contract-like healthcare system can be illustrated by the transition from nursing home care to home care, which in many European countries is an important policy in elderly care: care 'in the community'. Although this policy may appear to increase the autonomy of the elderly, in the negative sense of being free from intervention, they may as a result fall into a 'black hole' of loneliness and neglect.

In healthcare ethics, the concept of autonomy is based on the philosophical concept of the person, particularly the concept of the person as advocated by Immanuel Kant. According to Kant the person is a rational and free being who can determine his own actions, independent of both his natural circumstances or the desires and inclinations of his own body. Freedom, Kant says, is the following of duty. This means that man should act according to duties which are unconditionally and at all times binding for every person (according to one formulation of Kant's 'categorical imperative'). When there is no respect for the freedom of the person, one loses the possibility of acting morally.

In healthcare ethics, we are often encouraged to follow Kant in considering the person as an individual and rational being, whose autonomous decisions should be respected. However, there is an important difference between Kant and contemporary health ethics. While Kant sees the freedom of the person as embodied in acting from duty, in healthcare ethics freedom is merely seen as a freedom to decide on one's own body and mind, without any reference to a universal duty. Thus, the difference is between autonomy as self-legislation (Kant) and autonomy as 'self-determination' (healthcare ethics).

ACTIVITY: Stop for a moment and consider this important distinction, which reaches out beyond healthcare ethics into our entire popular conception of freedom and autonomy. What implications does it have?

Ter Meulen is making a similar point to that raised by Tony Hope in his discussion of Mr A's 'freedom' to drive. Mr A interprets his autonomy as freedom to continue driving, regardless of the consequences for others. In ter Meulen's interpretation of Kant, this is not justifiable. The autonomous decisions which deserve respect are those which coincide with the categorical imperative, which is also formulated as 'Act according to that principle which you could will to become a universal law.' But if everyone behaved as Mr A wants to, there would be utter carnage on the roads. Autonomy means choosing one's wishes to conform with reason, not simply giving in to every passing whim – like Mr A's abrupt decision to buy a new car just to prove that he can do what he likes. Whereas Hope, however, had to rely on empirical evidence that most people recognize responsibilities to others – which might or might not have been true of Mr A before his dementia – ter Meulen is relying on a philosophical rather than an empirical argument. Now continue with your reading of ter Meulen's paper.

In healthcare ethics, the only limit to freedom is the autonomy or freedom of another person. That is, the choices which one makes may not result in an unacceptable or unreasonable limitation of another person's freedom to choose. In fact, this view on autonomy is closer to the liberal social ethics of John Stuart Mill than to the philosophy of Immanuel Kant. In healthcare ethics, autonomy is usually defined as the freedom to make choices, particularly the freedom to decide on one's own body and mind. The only limit to this freedom is the autonomy or freedom of another person. That is, the choices which one makes may not result in an unacceptable limitation of the freedom to choose of another person. In case of conflicts one should reasonably argue or negotiate to reach a mutual agreement.

ACTIVITY: Think about how this view of autonomy as limited only by harm to others is illustrated by the case of Mrs B's wandering. Bear this in mind as you continue now with your reading of the rest of the paper.

The individualistic and rationalistic concept of autonomy is inadequate because it ignores the social processes which underpin the appeal to negotiation and mutual respect. According to the German sociologist Norbert Elias, this concept of the person as an independent actor is a fiction, or as he himself puts it, 'an artefact of human thinking that is characteristic of a certain level in the development of human self-experience' (Elias, 1971). Elias conceives of the individual as someone 'who in his relationship with other human persons possesses a higher or lower degree of autonomy, but who will never reach total or absolute autonomy, who during his life is fundamentally thrown into a world with others and indeed is necessarily dependent on these others'.

The concept of autonomy then, needs to be corrected: the emphasis on autonomous individuality should be adjusted towards a social and relational concept of the person, which pays attention to the social context in which the person realizes him or herself. I want to mention three aspects of autonomy which are not recognized in contemporary health ethics, but which can be part of this broader concept: 'identification', 'identity' and 'sense of meaning'. Each of these aspects of autonomy requires a social context for its development.

In his study on autonomy in long-term care George Agich (1993) also makes a strong plea for a social concept of autonomy. According to Agich the view of the person as a rational and free individual is an abstraction from reality. In reality, individuals are not so much directed by rational decisions as they are by the image of themselves. Acting autonomously means that you identify yourself with your own actions and practice. This kind of approach does not see autonomy as a quality of an abstract rational self, but as the way individuals experience themselves in reality. In this view of autonomy, psychological processes like 'identification' play an important role. When I can identify myself with my behaviour or with the results of this behaviour, I feel autonomous. When I write an article such as this, and I can identify myself with its creation, I experience a certain degree of autonomy. This experience can also accompany the writing itself: the more I can lose myself in an activity, the more I experience myself as an autonomous being. Autonomy is in this view never finished or 'ready': it is a process, by which the person develops himself and realizes himself. Being autonomous means to develop oneself, not in the direction of an abstract ideal, but by way of a continuous identification with changing circumstances.

This means that care for dependent elderly people should be organized in such a way, that the elderly person can identify herself with her own behaviour and with her changing environment. Respect for autonomy should not be limited to dramatic medical treatments, for example non-treatment decisions at the end of life, but should be a continuous process in daily care. It means, for example, that elderly persons in a nursing home are given the opportunity to make meaningful choices, particularly regarding daily care and daily activities. Rosalie Kane and Arthur Caplan (1990) talk about 'everyday ethics': particularly in normal interactions and daily care, there are many possibilities and obstacles for the realization of autonomy. This can mean that people may make their own choices regarding 'sleeping and feeding' times or the clothes they want to wear. In every nursing home one needs a regime, but not at the expense of a social sphere in which individuals can express their own individuality.

One may wonder whether autonomy and dependency can co-exist. A chronic disease has in many cases a profound impact on the life of those who are afflicted by it. Life-plans are disrupted, while social relationships and everyday activities are often seriously hindered. These dramatic changes often have serious consequences for the experience of one's own 'identity'. Kathy Charmaz (1987) talks about a 'constant struggle': people who are suffering from a chronic or enduring disease have to fight continually for their own identity, adjusting themselves to their handicaps, pain and loneliness. The promotion of autonomy is not in contradiction with the dependency caused by chronic disease: in view of their chronic diseases, people who find themselves to be dependent and vulnerable need support in finding a new identity or readjusting the previous one. Particularly in those circumstances, they need to recognize themselves in the choices they make. Opportunities should be offered then to make these choices a reality. In this process of identification and of regaining or restoring autonomy, the relationship with caregivers is extremely important. Autonomy, conceived as development of one's identity, is a relational process. It requires the solidarity and commitment of the caregiver.

However, to safeguard or restore autonomy, one needs not only the commitment of the caregiver, but also a sense of 'meaning' of what it is to be old, particularly of being dependent. Individuals do have some sense of meaning, but it may be fragmented and not articulated. The articulation of this individual sense of meaning of life and old age is hindered by the fact that as a society we have great difficulty giving meaning to old age and dependency. While in former times ageing was considered a normal process of existence, in modern times it seems a practical problem which can be solved by scientific research and technology. We live in a society in which being young seems to be the absolute norm.

Of course, it is important to stay healthy and active as long as possible during the course of our life. However, we must realize that our lives do come to an end, in spite of all attempts at rejuvenation. We also have to realize that this end is often preceded by a period of debilitating diseases and disability. Because we value youth and activity in such a strong way, we are not able to give meaning to our dependencies. Yet the acceptance and integration of dependency is an important condition for realizing autonomy.

Here I want to refer to what the Canadian philosopher Charles Taylor has called the 'horizon of meaning' (Taylor, 1991). According to Taylor, we can realize our identity only when we experience ourselves as part of a whole, that is within a spiritual or cultural tradition. The influence of liberal ideology on our culture has resulted in greater political rights. However, it has also resulted in the disappearance of a horizon of meaning, a cultural framework of values which gives meaning to individual and societal experience. The price to be paid for this freedom is a sense of meaninglessness and triviality.

What we need, Taylor says, is an 'art of retrieval': an attempt to regain senses of meaning that have been lost during the past, particularly the meaning of old age. Such a horizon of meaning is a necessary condition for realizing our identity. By regaining a commonly shared horizon of meaning, there will be growth of mutual ties and a decrease of the fragmentation of society into separate individuals. A shared interpretation of ageing and dependency may prevent the relationships between carers and elderly care recipients from becoming impoverished as a result of the individualization process. Horizons of meaning are in this respect an important and necessary supplement to the one-sided and narrow interpretation of the concept of autonomy.

Ter Meulen stresses identification with one's actions, support from caregivers in adjusting to the new dependent identity, and realization by caregivers that our society loads unattractive and burdensome meanings onto old age. Above all, he sees autonomy as created in relationship – in contrast to the usual notion of 'finding oneself'. In practical terms – for example, the case of Mr A – ter Meulen's 'broad' concept of autonomy would suggest helping the patient to recover self-respect despite dependency, perhaps employing 'lateral thinking' like that demonstrated by the nurse in the case of the forgetful mourner. Clearly Mr A's sense of himself is intimately linked to mobility and to being in control: both, not so incidentally, characteristics of his old job. Although Dr B would not be betraying confidentiality if he reported Mr A to the licensing authorities – and indeed, in many countries his professional code would require him to do so – there also needs to be some consideration of how Mr A can adjust to the loss of mobility without the loss of autonomy in the sense of relational identity. Hiding the car keys – understandable response though it is – doesn't address this problem, and only makes Mr A angrier. Instead, it would seem that Dr B has to assist Mr A's wife and daughter more overtly in their consultations, in challenging Mr A's limited, egoistic view of autonomy and in negotiating other ways in which he can remain mobile without posing a threat to others.

The emphasis on the self as constructed through relationship, which emerged so strongly in ter Meulen's article, is shared with many feminist approaches to moral philosophy and medical ethics. Like ter Meulen's analysis, such feminist approaches emerge originally from psychology and psychiatry, particularly the work of the American psychologist Carol Gilligan (1982). Like ter Meulen's 'broad' model, they suggest

that autonomy is too often narrowly construed, with unfavourable consequences for those who do not fit the 'rational consumer of health services' mould. In the final reading for this section, Gwen Adshead, a psychotherapist, forensic psychiatrist and medical ethicist, discusses autonomy from this perspective.

Autonomy, feminism and personhood

Gwen Adshead[4]

Traditional views of autonomy involve a vision of individual personhood which is both separate from others and hierarchical. Full autonomy is linked with rationality, 'untainted by desire', in Kant's phrase – reflecting a view of reason which excludes *affects* and feelings and links those aspects of mental life with irrationality. Another traditional view appears to draw on Darwinian notions of the survival of the fittest, so that decisions which do not further one's own interests are perceived as being suspect, and only self-interest is natural. The link between the two lies in the understanding of emotions as being both irrational in themselves (and therefore tending to diminish autonomy) and causing us to take decisions which are biased and therefore irrational.

It is recent feminist theory which has mounted the most consistent and sustained attack on traditional notions of autonomy. Can feminist theory offer a better account of autonomy – one which preserves the aspect of protection from interference and oppression by more powerful others, but acknowledges the need for connection to others, especially those with whom we are in relationships? There are two areas of social relationship which are relevant to the concept of autonomy, and which have been subject to feminist analysis: power relations and caring relations.

A complete explication of power relations cannot be offered here. Most significantly, feminist theory questions unequal distributions of power (especially between the sexes) and the devaluation of those who are deemed to be 'different' from the status quo, as defined by status quo setters. In addition feminist writers have questioned the devaluing of those who are deemed to be powerless. Where there is a strict hierarchy of power, those who have none are devalued: first because they have no power in the sense of agency, and second because they are perceived to be lower in the hierarchy, and thus vulnerable.

ACTIVITY: How might these points be particularly relevant to long-term care? Clearly elderly people receiving long-term care are one of the most vulnerable groups in society, and are one with little power. It is also true that a high proportion are women. Furthermore, given the earlier demise of men and the typical pattern whereby women marry men older rather than younger than themselves, women are less likely to be cared for by a spouse than men are.

Women, of course, are not *essentially* vulnerable, unless both difference from status quo holders (male) and biological difference are taken to define vulnerability and indicate reduced agency at any number of levels. But feminist questioning of traditional power structures has allowed the asking of another question: is vulnerability a problem? Or is it an essential part of human experience, without which we might not be human?

The question of vulnerability raises the area of caring relationships. Traditionally, the feminine gender role is associated with caring (Showalter, 1987), so that being female implies principal responsibility for the care and maintenance of relationships, and the protection of dependency and dependants. Gilligan (1982) has found some evidence that different *ethical* perspectives may be associated with gender role: a 'masculine' rights-based perspective and a 'feminine' care-based perspective in females. Gilligan presents these two perspectives on ethical reasoning as complementary and not mutually exclusive.

A more connected vision of autonomy, which addresses dependency needs, is not a sexist one, which applies only to women. Men also are dependent, and it is likely that some sexist practice is related to male gender role escapism and intolerance of dependency. For men and women alike, we might argue for a wider conceptual revision of the traditional view of autonomy. We might see autonomy as 'interstitial' (Agich, 1990) in the gaps between people and within their relationships. Accounts of autonomy need to include the concept of dependency and its effect on identity.

To be fully autonomous is to be located in a network, rather than an isolated dot in the universe. This accords with notions of best psychological health, where mutual interdependence is seen as being a goal of mature development, and detached isolation in terms of self is seen as being potentially pathological. If personal identity were understood in this way, then a richer account of autonomy might be possible. Autonomy, and the exercise of autonomy, would include accounts of the self as embedded in relationships. Agency would recognize the connections between persons in relationship, and understand those as relevant to ethical decision-making.

ACTIVITY: As your final exercise in this section, ask yourself how Adshead's statement that 'to be fully autonomous is to be located in a network' might apply in the case of Mr A.

One point which occurs to us is that although Mr A is exercising his 'individual right' to drive at the expense of his family's mental wellbeing and the safety of the public, he uses his car to drive to reunions. The car symbolizes connection as much as individual independence. Another point might be that Mr A is so fierce in his 'independence' because at some level he recognizes that he is in fact dependent on his daughter, in whose house he lives. Adshead urges us to reflect on people like Mr A within their 'network' – and as such she advocates revisions to the key notion of autonomy. In the next section we will build on this theoretical and practical reconstruction, with further development of the idea of narrative in ethical issues about long-term care.

Section 3: Ethics in relationships

The case of Lisa and Martin

Lisa and Martin are elderly residents in a residential home which caters for people who suffer from dementia. In general both Lisa and Martin seem to be happy and this appears to be largely the result of their relationship with one another. During the day Lisa and Martin are inseparable. They sit holding hands, they flirt with each other and talk or cuddle for most of the time.

However, despite the genuine happiness both Lisa and Martin experience the staff at the home are concerned about their relationship. It is apparent that Lisa falsely believes that Martin is her husband and that Martin, also falsely, believes that Lisa is his wife.

This poses several problems for the staff. On the one hand there is the ethical question raised earlier in the first section of this chapter of whether they ought to adopt a *reality orientation* approach or one based on *validation*. That is, should they encourage the two residents to confront the truth about their relationship or should they respect and validate their feelings and the meaning the relationship has for them? On the other hand, in the case of Lisa and Martin there is a much more pressing ethical dilemma for the staff. For whilst Lisa's husband is in fact deceased, Martin's wife is not and comes to visit him on average once a week. This causes practical as well as ethical problems for the staff.

When Martin's wife visits him he sometimes recognizes her, but sometimes he does not. This naturally upsets his wife. Martin's wife does not appear to know about the relationship between Martin and Lisa. When she comes to visit, the staff who work in the home try to make sure that Lisa is out or engaged in some activity in another room in order to avoid a confrontation. The problem with this is that Martin and Lisa desperately want to be together and protest when they are separated.

The staff do not know what to do. This is not, they feel, simply a matter of whether or not they should keep Martin's wife in the dark; it affects every aspect of managing the home. At bed time, for example, Martin and Lisa want to sleep together. They have said this when their respective children have been to visit them and the children have told the staff that such behaviour cannot be allowed.

Thus far, the staff who work in the home have respected the wishes of the children and have separated Martin and Lisa at bed times despite loud protests. The staff find this very upsetting when they see just how unhappy Lisa and Martin are but find it very difficult to know what they ought to do.

ACTIVITY: Stop here for a moment and consider what ought to be done in the case of Lisa and Martin. Make a list of arguments for and against allowing Lisa and Martin to continue their relationship. When you have done this, go on to read the British psychiatrist and medical ethicist Tony Hope's commentary on the case, picking out the arguments he uses and adding them to your list. We will return to these lists at the end of the section.

Commentary on the case of Lisa and Martin

Tony Hope[5]

This case appears to present a conflict between the interests of Lisa and Martin on the one hand and the interests of their families on the other hand. The interests of nursing home staff, and other residents in the nursing home, should, perhaps, be a further consideration. Before discussing the case of Lisa and Martin directly, I will start by considering a different but related hypothetical situation, that of 'Carla and Stefan'.

Carla and Stefan meet at a conference on bioethics. They form a close sexual relationship. Both are married and have children. They continue their relationship after the conference and separate from their respective spouses. Their spouses and their children are very upset.

In the case of Carla and Stefan we would normally say that no one has the right to prevent their relationship even if we do not approve of what they have done. The understandable distress caused to their families does not provide a justification for others to interfere.

ACTIVITY: Do you think that there are any morally relevant differences between the case of Lisa and Martin and that of Carla and Stefan? We may be tempted to disapprove of Carla and Stefan's relationship but even if this were the case, we would most likely consider it wrong to tear Carla and Stefan apart. In the case of Lisa and Martin, however, the staff consider this an option. Why is this a possibility in one case and not in the other? Tony Hope goes on to compare the two cases.

There are two important differences between the situation of Carla and Stefan and that of Lisa and Martin. The first is that Lisa and Martin both suffer from dementia; the second is that the nursing home staff do have a relationship of care towards Lisa and Martin and thus have some special responsibilities towards them. What is the ethical relevance of these two differences?

The issue of the staff's special responsibilities does not seem to me to be critically relevant. Suppose that Carla and Stefan were physically handicapped (say, for example, that they suffered from spinal cord injury resulting in the paralysis of the legs) and required institutional care. If, nevertheless, they were fully competent, I cannot see that the healthcare staff would have the right to interfere in their relationship. They might have the right to restrict their behaviour whilst in the hospital or nursing home for the sake of residents and staff (for example, sexually overt behaviour in the public rooms of the institution): the institution would also be justified in preventing such behaviour between a man and wife. However, the relationship between Stefan and Carla is a matter between them and their respective spouses and not in itself a concern for the healthcare staff. The key difference between the two cases is the impaired mental state in the case of Lisa and Martin.

The concept of 'competence' is generally used to help clarify when it is right for healthcare staff to act against the apparent wishes of patients. In simple terms, a competent patient can refuse any treatment even when such a refusal is clearly against the patient's best interest. However, healthcare staff should generally act in the 'best interests' of incompetent patients. The question of competence is not always straightforward. One important aspect is that competence must be judged with reference to the specific issue. That is, the question should be: is this person competent to refuse this specific treatment – does she understand the aspect relevant to coming to a decision in this case?

Applying this kind of approach to Lisa and Martin then raises two issues: are Lisa and Martin competent to choose to develop this close sexual relationship despite being married to other people, and what is in their best interests?

It should be said, at once, that an analysis relevant to the question of refusing treatment is rather different from the situation we are currently considering. However, even if the analysis is in theory applicable, it is difficult to apply in practice. Consider first the question of competence. Lisa and Martin appear to be able to recognize each other and to have sufficient memory of the past to sustain their relationship with each other. What exactly does it mean, and what should the criteria be for judging that they are incompetent to sustain this relationship? The key point in doubting their competence would seem to be the fact that Martin only intermittently recognizes his wife, and presumably has no memory of his long-standing relationship with her, and Lisa believes that Martin is her husband. But it is by no means clear that this makes Lisa and Martin incompetent to carry on their relationship.

When we read this we found ourselves asking why competence should be so important here. One possible response to Hope's analysis of the case thus far would be to point out that engaging in sexual and deeply emotional relationships is never fully a question of competence. We might argue instead that the key question here is the authenticity or otherwise of the emotions felt by Lisa and Martin. But perhaps the two questions are related: if Martin were aware that he is already married, would he feel differently about Lisa? At the very least, his feelings for her would probably be more conflicted than they seem to be. If Martin held strong views about fidelity in marriage before his dementia set in, his 'authentic' feelings might even be revulsion and guilt about his attraction to Lisa. Hope goes on to suggest a similar argument and to examine whether 'best interests' should also be considered in this situation.

Ronald Dworkin distinguishes between 'critical interests' and 'experiential interests' (Dworkin, 1993). As applied to the situation under consideration, the experiential interests of Lisa and Martin would depend upon their day-to-day experiences. Since Lisa and Martin are, presumably, enjoying their relationship, and not suffering significantly from the distress which they are causing their family, it would seem to be in their experiential best interests for them to be allowed to pursue their relationship uninhibited.

Critical interests refer to those interests we have in the kind of person that we want to be, and our long-term aims or enduring wishes. Thus a vegetarian might have a 'critical interest' in remaining vegetarian after suffering from dementia, even if, once demented, the person has no memory or understanding of vegetarian principles. If asked to complete an advance directive, such a vegetarian might state that she wishes to be prevented from eating meat should she, at some stage in the future, become demented and no longer be able to voluntarily restrict her diet.

The strongest argument I believe for restricting the relationship between Lisa and Martin lies in an argument along the following lines. Supposing Martin (or Lisa) had been asked, before the onset of dementia, what he would want to happen if, at some stage in the future, he suffered from dementia and the situation as described in this vignette occurred. Suppose he then said that his relationship with his wife was of great importance to him (a 'critical interest') and that for two reasons he would want those looking after him to prevent his developing and enjoying another relationship. The first is that the mere development of such relationships spoils his conception of his relationship with his wife; and secondly it would distress him greatly to think that he might cause such pain for his wife.

In the present situation, there is no such clear statement. So Hope first considers (again by the use of a thought experiment) what should be done were there good evidence that Martin had made such a statement. Hope starts by asking us to imagine a third case, involving another couple, 'Robert and Catherine'.

Robert is happily married. He is shortly going off to a bioethics conference without his wife. He says to several of his friends that he is worried that he might start to develop a relationship with someone at this conference. He says to his friends that if this were to happen he would want them to do everything in their power to stop such a relationship. Robert subsequently goes to the conference and develops a relationship with Catherine. When his friends learn of this and try to prevent his relationship with Catherine, he tells them to stop interfering.

ACTIVITY: The use of thought-experiments of this kind in philosophy is designed to throw new light on a philosophical problem (in this case an ethical one) by analogy. What are the similarities and the differences between the case of Robert and Catherine and Lisa and Martin? Continue reading and, as you do so, consider whether or not the use of thought experiments of this kind are useful here and whether this particular one works.

Unless there are some extra special circumstances I think that Robert's *most recent* view has to be respected. Although friends might reasonably try to persuade him, they could not go any further than this.

In the case of Lisa and Martin, there are further circumstances, the critical one being that Martin is now suffering from dementia. It seems to me that this fact of dementia is potentially relevant in two ways. The first comes back to the question of competence. That is, a reason why we should respect his previous and not his current wishes is that his previous wishes were made when competent. This raises problems to do with establishing what exactly competence means in these circumstances. The second difference is to say that he is now ill and his relationship with Lisa is a direct result of the illness. In order for this to be a reason for countermanding his current desires it would have to be further argued that the illness has interfered with his 'true self'. On this analysis his views prior to dementia represent his true views which have been obscured by the dementia.

In the present case we do not have this clear evidence of what Martin's and Lisa's views about the current circumstances would have been. We might try to establish what their views would have been, although, clearly the families' accounts are unlikely to be objective on this matter.

So where does this leave us with regard to what the staff should do? I think what it shows is that, in order to justify interference with the relationship between Lisa and Martin all of a number of statements would need to be considered true:

(1) That Lisa and Martin would have wanted their relationship to be broken, had they been asked about this situation before the onset of dementia.

(2) That such 'critical interests' should trump experiential interests.
(3) Either that Lisa and Martin are now incompetent with regard to the understanding of their relationship with each other; or that sense can be made of a distinction between a true self and a false self, and that the true self is represented by their pre-dementia state.

Each of these statements is problematic, and I think therefore, the balance lies on the side of allowing the relationship to continue (whilst trying to minimize the distress to the family).

An issue which I have not considered is what should happen if the analysis leads to a conflict between the interests of Lisa and Martin: that is, where on the above analysis we decide that (let's say) Lisa's interests are served by a continuation of the relationship whereas Martin's are not.

ACTIVITY: Return to the list you prepared earlier after your first reading of the Lisa and Martin case. Look again at your two lists of arguments, those for allowing the relationship to continue and those against it. In the light of the above commentary, what is your position?

Four types of practitioner–patient relationship

The conflicts experienced by the nursing home staff in the case of Martin and Lisa raise important questions about the nature of the practitioner–patient relationship in long-term care. We would now like you to consider four models of that relationship, as described below by Guy Widdershoven in the continuation of his article 'Truth and truth-telling'.

Four types of professional–patient relationship The perspectives on truth-telling discussed earlier imply different views of the professional–patient relationship. In each of the various approaches one may recognize the four models of the physician–patient relationship described by Emanuel and Emanuel (1992). The first is the *paternalistic* model. In this model the doctor decides, acting in the best interest of the patient. In this model the doctor is the guardian of the patient. The second model is the *informative*, or consumer model. It is based upon the autonomous choice of the patient, after being informed by the doctor. The values of the patient are considered to be given. In this model the doctor is the technical expert. The third model is the *interpretive* model. It aims at interpreting the patient's values and implementing the patient's selected intervention. The values of the patient are seen as inchoate and conflicting, and in need of interpretation. In this model the doctor is a counsellor or adviser. The fourth model is the *deliberative* model. It is based upon the presupposition that the patient's values are not only in need of interpretation, but also of discussion and deliberation. The doctor is regarded as a friend or teacher. This model is the most radical.

> The conception of patient autonomy is moral self-development; the patient is empowered not simply to follow unexamined preferences or examined values, but to consider, through dialogue, alternative health-related values, their worthiness and their implications for treatment.
> (Emanuel and Emanuel, 1992, p. 2222)

ACTIVITY: How did these models conflict in the case of Martin and Lisa? For example, we might identify the informative or consumer model as influencing the carers' feelings that they should not interfere with the couple's relationship. Given doubts about the autonomy and competence of the couple, however, would a paternalistic prohibition on their relationship be justified? Do the interpretive and deliberative models offer a way out of this conflict in the case? Widdershoven suggests that this may be true more generally.

According to the principlist approach, the professional can choose to follow the principle of beneficence, which means that he or she acts in the patient's best interest, or to respect the patient's autonomy, which means that the patient is regarded as a client whose wishes are to be responded to by the professional. In the first case, the professional–patient relationship is paternalistic; in the latter case, it is informative.

The therapeutic approach is in line with the interpretive model of the professional–patient relationship. The professional does not take his or her own views of the situation of the patient for granted (as in the paternalistic model), nor does he or she restrict himself to giving information and executing the patient's wishes (as in the informative model). Rather, he or she acknowledges that the patient's views are not clear and have to be interpreted. The patient's perspective is central, as in the informative model, but this perspective is not considered to be given. It has rather

to be elaborated by the professional. The professional has to listen carefully to the patient's utterances and help the patient to give meaning to the situation, without imposing his or her own views.

In the deliberative model of the professional–patient relationship, the professional and the patient both bring in their view of the situation and engage in a dialogue about what should be done. This model fits the hermeneutic perspective on truth-telling. Both the care-giver and the care-receiver play an active role. In a process of deliberation, the views of the care-giver and the care-receiver confront one another. The aim is to reach a common understanding of the situation, in which the views are no longer opposed to one another, but merge into a shared perspective,

The Emanuels (1992) use the table below to describe and summarize the four types of relationship and their implications.

	Informative	Interpretive	Deliberative	Paternalistic
Patient values	Defined, fixed and known to the patient	Inchoate and conflicting, requiring elucidation	Open to development and revision through moral discussion	Objective and shared by the physician and patient
Physician's obligation	Providing relevant factual information and implementing patient's selected intervention	Elucidating and interpreting relevant patient values as well as informing the patient and implementing the patient's selected intervention	Articulating and persuading the patient of the most admirable values as well as informing the patient and implementing the patient's selected intervention	Promoting the patient's wellbeing independent of the patient's current preferences
Conception of patient's autonomy	Choice of, and control over, medical care	Self-understanding relevant to medical care	Moral self-development relevant to medical care	Assenting to objective values
Conception of physician's role	Competent technical expert	Counsellor or adviser	Friend or teacher	Guardian

They conclude their paper in the following way,

> Over the last few decades, the discourse regarding the physician–patient relationship has focused on two extremes: autonomy and paternalism. Many have attacked physicians as paternalistic, urging the empowerment of patients to control their own care. This view, the informative model, has become dominant

in bioethics and legal standards. This model embodies a defective conception of patient autonomy, and it reduces the physician's role to that of a technologist.

The essence of doctoring is a fabric of knowledge, understanding, teaching, and action, in which the caring physician integrates the patient's medical condition and health-related values, makes a recommendation on the appropriate course of action, and tries to persuade the patient of the worthiness of this approach and the values it realises. The physician with a caring attitude is the ideal embodied in the deliberative model, the ideal that should inform laws and policies that regulate the physician–patient interaction.

Finally, it may be worth noting that the four models outlined herein are not limited to the medical realm; they may inform the public conception of other professional interactions as well. We suggest that the ideal relationships between lawyer and client, religious mentor and laity, and educator and student are well described by the deliberative model, at least in some of their essential aspects.

(Emmanuel and Emmanuel, 1992, p. 2226)

ACTIVITY: Think of a case from your own practice or experience which confronted you with an ethical dilemma. Can you identify which of these models you adopted and why?

In response to this activity one of our critical readers, Mark Wicclair, wrote,

In addition to the questions you raise, I would raise the following: there may not be one model to fit all patients. Accordingly, the informative model might be appropriate for patients who have clear preferences and values; the interpretive model may be appropriate for patients who do not have such clearly defined values and preferences; the deliberative model may be appropriate for patients who are conflicted; and the paternalistic model may be appropriate for demented patients or patients who prefer to defer to healthcare professionals. Different models might even be appropriate for different choices by the same patient.

Section 4: The meaning and ethical significance of old age

In this final section we will consider, in the light of our reflections of the importance of relationships, whether

there is anything unique about ethics in long-term care. Although we will take old age as our focus, we must remember that not all long-term care involves the elderly; as you read through the section, you might like to consider the similarities and differences between long-term care of the elderly and long-term care with other groups.

ACTIVITY: As you read through the following case study, consider the kinds of relationships being described and how such relationships can have implications for the 'meaning' of a person's life both for themselves and also for others.

The case of Emmi

Emmi is 85 years old and lives in a nursing home, suffering from the effect of two serious strokes. She has always been very particular about her appearance. Even now she continues to wear nice clothes and make up, despite the weakness in her left side.

Recently she suffered a further stroke which left her with a lasting paralysis of the throat. It has become necessary to change Emmi's diet and to feed her only pureed food. Despite this the food still often gets caught in her throat. Emmi feels ashamed about this and about the way she appears when eating in company with the others who live in the home.

At a recent staff meeting, one of the workers thought it might help if Emmi could be fed in her room. Other workers felt, however, that she should come out and eat with the others, as not to do so would mean isolating herself. It was decided that the head nurse would speak to the other residents. They said that they thought it was 'disgusting' when Emmi coughed at the dinner table and that she had difficulties with swallowing. The result of this discussion was that Emmi started to sit off to the side and sometimes even to eat in the nursing home's kitchen. For practical reasons, it was not possible for Emmi to eat at a different time to the other residents. The nurses cannot afford to spend any more time over meals than they already do as there are not enough staff. The other residents continue to say that they are disgusted by Emmi.

Emmi's doctor and the nursing home staff are considering using a new artificial and medically assisted type of food provision for Emmi. However, Emmi makes it clear to the nurses that she will refuse any and every form of artificial food and fluid administration.

Commentary on the case of Emmi

Chris Gastmans[6]

Caring should always be considered as an inter-human endeavour. It is not only the nurse, but also the resident, nursing colleagues and doctors, who play essential roles in the caring process. All of these participants have their own ethical and practice-based intuitions concerning the essential meaning of 'good care'. In the case of Emmi, the ethical intuitions of all are being tested. The interdisciplinary team of doctors and nurses is being challenged to clarify and justify their opinions about 'good nutritional care'.

It is worth mentioning that it is not very common for nurses and patients to talk about problems such as those described in this case. The day-to-day aspects of work in a residential home mean that nurses have very little time available for this kind of activity. There is not much time left for reflection on the human quality of the care provided. Residents like Emmi are often ashamed to ask for more attention from the nurse, and it is therefore up to the nurses to take the initiative and to adopt an attitude that invites con-fidences within the limits of time and resources available.

I would like to give some short suggestions on how to come to an ethically 'acceptable solution' in a case like that involving Emmi.

Firstly, as much information as possible about the case has to be collected. Informing ourselves about the technical and factual aspects of the problem is the first step in the ethical reflection process. If the prob-lem is described in a one-sided, incomplete or even inaccurate manner, then the ethical question itself and the solution we give to the question will be distorted.

Which possible ways are there in which we could help Emmi with her eating and drinking problems? Is there enough attention in the way nurses deal with the difficulties Emmi faces with eating and drinking? Is there enough space and time provided to help Emmi during meal times? These and many other questions have to be answered if we are to gain an insight into the real problem described in the case of Emmi.

Secondly, the emotional and intuitive reactions of all those involved in the case have to be clarified. This is important because whilst ethics is generally represented as a rational endeavour, to see it as such inevitably excludes emotions from the ethical dis-cussion. I want to deny this option. In my opinion, emotions are the 'feelers' with which ethical prob-lems can be detected. The emotional reactions (e.g. disgust) of the elderly residents make it clear that there is a (value-laden) problem with Emmi. The other elderly people experience the life situation of Emmi as a contradiction to human dignity. It is also important that the emotions and the quite unclear attitudes about 'good nutritional care' of all people involved in Emmi's care should be clarified. What are the real motivations for Emmi's refusal of every type of artifi-cial food and fluid administration? What are the atti-tudes of the nurses towards eating and drinking disorders? Are there any religious or cultural perspec-tives on meals expressed by Emmi, nurses, doctors and other residents? What kinds of personal experi-ences have the nurses themselves had with meals?

If this clarification doesn't take place, emotional reactions threaten to dominate or even block the ethical discussion altogether. The ethical debate, however, should not only be based upon emotions. Emotions and intuitions fulfil an important role in the detection of unethical situations, but in the discussion of ethical problems, the emotional level has to be transcended. For we have to evolve towards the level of rational ethical argumentation.

Thirdly, during the ethical clarification process various alternative solutions must be evaluated. This evaluation consists of a clarification of the moral values (advantages) and disvalues (disadvantages) which are inherent in each alternative.

At first sight, two alternative solutions might be distinguished. The first of these would be to force Emmi to be fed in an artificial (medically assisted) way. This 'solution' possibly brings a higher level of physical wellbeing for Emmi, which can be seen as a value (a quality which we spontaneously view in a positive way). Nevertheless, ignoring the wishes of Emmi is undoubtedly a 'disvalue' (something we condemn spontaneously). The second possible solu-tion would be for the nurses to continue feeding Emmi in a natural way, despite all the difficulties (e.g. isolation during meal times). As the most impor-tant value, we have to consider in this regard the respect for Emmi's autonomy. On the other hand, there is another disvalue which surfaces, namely the disruption of Emmi's chances of a higher level of physical and social development.

ACTIVITY: Gastmans, a Belgian professor of med-ical ethics, here emphasizes the meaning and symbolic significance of feeding and inter-personal relations in long-term care. Two alter-native solutions appear to emerge: either to force Emmi to accept artificial nutrition or to continue feeding her as 'naturally' as possible despite the difficulties this presents. What are the arguments in favour of and against each of these 'solutions'?

After having conscientiously weighed up the values and disvalues which are inherent in both alternative solutions, I have to admit that neither of these 'solutions' is acceptable to me. Moreover, I feel uncomfortable seeing Emmi losing the battle of being right between the doctor and the nurses. The important ethical question is not 'who is right?' or 'who may decide?' but 'what is good for Emmi?'.

With that last question, we return to the essence of our case. What should the nurses do with Emmi? Should they introduce artificial food and fluid administration or not? The answer to this question has to be the result of an interdisciplinary consultation including all those involved in the case. In our opinion, this case requires an individualized approach. Maximum attention should be given to the development of a relationship based on trust between the nurses and Emmi. They have to search together for the 'most humanly possible' outcome which can be realized in this (not ideal) situation. The autonomy of Emmi should be promoted by maintaining and supporting the natural feeding process. To realize this ethical option in the case of Emmi, a high level of competency, creativity and devotion will be required.

It is my opinion that the question of the artificial administration of food and fluids should only be taken into account when the capacity and the will of Emmi to continue the natural feeding process are undermined, and when all medical and nursing means to postpone or avoid the artificial fluid and food administration fail. Emmi unambiguously expresses her will to eat and drink in a natural way. Taking into account her capacity to achieve this, nurses have to analyse the ways in which they might be able to support and even promote Emmi's ability to do things independently as much as possible. In my opinion, supporting Emmi in her natural feeding and drinking behaviour, adopting an attitude of respect and patience, seems to be the most responsible ethical caring behaviour that nurses can show. If nurses do their best to put this ethical option into practice, they consider themselves as persons who are supposed to accept a certain amount of responsibility (moral agents), rather than as victims of circumstances beyond their control (in this case, the shortage of staff).

ACTIVITY: As we near the end of this chapter it is clear that there is a range of ethical questions which occur in long-term care, some of which appear to differ considerably from those we encounter elsewhere. To what extent do you think that long-term care, and cases like Emmi's, require a unique approach, distinct from standard 'principlist' approaches?

What is special about old age?

Guy Widdershoven introduced the idea of ethics as concerning the meaningfulness of relationships, and he used the Emanuels' schema for analysing the moral dimension of different types of patient–doctor relationship. Ultimately, he argued that the deliberative model is the best approach because it respects and enhances meaningfulness and meaning-making in some way, i.e. it allows and enables both patients and physicians to engage in the joint process of 'making sense'.

One question which has not been addressed directly, though it has been a theme running through this chapter as a whole, is that of the meaning of old age itself: whether this period of life is distinct in any morally significant way. An approach based on the meaning and significance of relationships must surely require some consideration of the differences (if indeed there are any) between the meaning(s) of different stages of life.

Yet it is not necessarily the case that there is a distinct stage of life which we might call 'old age'. Socially constructed understandings of 'old age' can be challenged, particularly when, in much of the developed world at least, populations not only live but also remain active for longer – a trend which is neatly captured by 'older and bolder' campaigns. However, we might still agree that there are features of life as it comes to its end which are distinctive. It seems likely that many of us as we reach the later years of our lives will reflect more on the nature of our decline and death than we did when we were younger and will perhaps begin to reflect increasingly on the nature of our lives as a whole.

It remains the case, however, that we are reluctant to talk about these things publicly. The US bioethicist Daniel Callahan, in his book *Setting Limits* (1987), argues that there is an urgent need for a public discussion of the values and distinctive characteristics of old age. He suggests that modern patient-centred medicine (the bioethics approach described by Widdershoven earlier) has tended to undermine the meaningfulness of old age by its emphasis on individualism and life-extending treatments. He suggests that it is tempting for us to avoid a consideration of the meaning of old age and to be fearful of it. Modern medicine and modern individualistic society tend to consider old age as if it were an inferior version of earlier stages of life. Callahan rejects this conceptualization and demands that we take the distinctive features and values of old age seriously. He asks:

> What kind of sense can be made of old age, of the fact that our bodies change and decline, sicken and decay, and then die? Even if we distinguish between growing old and becoming ill, between becoming old and becoming stale, between chronological and biological age, or between our externally assigned social role and our internal sense of place – even if, that is, we make all of the distinctions recommended in the professional literature on ageing, in the end death happens, and we exist no more. While old age and death are obviously distinguishable, death comes at the end of old age. How should we prepare for that moment, and what should we think about it?
>
> (Callahan, 1987, p. 31)

ACTIVITY: Read the following descriptions of the importance and distinctiveness of old age and reflect on how these differ from or reinforce your own view.

Three pictures of old age

Cicero (44 BC)

> Old men ... as they become less capable of physical exertion, should redouble their intellectual activity, and their principal occupation should be to assist the young, their friends, and above all their country with their wisdom and sagacity. There is nothing they should guard against so much as languor and sloth. Luxury, which is shameful at every period of life, makes old age hideous. If it is united with sensuality, the evil is two-fold. Age thus brings disgrace on itself and aggravates the shameless licence of the young.
>
> (Cicero, 1951, p. 47. Quoted in Callahan, 1987)

Simone de Beauvoir (1972)

> The greatest good fortune, even greater than health, for the old person is to have his world inhabited by projects; then busy and useful, he escapes both from boredom and decay ... There is only one solution if old age is not to be an absurd parody of our former life, and that is to go on

pursuing ends that give our existence a meaning – devotion to individuals, to groups or to causes, social, political, intellectual or creative work. In spite of the moralists' opinion to the contrary, in old age we should still wish to have passions strong enough to prevent us from turning in upon ourselves.
>
> (de Beauvoir, 1972, p. 28. Quoted in Callahan, 1987)

Daniel Callahan (1987)

> Old age has to find an integral place in the lives of those who ... become old. An old age lacking in meaning is not, save for the rarest person, a humanly tolerable condition. Yet, even if there is some agreement that the search for a common meaning would be valuable, it requires the complementary help of a reinvigorated theory of the life-cycle (including old age) ... Our civilisation has repudiated the concept of the whole life .... A concept of a whole life requires a number of conditions (such as) that life [is seen to] have stages ...
>
> (Callahan, 1987, p. 40)

Aristotle

Callahan's emphasis on the fact that the meaning of old age (or of any other stage) can only be grasped or worked out within a conception of the life as a whole, follows Aristotle, who argued in relation to ethics that:

> The good for man is an activity of soul in accordance with virtue, or if there are more kinds of virtue than one, in accordance with the best and most perfect kind. There is a further qualification: *in a complete life*. One swallow does not make a summer; neither does one day. Similarly neither can one day, or a brief space of time, make a man blessed and happy.
>
> (Aristotle, 1908, reprint 2002, p. 76)

This conception of ethics as both related to meaning and in particular to the meaning of the whole life seems to imply that old age has a very special status in relation to ethics. It is *only* at the end of life that we can reflect upon and consider our lives as a whole. Despite this, however, and in relation to the quote from Callahan earlier, the fact is that whilst old age might be ethically special, it is so if at all because we have to come to terms with some very difficult facts about ourselves and those around us, notably the inevitability of our decline and death. This in itself may mean that not everyone is going to be able to reflect or to engage in narrative, and this must be seen as a limitation of the narrative approach, which would seem to depend to at least some extent upon a range of cognitive capacities. Nevertheless, the narrative ideal, as expressed by Alasdair MacIntyre below, still has great appeal.

> Both childhood and old age have [mistakenly] been wrenched from the rest of human life and made over into distinct realms . . . it is the distinctiveness of each and not the unity of the life of the individual . . . of which we are taught to think and to feel . . . The unity of a human life [should instead be] the unity of a narrative quest.
>
> (MacIntyre, 1981)

Notes

1. Adapted with permission from Guy Widdershoven, 'Truth and truth-telling'. Paper presented at EBEPE workshop.

2. Reproduced with permission from Tony Hope, 'A commentary on the case of Mr A'. Paper presented at EBEPE workshop.

3. Adapted with permission from Ruud ter Meulen, 'Care for dependent elderly persons and respect for autonomy'. Paper presented at Seventh EBEPE workshop, Maastricht.

4. Adapted with permission from Gwen Adshead, 'Autonomy, feminism and psychiatric patients'. Paper presented at EBEPE conference.

5. Reproduced with permission from Tony Hope.

6. Reproduced with permission from Chris Gastmans.

7 Children and young people: conflicting responsibilities

Introduction

> States parties shall assure to the child who is capable of forming his or her own views the right to express those views freely in all matters affecting the child, the view of the child being given due weight in accordance with the age and maturity of the child … The child shall in particular have the opportunity to be heard in any judicial and administrative proceedings affecting the child, either directly or through a representative or an appropriate body, in a manner consistent with the procedural rules of national law.
>
> (Article 12) UN Convention on the Rights of the Child (1989)

To whom does the child care practitioner have responsibilities? Working with children and young people brings with it ethical responsibilities which may be different from those involved in work with adults. One answer to this question emphasizes the importance of listening to what children have to say. To a certain extent this child-centred approach can be said to reflect medicine's more general concern (particularly in northern Europe and the USA) with patient-centred care. It is commonly felt that practitioners ought to weigh up the value of a medical intervention solely in terms of the benefits and risks it is likely to have for the patient in front of them, in relation to that person's autonomy, and quite apart from the wishes of others such as the patient's family.

The patient-centred approach defines the relationship between the patient and the practitioner as the arena of care and hence of moral concern. The moral agents in such cases are assumed to be the patient and the doctor or other healthcare practitioner. But this approach does not resolve all of the particular difficulties faced by practitioners in their work with children. For, even from the perspective of children's rights it is often possible in such cases to ask oneself, 'Where do my responsibilities lie?' 'Who is the patient?' Is it the child, is it the child's family and parents, or is it some combination of these? Patient-centred care will have different meanings and different implications for practice in each of these cases.

Section 1: The child in the family

ACTIVITY: Before going on with the chapter, stop here for a moment and, in relation to your own experience, think about the practical and ethical implications of different possible answers to the questions raised above. What, for example, ought to happen in cases where there is or appears to be conflict between the practitioner's perception of the child's best interests and the parents' perception?

Please read the following case study and consider what ethical issues it raises about working with children and their families.

The case of Sean

Sean is 15 years old. He lives at home with his parents and a sister who is 12. His father is a senior civil servant and his mother is a healthcare professional. They live in a small town in an affluent part of Ireland.

When Sean's father first made contact with the therapist he said that he was looking for help for his son because the boy seemed to have a 'chip on his shoulder' and was always in trouble. He said that he had persuaded Sean to see someone. They arrived together for the first session but Sean was seen on his own.

Sean was anxious and uncomfortable, uncertain why he was there. He felt that he was being blamed for the tension that existed between his parents. It seemed that there had always been conflict between father and son; when Sean was younger he was frequently beaten for what he saw as minor misdemeanours. He said that his father would hit first and

---

possibly listen later. Sean felt that he could not rely on his mother to protect him from his father's anger. Sean had harboured fantasies for at least the last six years of 'getting his own back' by beating his father. He also constantly talked about wanting to be away from home.

Sean says that he has always felt that he is not good enough, that he has not achieved enough and is a disappointment to his parents. The transition from junior to senior school was a difficult one for Sean. In the senior school he associated with the boys in his class who smoked and took time off school. He felt that one teacher in particular was against him, because he constantly reprimanded and punished Sean for being cheeky. Two years ago there was a disagreement between Sean and the teacher during which Sean hit the teacher. Sean was then expelled from school.

His parents were very angry with him and immediately sent him away to boarding school. Sean was very distressed and refused to go but he was forcibly taken to the school and left there. In the first few weeks he was bullied by the other boys and ran away. He was apprehended by the police and returned to school where he continued to be subjected to frequent beatings. A little later he ran away again and managed to avoid being found by hiding in a derelict building. He then returned home, where he was surprised by his parents' acceptance that he did not want to return to the boarding school. Instead he was to attend as a day boy at a school nearby. Since then there had been no further conflict at the school he does attend.

Disagreements continue at home, however. Sean feels that his parents, his father in particular, are constantly spying on him. He is never allowed to be in the house on his own. Sometimes he is allowed to go out with his friends, but sometimes this is refused. He has continued to get into fights with other youths in the town and on one recent occasion was seriously assaulted. He feels bitter that his father did not find the youth and beat him up. He is nervous when he goes into town and recently has started to drink very large amounts of alcohol. This has caused more arguments at home, but Sean feels that his father has been hypocritical because he also drinks heavily on occasion.

Sean is confused about why he should need to see a therapist. He feels that his father is the cause of all his problems and is trying to offload the blame onto him. Sean's father wants his son to settle down to work at school so that he can go to university. He feels frustrated and angry about his son's behaviour and hopes that a few sessions with the therapist will 'sort him out'.

ACTIVITY: What do you think the therapist should do in Sean's case? In the light of the case study and your own experience, consider the following questions:

(1) What do you think are the practitioner's duties and responsibilities in cases such as the one above? To whom is the psychotherapist responsible in this case, and who is the patient? Clearly Sean doesn't want to be in therapy, though it might be said that he does appear to have a reasonably good understanding of *why* he is there. If you were the practitioner in this case, where would you see your responsibilities?

(2) Very often the interests of all the various parties (the young person, their parents, etc.) seem to pull in the same direction – but there are also occasions when they do not. If the best interests of the child are to be identified with remaining in the family, does this mean that the practitioner ought to follow the wishes of the parents, even when the young person does not request or accept treatment? Think of any cases from your own experience for a moment. Where would you as a practitioner place your responsibilities?

(3) Is it in fact always the case that the cohesion of the family is best obtained by respecting the wishes of the parents? Is it possible that by respecting parents' wishes a practitioner may not achieve it? Can you imagine a situation in which this might be the case?

The quotation from the UN Convention at the start of this chapter suggests that listening to the child's voice ought to be central to work with children. But is the patient-centred approach a realistic or workable model in all work with children? Surely to view the child solely as an individual is to exclude a large and important part of the child's world. It means leaving out those others who would seem to have a legitimate interest in the outcome of any intervention, such as the child's parents, siblings and other relatives. Whilst it is important to some extent for us to consider the child as an individual, being an individual is at most only part of what any of us are. We are also social beings defined by relationships and social interactions. The implication of this is that in at least some cases account will need to be taken of people other than simply the child and the healthcare practitioner.

To focus solely on the one-to-one relationship between practitioner and patient, in this case the child, is to ignore the fact that both patient and practitioner are inevitably part of wider social networks which are of crucial moral significance. In the case of children this often tends to mean their family and in particular their parents. There is usually a variety of interested parties in any case and surely these others ought to have their importance recognized. This is particularly the case with children and their families.

> It should not be forgotten that the child's interest [tends to] depend upon his well-being within his family. In this regard children teach us wisdom. They often minimise the conflicts of opposition ... A child who is hurting does not easily submit to treatment, particularly if this hurts his parents!
>
> (Hattab, 1996)

Hattab seems to be arguing here that when considering ethical questions relating to working with a child, it is essential to be aware not only of the child herself, but also of the social context in which she lives. What will the effects of an intervention be upon the child's family or other social relationships? If it will be in the child's interests in the short term but will destroy the family in the longer term, is it in the overall interests of the young person? It is also important to remember that the child is often but not always a member of a family, and that parents or guardians have a special form of relationship with and responsibility for the child.

ACTIVITY: What do you think about this point? Is there something special about the child's social location as compared to the adult's? Hattab's idea that the child is always the *child in the family* also raises important questions. One of these is once again the question of where the healthcare practitioner's responsibility lies in work with young people. Whom is the practitioner treating: the child, her parents or the family as a whole?

Is it always the case that the preservation of the family unit is in the child's best interests? If not, what alternatives are there, and what might be their ethical implications? Can you imagine circumstances in which a child ought to be treated without his or her parents' consent?

What do you see as the risks of seeing children as part of a family? Why might it be important to focus on the needs and wishes of the child as an individual rather than as a family member?

Hattab suggests that in practice children often place the stability of their family above their own immediate wellbeing. Can you think of any reasons why this might be?

There will obviously be cases where it is hard to say just where the practitioner's responsibilities lie when the child's voice collides with parents' preferences. In such cases we might want to say that the real responsibility is to act according to the *best interests* of the child or young person. 'Best interests' seems to be a middle position between uncritically accepting the 'child's voice', on the one hand, and equally uncritically, assuming that the child is always best served by respecting the parents' wishes, in the interests of family unity.

Now read the following two statements.

> The interest of the child, a consideration which appears in the Conventions and in other international instruments drawn up during the last forty years, is more than just a recurring theme, it is a true fundamental and universally shared idea.
>
> (Magno, 1996)

> In all actions concerning children whether undertaken by public or private social welfare institutions ... the best interests of the child shall be a primary consideration.
>
> (Article 3, UN Convention on the Rights of the Child)

ACTIVITY: What does the idea of the best interests of the child mean? The idea is framed in the UN Convention and in the national laws of many countries, but what does it mean in practice? In some ways these two statements might be seen to be on the same side of the fence, but in themselves and in the light of our consideration of the questions raised by Sean's case, they appear too simplistic.

Sean's case exemplifies the ways in which our sense of our responsibilities as practitioner to children and to their families or guardians might pull in opposite directions. But might we not also be pulled in other directions by other responsibilities such as those we have to other practitioners or to the law?

Take a moment to consider the various other responsibilities which might impinge upon the work of a practitioner in relation to children and young people.

The General Medical Council has issued guidance to doctors in England and Wales on assessing a child or young person's best interests, which contains the following points:

0–18 years: Guidance for all doctors (General Medical Council, 2007)

12. An assessment of best interests will include what is clinically indicated in a particular case. You should also consider:
    a. the views of the child or young person, so far as they can express them, including any previously expressed preferences
    b. the views of parents
    c. the views of others close to the child or young person
    d. the cultural, religious or other beliefs and values of the child or parents
    e. the views of other healthcare professionals involved in providing care to the child or young person, and of any other professionals who have an interest in their welfare
    f. which choice, if there is more than one, will least restrict the child or young person's future options.
13. This list is not exhaustive. The weight you attach to each point will depend on the circumstances, and you should consider any other relevant information. You should not make unjustified assumptions about a child or young person's best interests based on irrelevant or discriminatory factors, such as their behaviour, appearance or disability.

In England and Wales the paramount legal principle in deciding all questions about the child's upbringing, including health decisions, is the *child's welfare*. This is a form of the 'best interests' principle. As we can see in the General Medical Council guidance, the other two principles, the *child's voice* and *family cohesion*, are also considered to be relevant to the child's welfare, but they may be overridden.

In the Children Act 1989, 'welfare' is not explicitly defined, but courts are directed to apply a 'welfare checklist' of relevant factors. The 'ascertainable wishes and feelings' of the child – expressions of the child's voice – are one factor, and in fact they come first on the list (s1[3][a]). But the checklist also directs health- and social-care practitioners to consider the child's physical, emotional and educational needs; the likely effects of changes in circumstances (which would

presumably include any changes undermining family unity); harm which the child has suffered or is at risk of suffering; the child's age, sex and background. Another factor in the checklist also allows family unity to be overridden if that is in the child's best interests: 'how capable each of his parents ... is of meeting his needs'.

So the Children Act, the most all-embracing legislation on children in England and Wales, tells practitioners that their main responsibility is to uphold the child's best interests. But what sort of guidance does this provide in difficult clinical decisions? In the next section we will look at this question in greater detail.

Section 2: Consent to treatment and the child's best interests

In Section 1 we looked at three possible interpretations of the practitioner's principal responsibility:

- to listen to the 'child's voice',
- to maintain 'family unity', or
- to think first and foremost of the child's 'best interests'.

It will not always be easy to determine the child's best interests: as we saw in Sean's case, the child's own assessment of his or her interests might be quite at odds with that made by his or her parents, and there is also the physician's own assessment of the child's best interests to consider. Perhaps the doctor disagrees with both the parents and the child; perhaps he or she agrees with one parent more than the other. It is, perhaps, possible to argue that the crucial question here is not so much 'what treatment is in the child's best interests?' but '*who decides* what treatment is in the child's best interests?' A related question is this: who has the ultimate power to give or withhold consent to treatment?

ACTIVITY: Please read the following case study. As you read, ask yourself these questions:

(1) What conflicting interpretations of the child's best interests are illustrated by this case? Who has the ultimate power to give or withhold consent, based on their interpretation of the child's best interests?

(2) How does the child psychiatrist in this case interpret his responsibilities?

The case of Emilia

Emilia, aged four, had been brought to a child psy-chiatrist because she had regressed in her behaviour and speech. Since her parents separated, on the grounds of the husband's alleged physical violence against his wife, Emilia had been living with her mother. However, she had seen her father on regular access visits.

Clinical examination of Emilia revealed high risks of psychopathological disorders, but no current iden-tifiable pathology. Emilia's mother was concerned that the child's condition was worsening, and she attributed the child's problems to stress induced by fear of her violent father. She asked the psychiatrist to support her application for a court order discontinu-ing the father's access visits. The psychiatrist refused, stating that 'It is part of the therapy to side with the child rather than with either parent'.

After an initial period during which Emilia regu-larly attended therapy sessions, with reasonably good results, the mother renewed her request to the psy-chiatrist for an expert opinion to back up her court application. The psychiatrist again refused. There was no overt confrontation, but the mother stopped tak-ing Emilia to the therapy sessions.

In Emilia's case, considerations of her best interests quickly come to the fore – after all, given her age, we might think that Emilia's 'voice' is less relevant than in a case like Sean's, and, since her parents are already divorced, unity of the family is not really an option. However, determining Emilia's best interests is clouded by the fact that Emilia's mother's interpreta-tion of her child's best interests clashes with that of the clinician. Emilia's mother feared that regular access visits were harming the child; that harm, she judged, was the real cause of Emilia's speech and behaviour problems. She has the ultimate power to withhold consent to treatment on Emilia's behalf, but her power may seem rather hollow to her because it is only negative. It does not extend to success in persuad-ing the psychiatrist to give expert testimony against the access visits, which she views as the step most likely to advance Emilia's best interests.

The psychiatrist thought that therapy was pro-gressing favourably, and that the child's best interests lay in continuing it. He viewed the mother's refusal to continue therapy for Emilia as motivated by annoy-ance at her failure to win him over to her side in the court case, not by concern for Emilia's best interests. Yet in stating that 'it is part of the therapy to side with the child rather than with either parent', was the psy-chiatrist ignoring his responsibilities? There might be times when 'therapeutic neutrality' is not really in the child's best interests, either. If the mother was right – and she had reason to think that the father was violent, at least in her own case – perhaps the access visits really were the underlying cause of Emilia's problems, and no amount of therapy would work unless the under-lying problem was removed.

In Emilia's case, there was no possibility of forcing the mother to continue taking Emilia to therapy, it seems. But in other sorts of cases involuntary treat-ment does arise. In the extreme case, that might mean treating the young person against his or her will. Yet with adults, at least, consent to treatment is fundamen-tal in most legal systems. In English common law, for example, intervention in the absence of consent con-stitutes battery. What is true of common law in England – judge-made law, relying on precedents set down in earlier cases – is true of statute or constitu-tional law in other European jurisdictions. Article 32 of the Italian Constitution, for example, states that no one can be given treatment against his or her will, although in the case of minors the right to be informed is legally vested in the parents (Calzone, 1996).

Sean's case illustrates a comparatively mild exam-ple of treating the young person against his or her will. Sean is uncertain about whether or why he needs psychotherapy, and he feels scapegoated by his father. That raised issues about who was the 'real' patient: was the clinician in Sean's case responsible primarily to Sean or to his father? However, Sean doesn't actually have to be forced to attend therapy – although there was a strong element of compulsion in his being made to attend boarding school by his parents. That, how-ever, is not involuntary medical treatment. Indeed, because Sean was being treated by a 'talking' cure, it's hard to see how forcible treatment could be present in his case.

Yet there will be occasions when we want, and need, to treat a child against their will, possibly even in very intrusive ways like enforcing feeding or admin-istering injections. The notion of treating children against their will can arise because in many legal sys-tems children are *presumed incompetent* to consent to treatment, whereas adults are presumed *competent*. As we just noted, the Italian legal system vests the right to be informed in parents rather than children, assuming that children are less than fully competent to give or withhold consent to their own treatment. Different legal systems may accord different possibilities for minors to prove that they are capable of giving or refusing consent to treatment. But whereas adults' refusal of treatment is generally taken at face value, that of children and young people may not be. Even where a child or young person consents to treatment, perhaps we ought to think about this question: what does it mean for a child to give consent, if a child cannot legally refuse treatment? In other words, can a child genuinely consent?

It is especially important to consider cases of involuntary treatment, against the child's expressed wishes but in the name of his or her best interests – because they raise in the starkest form the conflict between the child's autonomy and the physician's duty to act in the child's best interests of beneficence. What are the practitioner's responsibilities if the child refuses treatment?

ACTIVITY: Stop here for a moment and think what sorts of cases these might be. Have you encountered any in your own experience? Have any come up in your national press? If you can think of more than one case, were there any common threads? You might also like to reread the case of W in Chapter 5 on mental health, which raised similar issues concerning a young woman suffering from anorexia nervosa.

The 'best interests' of the patient, and how we are to understand and interpret this concept, is likely to be one of the key themes arising in cases involving young people who decline to accept the treatment recommended by their carers. Sometimes the young person's opinion might stand in stark contrast to the consensus view adopted by his or her doctors and other professional carers. But sometimes there might be more than one clinical interpretation of what is 'really' in the child's best interests; 'best interests' is not an objective, agreed criterion that puts an end to all dispute. And to the extent that the young person is more likely to comply with a treatment regime that fits her own wishes, 'best interests' and 'the child's voice' converge.

Yet the young person's best interests might encompass more than this. We noted earlier that family unity can be an important goal, albeit one which raises the question of who the patient is: the young person or the family. But in some cases, the family unit may have broken down – for example, W's parents were entirely absent, and she was in local authority care. Are the clinician's responsibilities different in

such a case? We no longer need to consider the family, it seems. But if the child's interest does not then depend on her wellbeing in the family – as Hattab claimed – what does it depend on?

Amongst the most troubling cases are likely to be those in which the young person's decision appears to put his or her life in jeopardy. Does this mean that the responsibilities of the practitioner are more serious in a case like this than in, say, Sean's case? Should practitioners automatically give preference to the treatment which has the best chance of keeping the patient alive, even against his or her wishes? What could be more truly in the child's best interests than keeping him or her alive, after all? One case in which these questions might arise involves the young person who refuses treatment on religious grounds, such as a Jehovah's Witness. Jehovah's Witness parents would not see their child's 'best interest' as mere continuation of life, but as eternal salvation. Because blood transfusions may be regarded as an offence which carries the risk of eternal damnation, the real 'best interests' of their child, they might argue, lie in refusing consent to transfusions – even if that means death.

ACTIVITY: Now please read the following Dutch case study concerning a 12-year-old Jehovah's Witness boy with cystic fibrosis. As you read, ask yourself these questions:

(1) Was this child competent to give or withhold consent to treatment?
(2) How relevant is the child's age in this case?
(3) What would have been the consequences of taking custody of the child away from the parents and imposing treatment in the name of the child's best interests?

The case of JW

JW was a 12-year-old boy who had cystic fibrosis. Since his condition had been diagnosed JW had been visiting the same hospital and physicians regularly for many years. Both he and his family were well known to the staff there and enjoyed a good relationship with them. In recent months, however, the boy's condition had become very serious. He had developed extensive varices of the oesophagus which brought with them an accompanying risk of serious bleeding which would put the boy's life in danger.

When the doctor informed the family that the seriousness of the boy's condition might require a blood transfusion in order to save his life, both the boy and his family refused to consider such an option because of their faith. For the whole family were devout and active Jehovah's Witnesses.

The paediatricians involved in the case disagreed about how they ought to proceed and asked a child psychiatrist to assess the child's competence to make the decision to refuse treatment. One possible option which was considered was to make an application for a court order to take custody of the boy away from his parents in order to allow the transfusion to take place.

The psychiatrist reported that the boy was intelligent and sensitive, that he was in no sense emotionally or socially disturbed and that he had a good relationship with his parents. He also had a clear understanding of his illness and of the treatment and was conscious of the consequences of his decisions to refuse a blood transfusion. He stuck to his decision and said that his parents had exerted no pressure on him. He simply wanted to live according to the principles of his faith.

After interviewing the parents as well, it seemed clear that they cared very much for their son and indeed for all of their children. On the whole they were rational about the decision to refuse the transfusion and appeared, as the boy himself had said, not to have put any explicit pressure on the boy to refuse the treatment.

It seemed clear that this was a caring family who, in the light of their religious beliefs had come to a reasoned decision to refuse this particular form of treatment.

In this case the child's competence appears quite plausible, so that the 'child's voice' arguments appear well-founded. But although the child did seem able to judge the consequences accurately, we are also told that he was still young enough to be very dependent on his parents and their opinion. They, in turn, were not entirely autonomous, but perhaps under pressure from their religious community. So the 'child's voice' and 'unity of the family' positions both argue in favour of allowing the boy to refuse transfusions, but should they take precedence over the child's 'objective' best interest in longer life? That question is complicated in this case by the boy's cystic fibrosis. Although cystic fibrosis sufferers whose condition is detected and treated early in childhood do now survive into adulthood, late adolescence was frequently the limit of their lifespan in the past. So there is no straightforward contest between extended life and religious belief in this case; it may be well be that the boy's long-term survival is doubtful in any case.

English law allows adult Jehovah's Witnesses to refuse blood transfusions, but does not extend the same right to young people. However, there has been at least one case (*Re E* [1993]) in which a Jehovah's Witness boy with leukaemia, whose refusal of a transfusion had been overruled when he was 15, elected to refuse further transfusions as soon as he turned 18, and then died.

It is worth bearing in mind when considering cases involving Jehovah's Witnesses that the question of acceptable surgical techniques is changing quite rapidly (e.g. the use of the bloodless stem cell transplant; Sloan and Ballen, 2008) and that whilst such cases are useful for raising ethical questions, practice in these cases and the view of the Jehovah's Witness community is more subtle than is usually assumed.

Now please read the following article by John Pearce, a specialist in child and adolescent psychiatry based in England.

Ethical issues in child psychiatry and child psychotherapy: conflicts between the child, parents and practitioners

John Pearce[1]

Children are not given the same freedom as adults to give consent to treatment and to make ethical decisions. These are not simple decisions. In fact the distinction between what constitutes a child and what makes an adult different from a child is extremely blurred. Every adult is also somebody's child. And all children have similar qualities of character, mental function and physical activity to those that adults have. What differences there are between children and adults are concerned almost entirely with maturation and development – with quantity and complexity.

There is no absolute definition of what a child is. Whatever age is decided upon to distinguish between childhood and adulthood will always be open to debate. In any case it is more appropriate to use a child's stage of development rather than the chronological age when making this decision.

In spite of the problems that arise from thinking in terms of absolutes, a line does have to be drawn somewhere and ethical decisions have to be made.

Nevertheless, there will invariably be scope for disagreement as to exactly where or how the distinction should be made, and conflicts between children, parents and clinicians may be difficult to avoid. One way in which people have attempted to resolve conflicts about ethical issues in relation to children is to make decisions that are always in the best interest of the child. This sounds ethical and inherently right. However, there is still plenty of scope for disagreement and conflict even with this praiseworthy goal in mind. For example, in the case of an emotionally abused child – is it best to remove the abusing parent from the home of the child, or the child from the abusing and rejecting home?

Although it is clearly difficult to make ethical decisions and avoid conflict, a good starting point is to clearly recognize that making absolute distinctions will inevitably give rise to problems and confusions. The process of ethical decision-making will be enabled and the likelihood of conflict will be reduced if the following factors are taken into account:

(1) *The child's stage of development*. It is essential to recognize the ever-changing needs of children that are influenced by the stage of development that they have reached. Thus a knowledge of child development is central to ethical decision-making in relation to the clinical treatment of children.
(2) *Relationships between children and significant others*. Decisions about clinical treatment and the ethical issues that arise must be considered in the context of the relationships that the child has with significant figures such as their parents, their clinicians, relatives, teachers and peers. The child who has a poor relationship with his or her parents may reject a recommended treatment merely to make the parents angry and upset. This can present the clinician with the ethical dilemma whether or not to override the child's refusal to consent to treatment. Positive relationships make conflicts in clinical decision-making much less likely to occur.
(3) *Taking time to make decisions*. Because children's needs are constantly changing, it is usually best to take time before arriving at treatment decisions involving ethical issues where there is the likelihood of conflict between the child, the parent or the practitioner. It takes time to assess the stage of development that children have reached and

the nature of their relationships, as well as to gain an adequate awareness of their various needs. A child who has refused to consent to a particular treatment on one occasion may reverse that decision several days later, in the context of their developing awareness or their changing relationships.
(4) *Rights and responsibilities must be considered together*. If children are given rights without considering who takes the responsibility associated with these rights, this can easily lead to children being exposed to having to make decisions for which they are not in a position to take responsibility. Although every human being has equal rights, they may not have equal responsibilities. The responsibility for babies' rights or the rights of the person with learning disabilities has to be taken by the primary caregiver. In clinical practice these responsibilities are shared between the child, the parents and the clinicians. A recognition of this shared responsibility for decision-making is probably the most important factor that can reduce conflict in ethical decision making.

In conclusion, the conflicts that arise in clinical decision-making between children, parents and therapists are firmly rooted in the natural tendency to think in terms of absolutes with a clear line drawn between opposing views. Such polarization of opinions puts children at risk of inappropriate and possibly dangerous decisions being made. The chance of harmful conflict can be reduced by an awareness of the central importance of child development and supportive relationships. Agreement on clinical and ethical issues is much more likely if sufficient time is allowed for a decision to be made.

Pearce concludes by warning against 'the natural tendency to think in terms of absolutes with a clear line drawn between opposing views'. This is a useful reminder at our current point in this chapter. For clarity in analysing decisions, we've separated out best interests, the child's voice or rights and family unity. Pearce, however, reminds us that the effective making of ethical decisions involving children must involve all three.

In Section 1 we looked at Magno's idea that 'the interest of the child … is a true fundamental and universally shared idea'. That may seem attractive at first, perhaps intuitively true. But trying to work out what the child's best interests mean *in practice* is a great deal more difficult, even if we accept that the child's interest is the primary concern and even if it is clear that the child is the 'real patient'. As Pearce says, the balance is hard to achieve. A further case study from Finland illustrates some of the problems.

ACTIVITY: Please read the following case study about 'Pekka'.

The case of Pekka

The Finnish Act on the Status and Rights of Patients (enforced in 1993) offers a minor who is mature and capable enough the chance to make decisions about his or her own treatment, but in practice parents make decisions for children under 12. According to Finnish mental health legislation, at 12 a child can himself appeal against a compulsory treatment decision to an administrative court; the parents also have a parallel right to make a complaint. A child is an independent subject in his or her own right; the child's interests can be separate from and even contrary to the interests of his or her parents. For example, Section 7 of the Finnish Act on the Status and Rights of Patients states that,

'The opinion of a minor patient on a treatment measure has to be assessed with regard to his/her age or level of development. If a minor patient ... can decide on the treatment given to him/her, he/she has to be cared for in mutual understanding with him/her.'

This strong line on children's autonomy goes beyond law and practice in other Nordic nations, such as Sweden. However, while a child is *said* to be a subject in his or her own right, children usually lack resources and means to put their own rights into *practice*.

Despite this strong 'child's voice' stance, a 1995 case illustrated that these legal criteria are sometimes flouted. A boy of 11 – call him 'Pekka' – was treated under a compulsory psychiatric order for ten months, against his and his mother's wishes. She managed to arrange his escape from the institution where he was being treated and sent him to live secretly with relatives in Estonia. He only returned after his 12th birthday, when by law his own opinions had to be heard. Even more important than the legal position, however, were institutional rules. The psychiatric hospital where the boy had originally been treated did not take children of 12 and over. The institution for young people over 12 diagnosed the boy as normal; he subsequently lived with his mother and attended a normal school.

ACTIVITY: In Pekka's case, it might be argued that, the state intervened against the wishes of both the child and his mother, despite the emphasis in law on the child's voice. Stop now for a moment and think about what you know of comparable legislation in your own country. Is there a similar requirement to take the child's own wishes into account in devising a treatment plan? What are the provisions governing involuntary committal of minors?

Do you agree with the interpretation given above of the case of Pekka? Are other interpretations possible?

Tony Hope, one of our critical readers, argues in response to this case that there are a variety of other possible interpretations which might be made (without further information about the case). He points out that any of the following might also be true: (1) the original diagnosis might have been wrong; (2) Pekka might have become well as a result of maturing; (3) the ten months in hospital might have helped Pekka a great deal; or (4) he is now in very bad psychological shape and would benefit from more enforced treatment. What this reminds us usefully is that it is important not to jump to conclusions about a case on the basis of limited information.

If we accept the interpretation above, however, Finland appears to set a high value on the autonomy of young people, in conformity with a pattern more typical of northern than southern Europe – at least in the usual stereotype (but see Dickenson, 1999b). Yet although there are real differences, sometimes the 'autonomy-minded North' is not really very good at protecting children's rights. Despite the emphasis in Finnish law on the minor's voice in making treatment decisions, the number of young people given involuntary treatment actually nearly doubled in 1991–1993.

ACTIVITY: Now please read the following extract (adapted from Launis, 1996). As you read, ask yourself why you think this situation arose, and whether there are any lessons.

Moral issues concerning children's legal status in Finland in relation to psychiatric treatment

Veikko Launis[2]

The Finnish Mental Health Act, which came into effect at the beginning of 1991, sets down a different criterion for the involuntary treatment of patients under 18 than for adults. Minors can be given compulsory psychiatric in-patient treatment not only on grounds of mental illness, but also because of a 'serious mental disorder'. That is, personality disorders, not normally sufficient grounds for the compulsory treatment of adults, are enough reason to hospitalize a minor. More precisely:

> The child may be sent into psychiatric hospital care involuntarily if, due to a serious mental disorder, he is in need of care, so that failure to commit him to care would significantly aggravate his illness or serious endanger his health ...

> (Section 8)

There are two different sets of questions which arise from this discrepancy between the treatment of adults and young people: ethical and practical. Each one in turn entails two more questions.

The child holds a special place in psychiatric ethics for at least two reasons. First, the child's actions are normally regarded as the responsibility of his or her parents. Consequently, psychiatric intervention in diagnosing or treating the child inevitably involves the parents. Second, the child's capacity for autonomous decision-making is not fully developed (Graham, 1981). However, we must ask whether and to what extent the content of the child's decision should be taken into account in evaluating his capacity to make autonomous decisions. According to a substantive conception of autonomy, some particular decisions (e.g. a person's decision to commit suicide or to use addictive drugs) cannot qualify as autonomous, no matter how they are made. A more formal conception of autonomy denies this, claiming that any given decision, regardless of its content, can qualify as autonomous – so long as it is made in the appropriate way (Dworkin, 1988; Husak 1992, p. 83).

In practical terms, the first question concerning the Mental Health Act's application to young people concerns the high level of involuntary treatment to which it has led. The level of compulsory treatment of minors of Finland has nearly doubled since the Act came into force, and a large proportion of this is accounted for by the tripled rate of committal under

the new criterion, 'serious mental disorder', between 1991–1993 (Kaivosoja, 1996, p. 200). This makes one ask whether at least some of these young people should have been helped through less severe measures to decrease the risk of stigmatization and medicalization of disorderly but otherwise normal conduct.

Second, the same study indicates that in 1991–3 only 50% of minors treated against their will were treated in units for minors only – despite the provision in Section 8 of the Act on the Status and Rights of Patients that 'Minors shall be cared for separately from adults, unless it is considered in the child's best interests not to do so'.

The Finnish example illustrates the difficulties of reconciling the three approaches to practitioners' responsibilities towards children: to listen to the child's voice, to maintain family unity, or to act in the name of the child's best interests. Legislation which explicitly values the child's opinion is further advanced in Finland than in many European countries, but in practice children and their families actually seem to have fewer rights against compulsory psychiatric treatment than they had before, in Launis's view. Nor is it clear that 'best interests' criteria are really being met, when children are being treated in adult facilities so frequently: it is hard to believe that this is really in their best interests 50% of the time. The example of Finland shows how difficult it is, even in a small and homogeneous country, to put a legally and ethically coherent policy concerning children and compulsory treatment into practice.

Summary

In Sections 1 and 2 we began with cases involving young people's consent to psychiatric treatment but broadened the discussion to include other examples primarily involving somatic medicine, such as those of the girl with anorexia or the boy with cystic fibrosis. Three possible interpretations of the practitioner's responsibility were examined:

- to listen to the child's voice,
- to uphold family unity, or
- to serve the child's best interests.

These three views relate to the question of 'who is the patient?'. Although listening to the child's voice is an important responsibility, enshrined in European and UN conventions, difficulties arise because it is not the only voice to which practitioners must respond. The demands of other family members, the requirements of the law, and 'purely medical' best interests must also be considered. But these, too, are rarely uncontroversial; even medically defined best interests are usually open to disagreement among clinicians. These conflicts come to a head in the example of involuntary treatment, based on the debatable but often legally valid assumption that children and young people are not fully competent to consent.

Section 3: Confidentiality and conflicting responsibilities

The Finnish Act on the Status and Rights of Patients also gives the under-age patient the 'right to forbid the disclosure of information about his health and care' (Section 9). That is, children are entitled to the same standard of medical confidentiality as adults. That implies a 'child's rights' or 'child's voice' approach to looking at *confidentiality* as well as at consent to treatment. This, too, raises possible conflicts with what is really in the child's best interests, or with what the family think is in the child's best interests. Maintaining a child's trust can be an essential feature of treating the child ethically, and this will require the preservation of confidentiality. But consider also the situation where a clinician withholds information about child abuse or neglect for reasons of confidentiality. There, confidentiality seems to protect the abuser rather than the abused child. So in a way in this kind of case we're back to this question: to whom does the clinician's primary responsibility lie? Confidentiality itself does not tell us the answer to that question. Instead, we have to know who deserves the first claim on our sense of responsibility in order to know who deserves confidentiality.

ACTIVITY: Read the following case study from France, concerning child protection. What were the confidentiality issues, as the practitioners – and the law – saw them? Why was there a conflict?

Case study: the Montjoie affair

Until the early 1980s most professionals working with abused children in France would invoke the 'Law of Silence'. In this era of silence abuses of discretion abounded. It was difficult to evaluate the number of ill-treated children, or even of fatal cases of abuse. The

percentage of abuse cases reported to the judicial authorities was very low. Yet the law did make it plain that doctors were to be released from their normal professional duty of confidentiality when, in the course of their work, they came to know of abuse and neglect of children under the age of 15.

In the early 1980s, however, a public campaign was organized around the slogan, '50 000 children are abused every year; speaking out is the first step'. Interministerial circulars of 1983 and 1985 informed practitioners of their responsibilities and specified procedures for hospital admission in cases of suspected abuse. This was followed up by legislation on the prevention of child abuse, in May 1989.

But difficulties about confidentiality remained. There was a basic discrepancy between an article of the criminal code which respected professional confidentiality and another article which allowed the criminal prosecution of anyone who 'having knowledge about abuse of a child under the age of 15, does not report the case to the administrative or judicial authorities'. While it was clear that the doctor may report the case of an abused child without fear of criminal proceedings for breach of confidentiality, it was less clear whether he or she had an active responsibility to report cases of abuse encountered in the line of professional practice. Doctors were free to report abuse, but were they obliged to do so?

In December 1992 these dilemmas came to a head in the 'Montjoie affair'. Damien, aged seven, and Mickael, aged 18, had been placed together in a foster family, but Damien's foster parents informed Mickael's educational psychologist that Damien had complained of being abused by Mickael. The psychiatrist on the team, Dr Bernard Chouraqui, was informed two days later that the psychologist wished to separate the two boys immediately, sending Mickael to another foster family. After discussion the team decided to wait 10 days before informing the judicial authorities so as to allow constructive therapy for Mickael, who was thought to be on the verge of a breakdown, which would be worsened by the threat of prosecution. The clinical team felt that he needed to be prepared to face the judicial consequences of his act.

The juvenile court was duly informed two weeks after the abuse had first been reported. In January 1993 the investigating judge charged the educational psychologist and the social worker on the team with not having reported the abuse. On the same day the psychiatrist, Dr Chouraqui, appeared before the juvenile court of his own free will to explain the situation. He was immediately charged with the same offence and imprisoned, together with the educational psychologist. Dr Chouraqui was not released to await trial for another two weeks; at his trial 10 months later, however, he was acquitted.

Naturally there was a furore in the medical world. As a result of the outcry over the Montjoie affair, the dilemma about whether doctors were obliged to report abuse or merely free to do so was resolved in favour of the latter interpretation. The Criminal Code now makes it plain that doctors are not breaking confidentiality if they report abuse of children under the age of 15 (art. 226–14) but reporting abuse is a personal decision (see further Michalowski, 2003, pp. 76–8). But isn't doctors' responsibility all the greater now that it is a personal, ethical decision, rather than a legal requirement?

ACTIVITY: Think about this last sentence. Are ethical responsibilities greater than legal ones? Try to think of other areas in which practitioners' responsibilities are primarily ethical rather than legal.

One example we considered was a case like W's, and the extent to which a health professional should respect a refusal of treatment issued by a competent young person. Such refusal might carry relatively little weight in law – yet ethical practitioners might be more willing to honour their patient's objection. Of course, the Montjoie affair represents an unusually fierce conflict between the clinician's ethical duty of care, as he interpreted it, and the law. Dr Chouraqui thought that it was in Mickael's best interests to give him some time to prepare for the idea of a court action. But the investigating judge charged him with failure to report the abuse immediately, and under the criminal code he was actually imprisoned.

This is an extreme instance; imprisonment is rarely at issue in conflicts between practitioners and the law. But it does raise in a very graphic way the question of responsibilities under and to the law, and also to other members of the clinical team: it was only after team discussion that the decision was taken to postpone reporting the abuse, so in a sense all members of the team were mutually responsible. Crenier (1996) adds that although 'the law of secrecy' no longer prevails in public, the confidential deliberations of clinical teams may constitute another form of 'abuse of discretion'. 'The doctor must feel free to share his doubts and uncertainties with other professionals without having

his professional competence questioned. Ultimately, going back to the issue of professional secrecy, one could examine the idea of 'secret' remaining such when shared within a professional team.'

So far we have mainly considered responsibilities to the child and to the family, but at this point we might stop and draw up a checklist of responsibilities to consider in making ethical decisions. Remember that these responsibilities may well conflict.

ACTIVITY: To whom or what am I responsible?

(1) To my actual patient, the child
(2) To the parents and other members of the family
(3) To the law
(4) To other members of the clinical team
(5) To my own sense of good practice, my professional standards and conscience.

Can you think of any less extreme examples from your own experience? What responsibilities did you feel to the child? To the family? To the law? To others in the clinical team? To your own professional standards?

In a child abuse case, it may well be the rightful function of the law to be very sceptical about confidentiality. Child protection must come first. But what about more general questions of confidentiality in working with children? Consider the following case, which arose in the English law courts (*R (Axon)* v *Secretary of State for Health* [2006]).

The case of Sue Axon

Sue Axon is the mother of five children, including two teenage daughters. She objected to guidance, issued in 2004 by the Department of Health in England, which permitted doctors to provide abortion advice or contraception to young people under 16 without the knowledge of their parents. The guidelines, she argued, served to 'undermine the role of parents'.

Ms Axon's claim was reminiscent of a well-known earlier case, which had led to a ruling in the highest English court, the House of Lords (*Gillick* v *West Norfolk and Wisbech AHA* [1985]). In that case, Victoria Gillick unsuccessfully argued that parents should have to provide consent before a young person could be prescribed the contraceptive pill. Ms Axon's claim was different: she was not arguing for the right to *consent* but, instead, the right to *know* if her child was seeking such advice or treatment. She claimed that she was owed an obligation under article 8 of the Human Rights Act 1998 (which brought the European Convention of Human Rights directly into English law); article 8 protects the right to respect for one's private and family life.

ACTIVITY: Stop here for a moment and consider whether, if you were the judge, you would agree with Sue Axon. Consider your reasons for your decision.

Like Mrs Gillick, Ms Axon failed to persuade the court. Mr Justice Silber, in the High Court, decided that a young person's right to confidentiality took precedence over parents' rights, at least where the young person was mature enough to understand the implications and therefore capable of taking the decision in question. The Department of Health guidance was therefore upheld as lawful.

The guidelines to which Sue Axon objected did not require the young person's right to have his or her confidences to be maintained at all costs:

> The duty of confidentiality is not, however, absolute. Where a health professional believes that there is a risk to the health, safety or welfare of a young person or others which is so serious as to outweigh the young person's right to privacy, they should follow locally agreed child protection protocols . . . In these circumstances, the overriding objective must be to safeguard the young person.

ACTIVITY: Stop here and spend some time trying to find out what professional or legal guidance there is available in your country on confidentiality and children. Under what kinds of circumstances ought one to be allowed to breach confidentiality? Under what circumstances does one have a duty (ethical or legal) to breach confidentiality? Look for example, at the General Medical Council's guidance for British doctors in *0–18 years: Guidance for all Doctors* (2007).

Section 4: The child in society

In the first three sections of this chapter we have explored a wide range of ethical conflicts which can arise when working with children and young people. We have explored the conflicting responsibilities practitioners feel to the child and to the child's parents or guardians. We have also explored a variety of different ways in which these conflicting responsibilities might be expressed, as the duty:

- to 'listen to the child's voice'
- to 'maintain family unity'
- to 'think first and foremost of the child's best interests'.

We have addressed the question of who is to decide what is in the child's 'best interests' and have explored the responsibilities practitioners might have outside of the family, to the law, to others in their clinical team and to their own practice. In this section we will begin to look more closely at how one might begin to develop ways of resolving such conflicts in practice. In order to do this we will widen our scope to consider the position of the child in society. We start with a case that came before the English judges (*Re C* [2003]).

The cases of C and F

C and F were two girls, aged three and nine years of age respectively, both of whose parents were separated. The children lived with their mothers, each of whom refused to consent to their daughters receiving a range of vaccinations, including the combined measles, mumps and rubella (MMR) jab. The girls' mothers were opposed to vaccination because they felt that it posed unacceptable risks – indeed, there had, at the time, been much media coverage of research which suggested an association between receiving the vaccine and developing autism and bowel problems (Wakefield *et al.*, 1998).

The girls' fathers were, however, in favour of them being immunized, because they felt that this was in the children's best interests. The fathers approached the courts for permission for the injections to be given and (although there were some differences in their situations) the two cases were considered together.

ACTIVITY: Stop here for a moment. Based on what little information you have, what do you think you would decide if you were the judge? Consider arguments both for authorizing the vaccinations and for prohibiting them.

Mr Justice Sumner, in the High Court, basically agreed with the girls' fathers: he ruled that it would be in each child's best interests to receive a range of vaccinations. He did recognize that the mothers (and their daughters) were owed the right to respect for their private and family life, but he further noted how these rights were qualified by the need to protect the health of the children. He also thought that, in time, the mothers would be able to come to terms with his decision, despite any initial upset they might feel.

The mothers decided to appeal to the Court of Appeal, but here too their case failed. This court ruled that the trial judge had been guided by the right considerations, since he had determined the best interests of the children by considering both the medical evidence and other factors relevant to the welfare of the children. However, the appeal judges conceded that Mr Justice Sumner had been particularly thorough in his consideration of the medical evidence, but they felt that this was entirely appropriate given the crucial importance of this evidence. Like the trial judge before them, the appeal judges felt that the balance tipped considerably in favour of the combined MMR vaccination and away from the unreliable evidence presented by the mothers' legal team – which was, said Lord Justice Sedley, 'junk science'.

This case touches on many of the themes that we have been considering throughout this chapter, including how we ought to assess the best interests of a child or young person and who should be making that assessment. It is notable, for example, that the judges made no reference to what the girls themselves wanted. Did they – especially nine-year-old F – have views on vaccination, and, if so, should the judges (and the doctors) have taken these into account? And what are we to make of the fact that the judges preferred the decision that had been reached by the girls' fathers? Recall that the mothers were the primary carers of C and F; what effects might such a ruling have on these families and how far should we expect the judges to take account of such effects?

Talk of one side 'winning' and another 'losing' is, of course, an unfortunate feature of adversarial legal proceedings, particularly when those proceedings concern the care of a patient. Perhaps we are better off describing the judge's task not as one of preferring one side or another but, instead, as one of ensuring that the best interests of the child are protected and promoted.

ACTIVITY: Do you think that a focus on the best interests of the child provides the key to working out what should be done in the cases of C and F? Are there any other ethical dimensions to these cases that you would wish to include before reaching a recommendation?

There is likely always to be some contest over how one interprets and gives effect to the best interests of a child, particularly when we are dealing with the issue of vaccination – in which it is not only the individual child whose health is at stake (Dawson, 2005). What we now want to explore is whether the 'best interests standard' therefore gives us the appropriate ethical prism through which to view a case like that of C and F. Richard Huxtable, commenting on their case, suggests that there can be more issues at stake than a (seemingly?) straightforward appeal to 'best interests' would seem to allow:

Should the best interests of this child (or, more accurately, these children) really form the paramount concern when the good of the public is also in issue? The judicial mantra maintains that the welfare of the individual child is indeed the paramount consideration. Yet, in cases of vaccination, there are wider concerns of justice that need to be considered. The problem of the 'free-rider', unwilling to undergo vaccination, but reliant on others gaining protection that will thereby protect him or her is one such worry (see e.g. Cullity, 1995). Evidently, when we are addressing public health measures, the individual is not strictly or solely our key unit of concern. (see further Pywell, 2001: esp. 300–6)

Perhaps, then, there is a case for determining the immunisation question at the state level. The Department of Health has made clear its support for the triple vaccine (UK Department of Health, 2003), so perhaps that should be the end of the matter: the parent should have no autonomy in this regard. That may be a valid solution if there is, for example, a real threat of an epidemic, given low take-up of the vaccination (regarding fears of a measles epidemic, see Pywell, 2001: esp. 316–19; Murch, 2003). Of course, this would still be offensive to many in society, since it smacks of paternalistic meddling. (Huxtable, 2004)

Huxtable is here referring to the 'herd immunity' effect of vaccination, in which vaccination of the many can mean that protection is also conferred on the few who did not receive the vaccine. Note, however, that competent adults are entitled to decline vaccination and indeed any medical procedure: for example, I cannot be forced to finish my course of antibiotics if I foolishly break off halfway through, even if my action increases the risk of multiple-antibiotic-resistant disease developing in the population as a whole. Children might not enjoy such a right. Can we defend such a distinction? One might think that the issues about individual choice versus benefit to society are the same irrespective of age, so our conclusions too should be consistent regardless of the patient's (im)maturity. As Huxtable continues, the issue of community immunity is surely one for consideration by society as a whole:

And there are further complications at the state level. General practitioners, for example, are offered financial incentives for delivering a particular proportion of vaccinations: is this appropriate? As Pattison observes,
'This again raises the issue of whether doctors are acting in the best interests of the individuals or whether they are dancing to a financial tune. We need to ask whose interests do and should clinicians serve – do they focus on individuals, or is their job to deliver centrally determined, scientifically informed, health policy?'

(Pattison, 2001: 840)

Presently, of course, the individual child is the focus of the courts' concern, and the case law offers little opportunity for recourse to the interests of others [although] there are cases in which procedures on incompetent patients have been authorised, despite the absence of any direct benefits thereto (e.g. S v S; W v Official Solicitor [1970] (blood test determining paternity) and Re Y [1996] (harvesting of bone marrow to treat a sibling)). These cases may hint at a rather broader conception of best interests, one that is alert to the realities of family and community existence, but they do not yet bridge the gap between the individual and the community at large. Certainly, this writer would not wish to see the rights and interests of the individual entirely engulfed by the rights and interests of others ... Nevertheless, one is left feeling that these broader topics do need a fuller airing.

(Huxtable, 2004)

Huxtable here only sketches some of the wider issues that arise in the context of vaccination, but he rightly reminds us that the child and his or her family do not exist in a vacuum – they are part of a wider community.

ACTIVITY: What is the ethical significance of saying that someone is part of a 'community'? Consider the duties and rights that come with membership of a community, and consider particularly the ethical issues that might arise for children and their families.

For Michael Parker, one's community encompasses those people with whom one must find meaningful ways of co-existing (Parker, 1995a). Such meaningful co-existence requires negotiation, as Parker elaborates:

Within the family, people enter into complex and extended negotiation about a whole range of aspects of how to live meaningfully together (or separately) as a family. There is often a great sense of reciprocity here, even in disputes, and feelings of community within the family are often by far the strongest sense of community many people are likely to experience.

(Parker, 1995a, p. 64)

However, Parker acknowledges how the 'wider' community also surrounds the community constituted by one's family. In other words, individuals will have a sense of belonging not only to their families, but also to other communities, including the community 'at large'. Membership of a wider group like this also requires negotiation: for example, when we decide whether or not to recycle our refuse, advocate for action on pressing social issues (like climate change), donate to charity, and so on.

Parker's concern with reciprocal relationships and negotiation as the defining characteristics of community membership therefore differs from the usual approach, which focuses on the fact that people share certain attributes, interests or location. This approach has its merits – for example, it helps to explain why we might feel more of a sense of community with people (such as our extended family) who are distant from us than we do with our neighbours. Such ties appear to matter and so too, it would appear, do the communities constituted by these ties.

However, this is not to say that membership of a community is in and of itself a 'good thing', and nor is it to say that community per se should be our primary value, to which all other goods, duties and rights must be sacrificed. Sometimes we will need an ethical approach that protects the individual from their community (Bell, 1993). Parker is alert to this need and acknowledges 'the very real dangers' of an overemphasis on community at the expense of the individual (Parker, 1995a, p. 65). However, he argues that:

By defining 'community', as I did above, as consisting of those with whom I enter into negotiation about how we are to live meaningfully together ... I tie it to both the importance and the meaningfulness of an individual life and to the importance ...

163

This enables my conceptualisation, I believe, to avoid the very real dangers of an overemphasis on community.

(Parker, 1995a, p. 65)

Parker recognizes that the notion of universal human rights is capable of playing an important role in protecting individual citizens from the 'dangers of an overemphasis on community' to which he refers. The language of rights is increasingly familiar in contemporary politics and law – although it also has a long philosophical tradition, dating back to the Stoic philosophers in ancient Greece who referred to universal (non-relative) 'natural law' in pointing out the deficiencies of the actual laws of the State (Almond, 1991). Although mindful of this history and the pragmatic power of rights discourse, Parker nevertheless queries whether it makes sense to view human beings, and therefore their rights, as somehow transcending – or stepping outside – their community. Parker doubts that there is an 'inner person' who exists independent of social context, whose needs might come into conflict with those of the community. As he explains,

[T]he problem with any approach which demands the radical detachment of the person from his or her community and consequently from all meaningful interaction with others, is that it requires one to lose sight of the fact that human concerns are concerns for us just because of our social embeddedness, because we are human and because our humanity is framed by the fact that we share in ways of life with other people out of which we draw our identity. It is our social embeddedness which makes it possible for us to be individuals.

(Parker, 1995a, p. 66)

ACTIVITY: What do you think of Parker's attempt to say that we can have an ethics which values communities and also, at the same time, an approach which is based upon respect for individuals? Make a list of the tensions between respect for individual children and respect for the values which support families.

Parker believes that the way forward lies in recognizing that rights are not located in the individual, and nor are they located in the community, but they are instead located in the nature of the ethical negotiations between the two:

Ethical problems arise with respect not simply to individuals or communities in themselves but to the forms of negotiation they undertake, to work out meaningful ways of living together; that is, the

ways in which they treat each other. This means that if there is to be a justification of the use of a vocabulary of rights, this cannot lie in a commitment to the existence of an abstract 'individual' but must lie instead in a commitment to particular ways of living with others, to particular 'ethical' ways of living. The best expression of this kind of commitment, it seems to me, is Kant's maxim that we should treat each other not solely as 'means' but as 'ends' (Kant, 1909). One can see how such a commitment might lead, in a fruitful way, to a different analysis of rights, in a more socially embedded language, and comprising, on the one hand, a positive right to have an active role in the creation of a meaningful identity for oneself in one's negotiations with others, and on the other hand, a complementary negative right not to be objectified in such negotiations; that is, not to be fixed by it despite oneself.

(Parker, 1995a, p. 66)

Taking this approach, Parker believes that we get a more coherent understanding of the nature of rights and duties, since these emerge as more clearly tied to the nature of our relations to those with whom we must find meaningful ways of co-existing; in other words, with our community. The community in question may be small or large, and may permit of degrees; there may also be more than one community to which we feel attached and, accordingly, responsible. What is vital, according to Parker, is that we move away from an individualistic understanding of rights, towards concepts like the 'social embeddedness of individuals', 'community' and the 'negotiation of meaning', since this new focus 'leads not to the call for freedom *from* community but to the call for the right to a *voice within one's community*' (Parker, 1995a, p. 67, original emphasis).

Parker then explains how his approach has direct relevance to our dealings with children and young people:

Children, indeed all people, ought to be able to participate, that is to have a voice, in the everyday processes of dialogue which constitute the means by which people work out meaningful ways of living together and out of which they draw their identities. What is required, it seems to me, is the establishment, at many levels, of fora where children will feel safe and where they will be able to begin to participate in the dialogues which frame their lives. Perhaps the true measure of whether or not one's work with a child, or a parent (or anyone else for that matter), has been ethical is the extent to which they come through the experience feeling that their story has been heard and that they have been taken seriously.

(Parker, 1995a, p. 68)

Parker introduces some fairly dense philosophical reasoning into our consideration of how we should work with children. He offers us an approach to the child's voice which avoids some of the problems that we considered earlier and which, Parker believes, helps us to resolve some of the ethical issues relating to work with young people.

> **ACTIVITY:**   Parker discusses in some detail the concepts of community, ethics, rights, individuals and relationships from a philosophical point of view. Go back to the case of Sean, which opened this chapter, and try to apply Parker's arguments by making a list of the principles which you think ought to govern a meeting between Sean, his parents, the child psychotherapist and a social worker. (Philosophical reasoning can often seem very difficult or impenetrable on first reading, so you may find it helpful to re-read Parker's arguments before undertaking this activity.)

Parker argues that the resolution of ethical dilemmas in practical situations can only happen ethically in a situation where the participants, those with a legitimate interest in the matter at hand, can all participate and have a voice. He is also saying that the real test of whether one's work with children has been ethical is the extent to which they come through the experience feeling that they have been taken seriously and listened to. So it might seem that he is saying that our primary responsibility is our duty to respect the child's voice. But Parker has subtly changed the debate so that an emphasis on listening to children is no longer couched in individualistic terms. The child has to have a voice in balance with the legitimate voices of others. That is, she has to be able to participate in the decision-making process with those who have a legitimate right to be involved. He also suggested that the orientation of such participation ought to be towards the search for agreement about what constitutes the best interest of the child. Finally he has suggested that this can only be achieved by the creation of decision-making fora governed by certain practical ethical principles to guarantee the participation of young people in decision-making.

However, whilst Parker's proposal helps to provide us with a theoretical framework for working with young people, it is still quite abstract, and so in the next section we will develop further the practical ways in which we might work ethically with young people.

Section 5: Making 'the child's voice' meaningful

We began this chapter with the statement in article 12 of the UN Convention on the Rights of the Child that 'the child who is capable of forming his or her own views' should have 'the right to express those views freely'. Article 12 requires that the child's voice should be 'given due weight in accordance with the age and maturity of the child'. In many European countries Article 12 now has legal force: France, for example, passed legislation in 1993 which requires French law to conform to its prescriptions (Heller, 1997). The British government, too, has formally adopted the Convention. What then does it take to make this notion of 'the child's voice' not just a hollow legal concept, but a meaningful notion in practice?

> **ACTIVITY:**   What problems in making 'the child's voice' a reality have been suggested so far in this chapter? Make a list of some of the difficulties so far encountered. Then draw up a second list of the most frequent problems you encounter in your own practice, in this respect. How do you decide what to do in your own practice, if there is a conflict between the 'child's voice' and your professional responsibilities?

So far the chapter has considered some of the following problems in fulfilling the requirements of Article 12:

- A child-centred approach is not universally accepted throughout Europe. It stems from an individualistic discourse of rights which is usually associated with the USA and northern Europe (although that stereotype didn't seem to fit the Finnish case of Pekka). This may or may not be a realistic model in working with independent children.
- If the child is considered primarily within the family, as tends to be the case in southern Europe, the 'child's voice' is not necessarily separate from that of the family. But this creates problems for the practitioner who disagrees with the family's opinion of what will benefit the child. Think, for example, of the example of Emilia, a case which comes from Italy.
- In such cases, the child's voice may not be consistently expressed. Children's views also

change as they develop and mature; at what age does 'the child's voice' represent the child's true wishes?

- Likewise, the family is not always of one voice; in the vaccination case, for example, the mothers and the fathers disagreed about the appropriateness of vaccinating their daughters. Although we do not have a record of the daughters' own views in that case, we should be able to appreciate that in cases like this the 'child's voice' may be the voice of either parent, or none.

- Who is the patient? Sometimes, as in the vaccination case of C and F, we might think that the patient is actually the 'community'. Even if the answer is definitely 'the child', it may not be possible to treat the child independently of the family. If family members do not comply with the prescribed treatment regime, they could undermine a decision made according to the child's expressed wishes or the practitioner's opinion of the child's best interests, assuming either of those conflicted with the family's opinion.

- 'Best interests' and 'the child's voice' may be in conflict; however, what the child wants may be inconsistent with what you as a practitioner think would really be best for her. If the decision concerns life-prolonging treatment, involves a once-and-for-all judgement or entails serious risks of any other sort, is it right to let 'the voice of the child' be the only criterion? Most practitioners would find that seriously irresponsible, a denial of their professional duty of care. The case of the 12-year-old Jehovah's Witness boy with cystic fibrosis illustrated this difficulty.

- 'The child's voice' can only be a reality if it is the child or young person who has the ultimate power to give or withhold consent to treatment. If other agencies also have some power to decide – social services, for example – might the child's voice be lost in the welter of conflicting opinions?

- The law typically regards children as 'presumed incompetent' to withhold consent to treatment. Again, this is a serious constraint on making the 'child's voice' a reality. Even competent young people under 18 may be denied the right to refuse a particular treatment regime, as we saw in the case of W.

- Although the rhetoric of 'the child's voice' is widely accepted, in practical terms children's rights often seem to be diminishing rather than increasing.

An example of this was the huge increase in involuntary psychiatric treatment for minors in Finland, a country which might be expected to take rights seriously. Legislation which explicitly values the child's opinion is quite strong in Finland; so why is it so difficult to translate new legislation into practice – there and elsewhere? However, once again it is important to remind ourselves at this point that such statistics can easily be misleading and it may be (for example) that the system is now managing to identify correctly and treat patients who were previously slipping through the net in some way.

- Confidentiality may also be an arena of conflict. Does 'the child's voice' extend to 'the child's right to silence' – for example, in keeping records of treatment decisions from his or her parents, in the manner that Sue Axon opposed? In the Montjoie affair, we saw that professional norms of confidentiality failed to protect abused children, stifling their 'voices'.

This long list of impediments to making the child's voice count could well be discouraging. None the less, the notion of the child's voice is important in practice, ethics and law, marking what has been called 'a reconsideration of the child's status, now seen as a subject of rights and not simply an object of protection' (Heller, 1997).

In this final section of the chapter, we want to consider practical ways to resolve the conflicts introduced in the earlier sections, moving beyond the difficulties into conflict resolution in practice.

One crucial issue to resolve is that of competence. It is good practice in determining competence to listen to the child's voice wherever possible: as one surgeon put it, 'True competence is to answer me back and query things' (Alderson, 1992). But if the child is definitely incompetent to decide about treatment, he or she is unlikely to have the last word – as, for example, with very young children. We have already seen that in English law, at least, there is a presumption of incompetence in young people under 18. The case of W took this further by denying that even a young person who had been found competent could refuse treatment, so long as someone with parental responsibility consented on behalf of the minor. Competence, for someone under 18, is only competence to consent.

Many commentators (e.g. Devereux *et al.*, 1993; Huxtable, 2000) argue that this makes a nonsense of consent and weakens the voice of the child. If children are not considered competent to refuse treatment, how valid is their consent, given that they are not considered competent to say no?

It must be acknowledged, however, that this position finds support among some legal scholars (e.g. MacLean, 2008). Likewise, some practitioners such as John Pearce (1996) take a similar view:

> Devereux et al. have argued that there should be no difference between giving and withholding consent, because the right to give consent is worthless if it is not accompanied by the right to refuse consent. The logic of this position is clear enough, but it assumes that consent can be conceived in absolute terms and can be considered in isolation from the context in which it is given or refused. If a child declines to give consent for treatment, it might reasonably be assumed that treatment has been refused. However, the refusal could be due to the child's feelings of anxiety and anger, or related to a limited capacity to understand the nature of the request, or perhaps simply a misunderstanding about what is required. The consequences of withholding consent to treatment are usually much more significant and potentially dangerous than simply giving consent – unless one believes that most treatments are either unnecessary or are likely to be more dangerous than the condition for which they were prescribed.

ACTIVITY: Which of these two positions do you agree with? Pearce has given some counter-arguments to the view that meaningful consent is impossible unless the child has the right to refuse. Do you believe these counter-arguments are strong ones? If not, why not?

If best interests, the traditional paternalistic criterion, are no longer viewed as the sole prerogative of parents and clinicians to decide, does that mean that conflict will be endemic between doctors, families and young people? That would be unnecessarily pessimistic. Adolescents do not necessarily assert their rights at the expense of everyone else: the majority of both adolescents and parents agree that parents should be involved in deciding whether young people should participate in minimal risk research studies, although there is a greater perceived need for parental consent.

There is certainly evidence of movement towards greater acceptance of children's decision-making capacity on very major matters indeed, in reports from professional bodies such as the Royal College of Paediatrics and Child Health (2004). While stressing that the child's best interests remain the fundamental concern, the committee behind an earlier version of this report included the case in which the child *and/or* family feel that further treatment of progressive and irreversible illness is more than can be borne, as one of five situations in which withholding or withdrawal of curative medical treatment could be considered. A much-cited letter in the *British Medical Journal* from a practising clinician in child and adolescent psychiatry argued that children should be presumed competent from the age of five, rather than presumed incompetent until the age of 18 (Paul, 1997). To what extent is it true to say that the transition from incompetence to competence in young people is a general phenomenon, rather than one which may vary even in one person between different activities and decisions depending on experience?

The focus of this section, as has been noted, is to think about putting the ethical concepts you have encountered into practice, reflecting your own weightings of the importance of 'the child's voice', 'the child's best interests' and 'the unity of the family'. It is vital for clinicians to understand that ethics comes into small, everyday decisions in dealing with parents and children, for example, in creating a climate of openness and free discussion on the paediatric intensive care unit (Nelson, 1997). This can create genuine consent by both children and parents, rather than mere deference to the physician's technical ability in the hope of saving the child. If a child has a stable set of values, gained from experience of chronic illness, that should be taken into account, together with more cognitive criteria for decision-making capacity (Dickenson and Jones, 1995; Parker, 1995b; Harrison et al., 1997).

So to begin constructing a practical guide to resolving conflicts in working with children, you need to decide how you feel about whether treatment refusal should attract a higher 'tariff' than accepting treatment. If you accept that the two should be distinguished – and in English law, at present, they must be – your guide to practice might begin with this distinction:

- The nature of the decision: consent to treatment or refusal of consent.

A practical guide might also want to consider:

- The child's developmental maturity, considered in both emotional and cognitive terms (as required by Lord Scarman's opinion in the case of *Gillick* v *West Norfolk and Wisbech AHA* [1985]), which we mentioned in our discussion of Sue Axon's case), and including

- The child's ability to understand the consequences of both treatment and refusal of treatment.

Pearce calls this 'the central issue' in assessing the young person's ability to give or refuse consent:

> In order to give valid consent, children must have reached the stage of maturity where they have a clear concept of themselves in relation to other people, including an ability to recognise their own needs and the needs of others. Competent children will have an ability to understand the nature of their disorders and know why treatment is deemed to be necessary. They should be able to understand the significance of the risks and benefits of having or not having the treatment. In addition, the competent child will be able to understand these issues in relation to the passage of time and be fully aware of what might happen in the future as a result of having or forgoing the treatment.
>
> (Pearce, 1996)

This ability is usually absent in children under eight, he believes, but almost always present in young people over 14. Alderson (1994), on the other hand, has concluded that children younger than ten years old are able to understand the nature and consequences of treatment quite well.

While noting that these decisions mainly concerned elective surgery, Pearce concedes that:

> Alderson highlights the risk of underestimating children's ability to make wise and sensible choices. By excluding young people from the decision-making process, children as young as four or five years old may feel resentful and angry as they grow older and have to live with the consequences of decisions in which they had no involvement.
>
> (Pearce, 1996)

This suggests that one item which your practical guide to making decisions should not *necessarily* include is the age of the child. A functional test of competence – being competent to make this particular decision at this particular time – will go further towards making the child's voice count than a rigid age barrier.

ACTIVITY: You've now made a start on a practical checklist of what you would want to consider in deciding how to balance the child's voice, the child's best

interests and the unity of the family in making decisions about treating children and young people. Take some time now to add to your list. What else would you want to know? Then compare it with the 'consent checklist' developed by Pearce in the box below.

Factors to be taken into account when assessing competence to give or refuse consent (Pearce, 1996)

1. *The child's stage of cognitive development*
   Does the child have a satisfactory understanding of:

   The nature of the illness?
   Their own needs and the needs of others?
   The risks and benefits of treatment?
   Their own self-concept?
   The significance of time: past, present, future?

2. *The parent–child relationship*
   Is it supportive and affectionate?

3. *The doctor–patient relationship*
   Is there trust and confidence?

4. *The views of significant others* (*e.g. other family members and friends*)
   Whose opinion influences the child and how?

5. *The risks and benefits of treatment*
   What are the risks of treatment or no treatment?

6. *The nature of the illness*
   How disabling, chronic or life-threatening?

7. *The need for consensus*
   Is more time or information needed?
   Is a second opinion required?

ACTIVITY: Now apply both Pearce's list and your own version to the following case study (adapted from Alderson, 1994, p. 9 ff.).

The case of Danny

Ten-year-old Danny has neurofibromatosis, which required removal of a major fibroma in his left tibia when he was only two. (His mother had previously died of the disease.) Bone was taken from his right fibula in an attempt to strengthen the left tibia, but after 15 months in plaster, his lower left leg had to be amputated. His right leg was weakened by the surgery, and he then underwent two attempts at osteostomy to treat a valgus right foot (one that rolls over). Now he is undergoing limb lengthening of the right fibula. As he describes it, 'I'm going to have a bone graft in my right leg. Take a little bit from here (he touches his hip) and put it here (he touches his ankle) to fix it. And get a pin, just put it in and stitch it, then they wait till they heal it.' He smiles and jokes about the forthcoming procedure: 'Then I'll get a wheel-chair – be lazy all the time, I like that, better than crutches.'

Danny's parents are less sanguine: they have just learned that another large tumour has to be removed from his left leg stump. They feel that they have little choice but to consent to a further amputation if that proves necessary during the additional surgery, which will be done at the same time as the limb lengthening. They have not told Danny that his entire leg may have to be amputated. He knows about the new tumour, and has said 'I don't mind them taking the tumour, but I don't want them taking any more of my leg away'. Danny's father says, 'You feel that everyone is doing what they believe to be in his best interest, but they are tending to work a little bit blind'.

ACTIVITY: Stop at this point in the story and complete your checklist in relation to the limb length-ening of Danny's right fibula and possible left leg amputation. Has a meaningful consent been obtained? Has the child's voice been heard? What about the parents' position?

In the event it proved possible to save the remaining left leg, and the right leg grew well, although Danny suffered a great deal of pain from the limb length-ening procedure. Now the surgeons want to lengthen the small stump below Danny's left knee. Danny's stepmother explained to the boy that this will give greater leverage to the prosthesis, but Danny said adamantly, 'I don't want them doing that!'. He would not explain why; he looked tired and depressed now, with dark circles under his eyes and little of his former chirpy manner. The surgeon gave the family three months to think about it, though he hinted that 'It would be interesting to see how the leg responds'. Danny's stepmother was sceptical about the surgeon's motive: 'Is he really thinking about what's for Danny's benefit, or is he just curious?'

Danny's father replied, 'He genuinely felt that there was some advantage to Danny'. But Danny's stepmother argued, 'He's going to senior school soon, he doesn't want another six months in a wheelchair'.

In the end, the family refused consent for lengthening the left leg stump.

ACTIVITY: Do you think that a decision that respected the child's voice was made at the expense of his best interests? Again, compare the factors in this second decision with your own checklist and that used by Pearce.

There is some uncertainty about what would be in Danny's medical best interests in this second decision. His stepmother also points to the importance of his *social* best interests when she remarks that he is going to senior school soon and doesn't want to begin his time there in a wheelchair. This is an important factor which does not appear on Pearce's otherwise very complete checklist (unless it can be included under item 4, views of significant others).

Danny showed a great deal of cognitive maturity in the first part of his story: he has clearly grown up early, in the face of long familiarity with his illness. In the second part he may actually seem less mature insofar as he is adamantly unwilling even to consider the additional surgery; is this his pain and fear speaking? Alderson makes the important point that failing to listen to a child's fear, even if it seems irrational, is a form of ignoring the child's voice: 'Children can then be excluded and silenced, perhaps isolated within fears they feel unable to express.' This is a family with intimate and painful knowledge of neurofibromatosis, to which they have already lost one member.

They are perhaps less likely to accede to whatever the doctor says than patients with less experience of long-term illness. So it seems to us that the family's decision to reject further limb-lengthening is a reason-able resolution, one which the surgeon has facilitated by giving them plenty of time to think it over.

Limb-lengthening is not a life-or-death decision, but even in terminal illness professional opinion in many countries is beginning to swing round to the view that withholding or withdrawing curative treat-ment may be an acceptable extension of listening to the child's voice. In 1997, after taking submissions from religious representatives, professional and patient groups, and severely disabled young adults, the UK's Royal College of Paediatrics and Child Health Ethics Advisory Committee recommended that withholding or withdrawing curative medical treatment may be considered consistent with the paramount principle of respecting the child's best interests. The guidance, which you met in Chapter 1, refers to five situations in which it might be best not to treat:

(1) *The 'brain dead' child*: In the older child where criteria of brain-stem death are agreed by two practitioners in the usual way, it may still be technically feasible to provide basic cardio-respiratory support by means of ventilation and intensive care. It is agreed within the profession that treatment in such circumstances is futile and the withdrawal of current medical treatment is appropriate.

(2) *The 'permanent vegetative' state*: The child who develops a permanent vegetative state following insults, such as trauma or hypoxia, is reliant on others for all care and does not react or relate with the outside world. It may be appropriate to withdraw or withhold life-sustaining treatment.

(3) *The 'no chance' situation*: The child has such severe disease that life-sustaining treatment simply delays death without significant alleviation of suffering. Treatment to sustain life is inappropriate.

(4) *The 'no purpose' situation*: Although the patient may be able to survive with treatment, the degree of physical or mental impairment will be so great that it is unreasonable to expect them to bear it.

(5) *The 'unbearable' situation*: The child and/or family feel that in the face of progressive and irreversible illness further treatment is more than can be borne. They wish to have a particular treatment withdrawn or to refuse further treatment irrespective of the medical opinion that it may be of some benefit.

In situations that do not fit with these five categories, or where there is uncertainty about the degree of future impairment or disagreement, the child's life should always be safeguarded in the best way possible by all in the healthcare team, until these issues are resolved (Royal College of Paediatrics and Child Health, 2004).

ACTIVITY: The Royal College Guidelines represent a practical attempt to lay down guidelines for clinical practice in a highly charged area. Do you agree with them? For your final activity, we'd like you to draw up a similar set of guidelines for withholding or withdrawing curative treatment which reflect your own conclusions, after studying this chapter. Try to make them as concrete as possible. Then do the same exercise for some of the other ethically difficult choices which we've covered in earlier parts of the chapter. You might want to include some or all of the following:

- Conflict with one or both parents
- Involuntary treatment
- Knowing when the child is competent to give or withhold consent
- Balancing the interests of the child against the interests of the community
- Confidentiality.

At the end of this process, you should have your own set of 'protocols', your own personal code of practice, which can be applied to some of the ethically contentious difficulties in working with children and young people.

Notes

1. Adapted with permission from John Pearce, 'Ethical issues in child psychiatry and child psychotherapy: Conflicts between the child, parents and practitioners'. Paper presented at First EBEPE workshop, Rome, 1996.

2. Reproduced with permission from Veikko Launis, 'Moral issues concerning children's legal status in Finland in relation to psychiatric treatment'. Paper presented at First EBEPE workshop, Rome, 1996.

8 Resource allocation: justice, markets and rationing

Introduction

Medical resources are inevitably limited, and decisions will always have to be made between the various ways in which such resources might be used. The amount of money spent on healthcare varies both between countries and within countries over time. Different healthcare systems exist – some more efficient than others. Nevertheless, despite this variation, decisions will always have to be made about the priorities of healthcare spending. This is a profoundly moral matter and raises a wide range of ethical questions: What counts as a just distribution of healthcare resources? How ought we to decide between the provision of different treatments and the treatment of different patients? Given limited resources, which treatments don't we offer? What criteria ought to be used for rationing treatments?

We begin this chapter with an everyday sort of case, about long-term care of the very old. The demographic 'crisis' throughout Europe means that resource questions about the care of older people will become increasingly important, although the elderly are not our sole concern in this chapter. The case of Mr K also highlights conflict over resources between health and social services, between chronic and acute services, and between families and service providers, with clinicians caught in the middle. In this case the individual and the social collide. We shall use the case of Mr K as a starting point in trying to work out what guidance can be offered to clinicians and other healthcare professionals over such wider issues of resource allocation.

Section 1: The problem of resource allocation

The case of Mr K

Mr K was a 95-year-old patient in a long-stay ward at Park Prewett Hospital, Basingstoke, North and Mid-Hampshire Health Authority (UK). Like many other hospitals, Park Prewett was under pressure to close long-stay wards and free up resources. Legislative changes meant that there was conflict between health authorities and social services departments over who should foot the bill for long-term care of the elderly. It was in both parties' interests, however, to transfer the responsibility to families, who were expected to pay privately for the care of their elderly members.

At a meeting behind closed doors, the health authority decided to bring forward the date for closing Mr K's ward by 21 months. Although the consultant in charge of Mr K's care had deemed him unfit to be moved, the authority brought in an outside psychiatrist while the consultant was on leave. The psychiatrist conditionally approved the transfer. Along with 23 other elderly patients, Mr K was discharged to a private nursing home – on the very day of the decision. Seventeen days later he died. Four other elderly patients also died within three weeks of discharge from the hospital.

Mr K's son-in-law brought a complaint against the health authority to the Health Service Commissioner, an independent authority established by the Health Commissioners' Act 1993, who has powers to investigate complaints which cannot otherwise be settled in a court of law. The Commissioner condemned the health authority for acting undemocratically. He stated that their decision 'fell far short of the standards of accountability which a public body should display'. Although the health authority had originally claimed that the meeting was 'informal' and therefore private, North and Mid-Hampshire officials now acknowledged that 'the only sense in which it was informal was that it was not held in public'.

The Commissioner declared that his decision should serve as a 'grim warning' to any health authority or hospital trust planning to transfer long-term patients to the private sector. He also expressed 'considerable doubt' that doctors' consent to the patients' discharge had been obtained – let alone that of patients and their families.

The authority's handling of the affair was also censured by a House of Commons Select Committee, which called on ministers to dismiss those responsible. This was a national issue, it was felt, because the authority had flagrantly ignored government guidelines. Eight months after the censure vote by the Commons committee, the authority's chair, Angela Sealey, offered her resignation.

ACTIVITY: Stop here for a moment and make a list of the conflicts you see in Mr K's case. We've mentioned the tensions between the National Health Service and social services over who should pay for long-term care of the elderly. What other conflicts are there?

If we use a broad definition of conflicts – to include not only overt conflicts between people but also more abstract conflicts of principle – conflicts between some of the following might have come to your mind:

- The health service and social services
- The family and the public providers (either health or social services)
- Private, for-profit nursing care and state-supported care
- Hospital doctors and hospital managers
- Clinical criteria vs. financial criteria
- Nursing home doctors and hospital doctors – over the issue of Mr K's requirements for hospital-based care
- The best interests of Mr K versus the good of others
- And, of course, the Commissioner vs. the health authority.

How typical is the case of Mr K, do you think? Are cases about resource allocation usually this blatant? In one sense it's very atypical: a particularly flagrant example, clearly an abuse of power by the health authority. And you may also think that the nursing home's professional practices are unusually lax – in accepting the transfer apparently without the clinical sanction of Mr K's consultant hospital physician. But even if Mr K's case is atypically bad practice, the sorts of conflicts which it illustrates occur everyday, even if they're not always this obvious.

ACTIVITY: Stop for a moment and think about a case of resource allocation which has recently been in the news. Did conflict occur? What about? Who were the parties to it? And how was it resolved?

Although the immediate background to Mr K's case was community care legislation in the UK, the resource issues it illustrates are by no means unique to British practice. The following commentaries on the Mr K case, from Greece and Sweden, show that resource conflict is a crucial and familiar issue in both southern and northern Europe.

Dimitrios Niakas (Niakas, 1997), of the Department of Economics at the National School of Public Health, in Greece, identifies four problems in Mr K's case:

(1) *The problem of accountability for providing services between social and healthcare authorities.* Given the scarcity of resources, and the fact that in many healthcare systems there is a division of these services, battle is joined between these two departments in attempting to save money and transfer responsibility. This conflict over the boundaries of services creates many problems for the elderly and other disadvantaged groups.

(2) *The efficiency problem for policy-makers, who are responsible both for saving money and for improving access to healthcare, reducing waiting lists.* Thus, the replacement of long-stay wards in hospitals is necessary, if more patients with acute problems need treatment and care. The transfer of long-stay patients, including the elderly, to other settings (such as nursing homes and home care) seems to be a necessary step for efficiency.

(3) *The ethical problem for the clinician who has to give permission for the transfer, although he or she may not know whether the conditions in the new setting will be appropriate to the patient's particular needs.* On the other hand, the clinician is under pressure from hospital management, and knows that many acute cases are waiting for admission as well.

(4) *The problem of implementation and social acceptance, even if changes were planned and rational.* There will always be losers under any change, but equally, lack of change may be unfair to others. Media coverage may be sensationalistic: for example, in this case Mr K's death was apparently blamed on the transfer, although nobody can provide evidence to prove that.

Marti Parker (Parker, 1997), of the Department of Social Work at the University of Stockholm in Sweden, confirms that Mr K's case could have happened almost anywhere in Europe:

The case is well chosen in that it is typical of what is happening in many places. Sweden is also closing long-term-stay institutions in an endeavour to decentralize and provide the minimal care necessary. There is also a hope among many politicians that the family will take over more responsibility. Because these decisions are now being made at the local level, with few central directives or standards to go by, and where there is often a lack of competence, there is a greater risk that the 'wrong' decision will be made.

One of the arguments we have heard for decentralizing has been to increase local democracy concerning local decisions. Unfortunately, democracy has actually suffered under decentralization, in my opinion. The case illustrates a similar process in the UK.

There are several issues here. The first is the issue of the decision itself – to move Mr K. A second issue is how the decision was arrived at and implemented – quickly, and without involving the family, or even informing them. A third, related issue is that of consent – of course, a very complicated issue in this age group.

The case, as presented here, does not take into account the fact that moving involves great risk to people in this age group. Any move, even to much better accommodation, increases the probability of death. The fact that five out of 24 persons in this age group died within a 3-week period may not be so remarkable, especially after a move. This is regardless of how the decision was made and of whether consent was granted. Even if the decision had been taken under the best, most democratic and humane circumstances, the transfers might still have resulted in the same mortality rate.

Obviously, the circumstances surrounding this decision were scandalous. The families and physicians should have been informed and involved in the decision. The information to the families should have included the risk involved in transfer at this age. The old people themselves should also have been involved to the greatest extent possible. However, the deaths cannot be said to be directly related to the undemocratic process which preceded the decision. We must be careful not to imply a latent causal effect.

Marti Parker's colleague, the Swedish social work professor Mats Thorslund, points out that so-called 'bedblockers' cost a hospital less than acute cases, and continue to decrease to the level of the hospital's 'hotel' costs of care. We must avoid the trap of assuming that decisions ostensibly taken on economic grounds are necessarily efficient!

The commentaries from Greece and Sweden both remind us not to assume that Mr K's death was directly caused by the authority's decision; but they also emphasize that conflicts over resource allocation extend to other areas than those we have already considered. Three more conflicts are suggested by Niakas and Parker:

- Between saving money and widening access to healthcare
- Between the media and health authorities or hospitals
- Between central and localized decision-making.

We also need to bear in mind the distinction between the *outcome* and the *grounds* of the resource allocation decision and the *process* by which it was made. The Commissioner did not so much criticize the *substance* of the health authority's decision as the *procedure*. He did not lay down an absolute prohibition on discharging long-stay patients, provided that doctors consent, decisions are made publicly, and sufficient notice is given. If the health authority had been willing to wait until the original date projected for the ward's closure, the case of Mr K would probably never have been made public.

After all, as both the Greek and Swedish commentators remind us, even an openly and fairly made decision might have resulted in Mr K's death. So judging by the outcome alone is inappropriate. This is particularly true because, of course, clinicians can't know the outcome of resource allocation decisions in advance. Judging by outcome tends to turn into judging from hindsight.

So what are the criteria by which we should judge the *procedures* behind resource allocation decisions? How do we decide? The second section of this chapter begins to formulate some answers to that crucial question. Before you go on to that section, however, please undertake this final activity.

ACTIVITY: Think of a decision about dividing resources fairly – but this time from outside the healthcare context. You could choose something as trivial as dividing a birthday cake, or something more complicated. How would you decide? What principles of fair distribution lay behind your decision? Make a list of the considerations you would take into account. We will ask you to refer back to this list at the end of the chapter, to see whether your ideas have developed or changed.

The usual presumption would be that *everyone should get an equal share* of the cake, unless they disclaimed it by saying 'None for me, thanks', or 'Oh, no, I don't want that much'. So *equality* is one obvious principle to use in decision-making. Some analysts would want to invoke it as what is called a *prima facie* principle. From the Latin for 'at first sight', *prima facie* means that there is a presumption in favour of that principle, in this case 'equality', unless proven otherwise.

However, other principles might also enter the equation: for example, a *medical* criterion that a person with diabetes shouldn't have any cake at all. Or a *first-come-first-served* principle might be relevant for latecomers who complain that they missed out on the division of the cake altogether.

This principle is the rationale for using a waiting list in healthcare resource allocation. What other principles do we use in everyday life to allocate resources fairly?

Section 2: Deciding by medical criteria

Considering how you would go about distributing things fairly in everyday life may give you some insights into the principles you would use in medical decision-making. But equally, you might well have objected to the exercise on the grounds that making everyday decisions – such as dividing up a birthday cake – is qualitatively different, precisely because they aren't medical decisions. True, medical criteria slipped in through the back door in the cake example, in so far as people with diabetes got no cake, on medical grounds. But, you might feel that this is atypical: most everyday decisions about sharing out scarce goods needn't consider health status.

Medicine also has the advantage over everyday decisions, one could argue, because it represents an objective, frequently quantifiable body of knowledge. In allocating scarce medical resources fairly, isn't the answer just to go by these objective medical criteria? In this view, evidence-based medicine (EBM) can tell us which treatments are the most effective. Those are the treatments to which we should devote maximum resources, EBM advocates might argue. Futile or ineffective interventions don't deserve our scarce resources, and it would actually be unethical to waste money on them.

On the face of it, this looks incontrovertible. Doing the best we can for patients – perhaps the most basic dictum in medical practice and medical ethics – seems to mean that we should give the most effective treatments to the cases that need them most. Medical criteria are often seen as a value-neutral 'trump card', which puts paid to any further debate about allocation of scarce healthcare resources. On this argument, doctors should stop providing treatment at the point when it becomes medically futile, and that is also the threshold at which the health purchaser – state, insurer or other purchaser – should stop purchasing. So deciding by medical criteria cuts short any further discussion about allocation of scarce healthcare resources, it is claimed.

This line of argument has a strong common-sense appeal, particularly to doctors who fear that they may be forced otherwise to provide treatment against their clinical consciences (Paris and Reardon, 1992), but we'd like you to think about possible complications in what may seem so obvious an argument.

> ACTIVITY: Stop here for a moment and write down three possible arguments against the view that we should decide questions of scarce resources by medical criteria, and medical criteria alone.

There are several sorts of arguments against the apparently attractive option of deciding purely on medical criteria (Biller-Andorno *et al.*, 2002; Dickenson and Vineis, 2002; Rogers, 2002). We chose the following three points.

(1) The terms are not clear

When advocates of EBM say that no money should be spent on 'futile' or 'ineffective' interventions, they assume that we can all agree on what is 'futile' or 'ineffective'. But, in fact, a range of definitions of 'futile' have been offered by different authors: among them are 'failing to prolong life', 'failing to achieve the patient's wishes', 'failing to achieve a physiological effect on the body', and 'failing to achieve a therapeutic benefit for the patient' (Halliday, 1997, p. 149). This is not merely a semantic quarrel: it reflects deeper disagreement over both the *utility* or value to be served by treatment (which, as we suggested in the first chapter, links with the value we place on human life), and the *probability* of success. In the long run, of course, we are all dead, and therefore all treatment is futile. In less facile terms, there may be disagreements among practitioners, or between practitioners and patients or their families, about what counts as futile, and things don't always turn out as predicted. Consider the American case below, that of 'Baby Ryan' (adapted from Capron, 1995).

The case of 'Baby Ryan'

Ryan Nguyen was born 6 weeks prematurely, asphyxiated, and with only a weak heartbeat. His clinicians also diagnosed brain damage following seizures, an intestinal blockage, and renal failure which meant that his kidneys failed to clear toxins, although they produced urine. Initially, Ryan was sustained through intravenous feeding and dialysis, but his clinicians doubted that he could be kept alive in this fashion until he was old enough for a kidney transplant, at about 2 years. They wanted to end treatment on the grounds of futility: it was argued that 'long-term dialysis would not only be inappropriate but would be immoral', since it would prolong Ryan's suffering with no chance of improvement.

Ryan's parents refused to accept withdrawal of treatment, despite the hospital's view that imposing 'virtually futile' treatment would be inhumane. The Nguyens sought a second opinion from a neonatologist at another hospital, but that, too, was unfavourable. Finally, they obtained an emergency court order, permitted under the legislation of their home state, directing the hospital to take whatever steps were necessary to maintain Ryan's life, including dialysis. The publicity surrounding the case attracted another hospital's attention, and this third hospital accepted Ryan for transfer. Three days later, surgeons there operated to clear Ryan's blocked intestines. He was shortly able to take nutrition by mouth, and at 3 months he was sent home, not having needed any further dialysis. At 1 year he appeared to be developing normally for his age, free of any permanent neurological deficit; his most recent CAT scan shows no structural problems.

---

(2) We cannot always get the necessary evidence

Evidence-based medicine gives a high priority to certain types of evidence, particularly from randomized clinical trials; yet such high-quality evidence isn't always available. This isn't just a matter of the evidence not being available *yet*, because not enough trials have been done – although that, too, is a problem. Drug treatments, for example, are more likely to attract the necessary funding for trials to be carried out – possibly funding from pharmaceutical companies. There might be some alternative treatment which didn't involve the use of drugs – but we would never know about it. 'This could result in some drug treatments being recommended and purchased, not because they are better than alternative, non-drug treatments, but because the *evidence* for effectiveness is better' (Hope, 1995, p. 260).

Outcomes for acute conditions are also easier to measure and test than those for chronic ones, which typically have fuzzier, longer-term parameters. This raises issues about *fairness*. The elderly might be more likely to have chronic conditions, for example; so deciding only to support EBM-approved interventions could inadvertently discriminate in favour of younger people with acute conditions.

Justice

Is such discrimination unjust, and how do we judge what counts as justice? Justice is often seen in terms of fairness (Rawls, 1971), of what principles of fair distribution we could agree to. This is *distributive justice*, the main concern of this chapter, though justice can also be considered in terms of respect for *rights and the law* – crucial in *criminal justice*. What the two branches of justice have in common is that both are concerned with ensuring that individuals receive the treatment that is proper or fitting for them (Miller, 1986). The classic formulation of formal justice is Aristotle's injunction to 'treat equals equally'. This does not mean treating everyone alike: in relation to healthcare, for example, the sick deserve different treatment from the well, and more resources. Indeed, Aristotle also specified that unequals should be treated unequally. It is substantive analysis of what counts as a *relevant inequality* which varies between different philosophical approaches, and, in relation to our concerns in this chapter, between different approaches to resource distribution.

In Section 5 of this chapter we will be going on to explore different approaches to the question of justice. However, it is already clear that we cannot escape ethical debates about justice by looking to allegedly scientific and objective medical criteria. Even if in principle it were possible to test every proposed treatment, some would argue that it might actually be unethical to run a randomized clinical trial with a particular population, particularly of patients who can't decide for themselves whether to enter a trial: very sick neonates, for example, or elderly people with dementia. This suggests a final point about why it is not sufficient to decide by medical criteria alone.

(3) Even if we had the necessary evidence, we might not want to make it the only criterion for deciding

Patient choice might be another factor to consider, for example. Even if we didn't want to allow patients to choose treatments that were patently and clinically *bad* for them, there might be a certain degree of latitude in letting them choose interventions which suit their particular circumstances, religious or cultural beliefs, or family preferences. In a democracy, shouldn't patient choice also be a value?

Clearly, there are limitations on patient choice, however, when there simply are insufficient resources to satisfy everyone's demands. In the example described below, the UK case of 'Child B', the child patient – or, primarily, her father – 'chose' an expensive treatment with a low probability of success. Evidence-based medicine would probably not have supported the treatment in this child's case. None the less, public feeling ran high, illustrating the point that evidence-based criteria are often unacceptable for particular classes of patients – notably very sick children. In this case, unlike that of 'Baby Ryan', the decision that treatment was futile turned out to be correct, in the sad sense that the child died. But were other values served by treating the girl? – not least, perhaps, society's sense of solidarity with other parents and children in this tragic situation.

The Case of 'Child B'

Child B (later publicly identified as Jaymee Bowen), aged 10, was acutely ill with leukaemia (*R v Cambridge Health Authority, ex p. B* [1995] 1 FLR 1055). A bone-marrow transplant had proved unsuccessful. Now both her own doctor and oncologists from London's Royal Marsden Hospital believed she had only a few weeks to live, with further treatment being futile. Although Jaymee's own views in favour of treatment were of uncertain validity – she had not been told how ill she was – her father refused to accept this decision. He located a professor at the Hammersmith Hospital who recommended a further course of chemotherapy followed by an experimental second bone-marrow transplant, which would have to be provided by Jaymee's younger sister. Primarily because the professor had acknowledged that this was experimental, non-standard therapy, and

secondarily because Department of Health guidance limited the funding of unproven treatment, Jaymee's Health Authority in Cambridge decided that 'the substantial expenditure on treatment with such a small prospect of success would not be an effective use of resources' (Herring, 2008, p. 57).

Mr Bowen brought a legal action to compel the Health Authority to fund Jaymee's treatment with the experimental procedure. His chances of success looked poor, despite a massive outpouring of public sympathy and extensive media coverage. Normally, English courts are reluctant to intervene in such matters unless it can be shown that the decision was taken in bad faith or was patently unreasonable. Although in a 1987 case (*R. v. Secretary of State for Social Services, ex parte Walker*) the Court of Appeal had stated that courts could strike down decisions about resource allocation, no court had actually done so.

Nevertheless Mr Bowen succeeded, at least at first. In the High Court the Health Authority's decision was quashed, and their powers to refuse treatment on grounds of resource shortage were severely limited. The Health Authority was ordered to reconsider its decision and to spell out its reasoning more clearly, allowing the father a chance to show that the decision had, in fact, been unreasonable. The burden was put on the Health Authority: its duty to recognize Jaymee's fundamental right to life required it to show compelling reasons why other patients should implicitly have priority over her.

However, the Court of Appeal overturned the High Court decision. Whether or not a treatment was life-saving, the Appeal Court held, had no bearing on the general principle that courts could not intervene to determine the merits of the dispute. Courts should not be drawn into resource allocation decisions. Nor should the Health Authority be forced to show where it planned to spend the money that would notionally be saved by not treating Jaymee. The Appeal Court's reasoning was based not primarily on resource shortage, however, but on the weight of medical evidence, suggesting that it was not in Jaymee's best interests to undergo the experimental procedure. So efficacy of treatment clearly *is* a proper legal consideration.

In the end, a private benefactor came forward, offering to fund Jaymee's experimental treatment. She appeared at first to be doing well after the procedure, but worsened after a few months and died. After her death, Mr Bowen reiterated his satisfaction that everything possible had been done, despite the tragic outcome.

ACTIVITY: Given that there will always be tragic cases, how can practitioners allocate resources fairly? How can we avoid being blown by the media winds into favouring the most emotionally gripping cases? – such as those of Jaymee Bowen. A Norwegian set of guidelines for practical use (from Elgesem, 1996) is instructive, setting out five levels of priorities for healthcare funding. These guidelines were intended to be realistic, reflecting what interest groups and the press would find acceptable – even if that might conflict with consistency of principles.

We would now like you to read through these guidelines and then undertake the following activity. Firstly, think of two further examples (in addition to those given below, by the Norwegian committee), which you think would fit under each level of priority. Secondly, having thus worked out what are the practical implications of each level of funding, ask yourself whether you agree with these rankings. Would you want to set priorities differently?

Priority level 1: Procedures immediately necessary to save lives in acute physical or mental illness. Examples: emergency surgery, emergency situations in psychiatric care and treatment of severely ill neonates.
Priority level 2: Procedures required to avoid longer-term harm to patients or groups of patients, where interventions are well supported by evidence. Examples: diagnosis and treatment of asthma or diabetes.
Priority level 3: Procedures with documented effects, but where the consequences of not treating are less serious. Example: treatment of moderately high blood pressure.
Priority level 4: Services which are in demand but where there is little or no physiological ill-effect from not treating. Examples: IVF and repeated ultrasound on request during pregnancy.
Zero priority: Services which are in demand but which have no documented benefits. Example: special health services for top athletes.
Note: Under this scheme, public funding would only be available for levels 1, 2 and 3.

How did you get on with evaluating these levels of priority? We found the zero-level rather puzzling: it seemed to us that the distinction being made was not

that the procedures were of no benefit, but that only an elite would benefit from them. And we thought that the refusal to fund IVF might be very unpopular – whereas the committee had said that it was taking public opinion into account. In Section 3 we will look in more detail at the issue of public response to rationing IVF treatment.

Underlying these five levels of priority in the Norwegian report were five criteria which the commission initially suggested for rationing scarce resources:

- Seriousness of the condition
- Equity in access to health services among all regions and classes
- Length of time patients have to wait for services
- Fairness to disadvantaged groups (defined as single elderly and disabled people, psychiatric patients and people with learning difficulties)
- The patient's responsibility for the disease, in terms of lifestyle.

It seems likely that equity of access to health services for all regions and classes collides with enforcing patients' responsibility for their own condition, in lifestyle terms. Smoking, for example, is typically more heavily distributed among members of the lower social classes than among the better-off. Smoking also illustrates possible conflict between seriousness of the condition and the patient's responsibility for it: should lung cancer and cardiac patients who have smoked be denied resources for their serious condition? An English consultant who refused to perform a heart bypass operation on a cardiac patient who was not willing to give up smoking was, in fact, required to perform the operation, despite his argument that the procedure would have been a waste of resources were the man, as seemed likely, to continue to smoke.

In the end the Norwegian report, in fact, omitted patient responsibility as too contentious a criterion. A later version replaced the five criteria with only three: seriousness of the disease, utility of the procedure and equity.

ACTIVITY: Do these three criteria cover the appropriate bases for making a decision about rationing resources, do you think?

We wondered if you have noticed the omission of one factor which appears very often in decisions about withholding scarce resources: age. Mr K's case is at the opposite end of the age spectrum from those of Baby Ryan and Child B, but perhaps both sets of cases are really explained by the operation of unexpressed age criteria in rationing. Age considerations, in reverse, explain the special importance society seems to attach to saving children at all costs – as we saw in the public reaction to the Child B case. That is not to say that deciding by age is ethically justified, of course.

Before moving on, we just want to emphasize the 'ordinariness' of resource conflicts. Mr K's case was a particularly flagrant example, but hospitals do have to make decisions every day about devoting resources to long-term care of the elderly. This is inescapable, but not necessarily a bad thing. In making judgements practitioners may improve their powers of reasoning, sharpen their skills of analysis and acquire better styles of communication. This is especially true, we would argue, if they can bring ethical analysis to bear in making these judgements. The skill of elaborating judgements about particular cases – what Aristotle termed *phronesis* – is consistent with making better clinical judgements, we think. We have emphasized particular cases in this chapter because we, too, believe in the development of *phronesis*.

The cases of Baby Ryan and Child B were more public and controversial, less common than that of Mr K, and they were also atypical in that they both wound up in court. Legal guidelines were laid down in the Child B case, for British practitioners, that do affect clinical work; but even in the absence of such legal guidelines, ethical analysis can help unravel the reasoning behind the kinds of priorities clinicians have. Some of the ethical values we have encountered so far have included:

- The notion of *distributive justice*, that is, how we can divide up resources fairly
- The concept of *equity* between classes, and of healthcare as a form of reducing social disparity
- The converse notion of *desert or responsibility*, for example, in the argument about whether people who are responsible for their own conditions deserve fewer resource
- The underpinning notion that we cannot escape from social and ethical judgements by taking refuge in medical criteria alone.

We will explore these concepts in greater depth in the remaining sections of this chapter.

Section 3: Using social and political criteria to decide on resource allocation

In Section 2 we asked you to consider a Norwegian model of resource allocation based on the use of priority levels. Whilst doing so, you may have noticed that the priority levels included what might be called 'social criteria' in addition to medical ones: for example, the terms 'equity in access to health services among all regions and classes' and 'fairness to disadvantaged groups' in the list of five criteria, along with more obviously clinical criteria such as 'seriousness of the condition'.

Running the two sorts of criteria together is something of a sleight of hand, even if an unintentional one. Social criteria for resource allocation at first appear much more problematic than medical criteria, although we have already argued that even evidence-based medical criteria cannot be entirely extricated from social issues, such as inadvertent discrimination against certain patient groups. Nevertheless, since the days of the Seattle 'God project', social criteria for resource allocation have had a dubious reputation. 'God project' was the derogatory term given to the early attempt by a committee deciding allocation of then-scarce kidney dialysis on the basis of 'social worth', including church membership and Scout leadership (Dickenson, 1995, p. 245).

Just because social values *do* often enter surreptitiously into clinical criteria does not mean that we *should* legitimize them in such blatant forms of discrimination. But often social and political criteria are much less easy to condemn, and much harder to disentangle from medical factors. The Norwegian attempt to rank various clinical interventions for funding priority often ran medical and social criteria together – for example, in allocating zero priority to services which had 'no documented benefits', when these interventions might actually have been effective enough but favoured privileged groups. The position of fertility treatment in priority level 4 – which was not to be funded – was justified on the basis that there was 'little or no physiological ill-effect from not treating'. Had the criteria taken *psychological* ill-effect into account, that argument would have been very much harder to maintain. Likewise, had the criterion been physiological *benefit* from treating, IVF should have been entered for consideration, although its comparatively low overall success rates might have told against it.

Medical futility, however, is rarely a black-and-white matter. It can certainly be argued that social criteria also influence the measure of futility which is selected. As we suggested earlier, various definitions of futility have contended for dominance, including 'failing to achieve the patient's wishes', 'failing to achieve a physiological effect on the body' and 'failing to achieve a therapeutic benefit for the patient'. Even unsuccessful IVF treatment may still satisfy the patient's wishes *for* treatment and also achieve a therapeutic benefit if the psychological pain of childlessness is weighted into the equation, since patients may feel that at least all has been done that could be done to treat their infertility.

In this section we will look at the example of public funding for fertility treatment as an instance where social and medical criteria both play a part. Underlying the example is the question of whether our society views infertility as a medical condition to be allocated the same priority as other medical conditions, or whether because it is not life-threatening, it is somehow less urgent. This judgement itself cannot be made on merely medical grounds: it is inescapably ethical and social. And the case study also raises troubling issues in which semi-medical criteria appear to be used as a 'front' for what are primarily political decisions about restricting IVF treatment, not only by women's age but also by more arbitrary factors.

In 2004 the UK's National Institute for Clinical Excellence (NICE), which is charged with producing criteria for resource allocation within the National Health Service, published a set of clinical guidelines on funding infertility treatment. These criteria 'provided an evidence- and cost-effectiveness-based approach' (Barlow, 2009, p. 293) which was intended to act as a national policy. The hope was to rectify what was widely seen as an unjust and uneven situation, whereby women in some areas received fully funded infertility treatment, while those in other regions received none. However, NICE recommendations are only advisory. In this instance, NICE had substantial difficulties in enforcing its recommendation – that all local health authorities should provide women aged 39 or under with three free cycles of IVF treatment.

ACTIVITY: Would you say that this recommendation is primarily based on medical or on social criteria?

You may have wondered where the figures of three cycles and 39 years came from. Professor David Barlow, who chaired the committee that drew up the NICE guidelines, has defended the first figure as evidence-based. 'The basis for the recommendation that three cycles should be offered was that the evidence base for the effectiveness of IVF in consecutive treatment cycles appeared most convincing for the first three cycles of IVF treatment' (Barlow, 2009, p. 297). Beyond three cycles, Barlow says, diminishing returns appeared to operate. Other European countries, however, offer more than three cycles, with six being the norm in Belgium (Pennings and de Vroey, 2006).

You may also have wanted to ask whether the age cut-off of 39 years is a form of unjust discrimination against older women, or whether it is medically justified. Ostensibly this age cut-off was rooted in medical criteria, but there's also what philosophers call a 'slippery slope' problem that suggests social criteria also play a part. 'There is no specific threshold age at which reproductive ageing becomes critical' (Barlow, 2009, p. 293). Obviously, we cannot say that a woman aged 40 years and one day is completely incapable of conceiving, unlike a woman aged 39 years and 364 days. But NICE deals in statistical probabilities for entire classes of patients rather than single individuals, and it also operates cost-effectiveness criteria based on 'value for money' for different treatments. It can equally well be argued that NICE intends to remedy the injustice of 'postcode prescribing', which can be seen, in Aristotelian terms, as a form of treating equals unequally. Couples who present with similar clinical criteria of male or female infertility should not be treated differently according to where they live; that's not a relevant inequality which would justify treating unequals unequally.

It is indisputable that female fertility does fall off rapidly in the second half of a woman's thirties (Hillier, 2009), and so the cut-off age of 39 is not entirely implausible in clinical terms. The NICE guidelines stated that women aged 40 years and over had a 6% chance of a live birth in one treatment cycle, but contrasted that with rates greater than 20% for women aged 25–35, 15% for women aged 36–38, and 10% for women aged 39. So in terms of 'value for money', the group of all women over 40 are a worse 'investment'; more pregnancies can be achieved for the same amount of money by concentrating resources on women under that age. Perhaps some people might feel so strongly about childlessness that they would want to say that all infertile couples should be treated whatever the cost, and that's entirely understandable – but it would inevitably mean that less would have to be spent in some other area of health funding.

What is more problematic is the way in which a medical criterion is intertwined with social judgements about 'value for money', which is more than merely an accounting question. In the case of infertility, that is primarily true because fertility treatment does not actually save lives, however vital it may be to the couples undergoing it. It creates new ones, true, but that does not factor so readily into the calculations on which NICE normally bases its resource allocation decisions.

The real issue, however, turned out to be the reluctance of local health authorities to fund infertility treatment at all. Although the NICE recommendation of three free cycles for women under 39 might rightly or wrongly have been accused of discriminating against older women, at least it would have provided women under that age with treatment, available uniformly across the country. Yet five years after the NICE guidelines were issued, most local health authorities provided at most one IVF cycle, and some provided none at all. As a result, two-thirds of IVF treatment in the UK had to be purchased from the private sector (Greenwood, 2009, p. 309).

Berkeley Greenwood, a political advisor to the UK National Infertility Awareness Campaign, has written a compelling case study of the way in which social and political factors interacted with medical ones as government ministers and NICE itself attempted to impose the recommendation of three free cycles on the local health authorities who would have to pay for them. We would now like you to read the following selections from his article. As you read, ask yourself what arguments about distributive justice were implicitly or explicitly used by each side.

Bang for the buck: what purchasers and commissioners think and do

Berkeley Greenwood[1]

Perhaps those who are wedded always to the need for a rigorous evidence base had better look away now.

To understand why we are where we are with the funding of ARTs [Assisted Reproductive Technologies], it is helpful to review the history of this issue. We will primarily review the situation in England rather than the UK.

The first IVF birth was achieved 30 years ago. In the years that followed, what had initially been presented by the press and media as a Star Wars-style technique gradually became a more commonplace and straightforward procedure. It started to become available in limited quantities on the NHS too. As so often has been the case, it was rapidly picked up and more readily embraced in the less conservative healthcare environments elsewhere in Europe.

Being a new area of medicine, there was absolutely no budget in existence for it in the NHS and so creating one meant taking money from elsewhere in what, throughout the past 20 years, has been a continually cash-strapped system. This has been the major challenge for campaigners in this area throughout.

In the early 1990s Ministers had difficulty in accepting that infertility comprised a health need at all. They were reflecting wider public opinion (indeed 'smug haves' or 'smug don't wants' can still be found loudly opining against NHS provision of such treatments at dinner tables, whenever this topic is discussed). After much campaigning, the Department of Health at last began to concede in correspondence around 1995 that infertility did indeed comprise 'an important health need'. But it still was not going to instruct anyone to fund it and the area remained outside the waiting list targets.

The improvements in service that took place in the 1990s from health authority to health authority were largely the result of enterprising groups of patients taking up the cudgels with local commissioners and forcing them to make some provision. This was backed by approaches to MPs at national level to try to persuade them to take issues up with directors of public health in their patch. Interestingly, this has always been an area that has commanded genuine cross-party support, amongst backbenchers at least, and Early Day Motions (EDMs) tabled as early as 1993 and as late as 2008 bear testimony to this. The arguments that came back were that infertility treatment wasn't a priority, wasn't successful and could be categorized alongside wisdom tooth extraction, breast reduction, varicose veins and sterilization in terms of its value.

Enter NICE and a way out of the conundrum. The then Health Minister, Yvette Cooper, after some arm twisting which was greatly aided by press stories about the gap between provision in the UK compared with everywhere else in Europe, referred infertility to NICE's clinical guideline process. Two years later, in 2004, out popped the NICE clinical guideline on fertility in all its 216-page glory. The guideline recommends that three cycles of IVF [in vitro fertiliza-tion] or ICSI [intra-cytoplasmic sperm injection] should be provided. It makes no *binding* recommen-dations as to eligibility criteria to define which patients should or should not receive treatment but does point the way on factors such as age, smoking and BMI [body mass index].

The guideline's publication was accompanied by a statement from the Secretary of State for Health, who at that point was John Reid. He asked PCTs [Primary Care Trusts] – as Health Authorities had now become – to begin to move towards implement-ing the guideline, over time, but initially by providing one cycle of treatment from April 2005. On the same day, the then Prime Minister, in the House of Commons, made it plain that he expected PCTs to implement the whole guideline over time.

The period that followed was perhaps the most cash-strapped period that the NHS has ever endured as, despite huge resources being poured into the Service, budget deficits accelerated. A Treasury-driven desire to balance the books meant that major efforts were needed to clear this debt. Anything that wasn't nailed down went over the side and, far from implementing one cycle, some PCTs actually began to disinvest.

It is an uphill battle, but one in which there is at long last evidence of success. More PCTs than ever before now fund at least one cycle and increasing numbers seem tentatively to be beginning to fund two. What is not clear is whether they are 'cheating' by providing more cycles to a smaller number of people, using widely varying eligibility criteria to nar-row down the numbers of people who will qualify for treatment. This is the next phase in the challenge that we face to ensure that ARTs are properly funded.

It is clear that the UK undertakes fewer cycles of ART per woman of reproducing age than most major European countries, including all types of funding. The major exception is Germany, which performs about the same, and this is a country that has seen its State provision slashed in the past few years, lead-ing to a significant fall in total cycles. It is reasonable also to assume that the UK lags behind other coun-tries in terms of State provision since examining the funding policies of various countries does, as a rule, show a more generous approach to funding ART by other Governments.

Ministers do not feel that they can simply order PCTs to do something that they don't wish to do. Exceptions to this are the central priority areas – CHD [coronary heart disease], cancer and mental health, the 'core' standards, which include elements

of those three areas amongst others, the mandated areas such as NICE technology guidance, and those areas of public health that are laid down in statute. The next layer down in terms of national priority are 'developmental standards', which are areas on which the NHS has to demonstrate that it is working towards achieving, and these typically include NICE clinical guidelines. But the rules are vague here about what constitutes 'reasonable progress'. So decisions on infertility continue to be made locally and Ministers have left themselves with limited weaponry with which to cajole reluctant funders into improving serv-ices for infertility patients.

Again, anecdotally, from discussions with PCTs it is clear that far fewer of them rely now on the argu-ment that infertility is not a health need at all. Most will also accept that a higher degree of priority now applies to this area than ever did in the past. Typically, those that do not fund or who have tried to cut services in the past couple of years, have cited budget restrictions as their reason for doing so.

So are any of the factors surrounding funding age-dependent? Clearly they are. Almost all, if not all, PCTs will apply upper age limits on women receiving treat-ment and some on men. Some also apply a lower age limit, which is 23 in many cases (in line with NICE) but can be as high as 30 or even 35.

There is one – scarcely believable-case of North Yorkshire and York PCT, which allows a window for treatment of just 6 months up to 40 years of age. This is about as unscientific, cost-ineffective, random and reluctant as it is possible to be. Why not simply offer a treatment to a left-handed, dark-haired woman, born on a Monday in June, and then only if you really have to?

Upper age limits may well be grounded in sensi-ble scientifically based reasoning, namely that the effectiveness of the treatment will fall with age. But lower age limits – at least down to 23, below which NICE says there is little available evidence – are surely only about budget restraint. What matters on clinical grounds is the duration of the attempt to conceive and the nature of the patient's problem. It hardly makes clinical, cost efficacy or social sense to delay treatment in, say, a 26-year-old, who is in a stable and long-standing relationship, has tried for three years to conceive and has a known cause of their infertility.

When NICE examined the question of infertility it used a fairly basic estimate of cost efficacy related to the numbers of cycles performed, their cost and likely success rates in various age bands. It did not attempt to perform a more sophisticated cost effective analy-sis resulting in a quality-adjusted life year (QALY) estimate, arguing that this methodology was more geared to life saved and quality of life gained, than to additional lives created. So there is no QALY provided for ART, certainly through any official process. One would imagine, though, that given the years of high-quality life that ARTs would create, it would look pretty cost-effective on normal measures.

ACTIVITY: Greenwood is referring here to the concept of the Quality-Adjusted Life Year, a resource allocation measure which analyses the cost and the utility of any proposed intervention. 'Instead of simply comparing how many life-years can be saved through various interventions, QALY analysis weights in how much value or utility people attach to a year in a particular status: complete freedom from pain, moderate pain, minor disability, major disability and so forth. The weights used reflect individual preferences, standardized between 0 and 1. The value of zero corresponds to death, whereas one equals perfect health. The results of such a cost-utility analysis are expressed in terms of the cost per QALY' (de Graeve and Adriaenssen, 2001). Do you agree with Greenwood that QALY analysis would favour assisted reproductive technologies? Whose life is he considering when he talks about the 'years of high-quality life that ARTs would create?' It's not clear to us whether he means that the lives of the couple will be enhanced through fulfilling their wish to have children, or whether he means that a new life will be created through fertility treatment.

Either way, that is not the usual clinical situation which QALYs are meant to analyse, where what is at stake is how much freedom from disability or pain a particular intervention can purchase for the patient on whom it is performed. As the NICE guidelines themselves noted, 'QALYs are intended to capture improvements in health among patients. They are not appropriate for placing a value on additional lives. Additional lives are not improvements in health; preventing someone's death is not the same as creating their life and it is not possible to improve the quality of life of someone who has not been conceived by conceiving them. Cost-utility analysis has little relevance to the management of infertility, where lives are produced and not saved' (quoted in Barlow, 2009, p. 297).

Now continue with your reading of the Greenwood article.

Into this calculation must come not only the life produced as a result of the treatment but the morbidity avoided in terms of depression, failed marriages, underperformance at work and other factors which are reported co-morbidities in some who are unable to have children. This is discussed in depth in the NICE guideline. Against this are the costs that arise as a result of ARTs and arising particularly from the increased incidence of multiple births and their consequences.

As mentioned earlier, the thorny issue of eligibility criteria is one with which the infertility world continues to have to wrestle. These vary widely from PCT to PCT and are strongly suspected by patients and some clinicians and politicians of being used primarily to ration services.

NICE partially addressed the issue of eligibility criteria and the British Fertility Society (BFS) has also taken a view. The main areas of criteria are age – which we have discussed above – body mass index (BMI), pre-existing children, previous numbers of cycles, duration of infertility and/or of the couple's relationship, history of sterilization and whether the couple are same-sex. Most PCTs specify an age range and stipulate a maximum and minimum BMI. In the latter case, if this can be seen to drive clinical success rate or the welfare of mother or child, then it may be seen to be reasonable.

Criteria with regard to secondary infertility are much more contentious and – arguably – inadvertently discriminate against older people, since these are more likely to be in second or third relationships as they get older. Denying a couple the chance of treatment if there is a pre-existing child from any previous relationship seems especially harsh, but is frequently applied. Other PCTs deny treatment to people only where the child is from the same relationship or from a previous relationship but living with the couple. This is often regarded by people in that situation as very unfair since it ignores the desire for the woman to have her own child or for the couple to have a child that is the fruit of their particular relationship. Some couples also say that the pain from secondary infertility is every bit as bad as that from primary infertility, not least because the couple now know the very real joy that a child brings.

There is also wide variation from PCT to PCT regarding their views on pre-existing relationships, duration of infertility and of previous cycles received either privately or on the NHS. Only on the question of previous sterilization does there seem to be agreement, with PCTs either barring treatment to those previously sterilized or (much more rarely) taking no view.

ACTIVITY: As your final activity in this section, make a list of the differentiating factors used to allocate infertility treatment, classifying them as medical, social or political. Which factors do you think are legitimate?

Section 4: Global justice, markets and healthcare rationing

You may be wondering by now whether we will ever come to a definite agreement about what the substantive relevant inequalities really are. If not – and agreement does seem unlikely – then why not bypass the entire attempt to find a philosophically satisfying set of criteria for rationing scarce healthcare resources? Why not let an impersonal mechanism such as the market determine the allocation of scarce healthcare resources? Is it necessarily unjust for infertility treatment to be allocated according to market criteria, for example – as we tended to assume in the last section, where it was pointed out that two-thirds of IVF treatment in the UK was paid for privately?

Perhaps letting the market decide, here and in other areas of medicine, would be actually fairer *and* more efficient than trying to intervene with principles of justice on which no ultimate agreement can be reached. If the market were the most efficient means of allocation – which is not a foregone conclusion – it would also be the fairest, insofar as there would be minimum waste and maximum efficient co-ordination on a national or even international scale. 'The crucial feature of the market as a co-ordination device is that it involves voluntary exchange of goods and services between two parties at a known price. Through a complex set of such exchanges the economic activities of people who are widely dispersed and who are entirely unaware of each other's existence can be co-ordinated' (Levacic, 1991).

To put it another way, so far our discussion has assumed that governments, health authorities, or other purchasers must intervene to allocate resources between competing recipients. We have conceptualized this as a problem in distributive justice, treating equals equally and unequals unequally. But according to proponents of markets in healthcare, such active

intervention is neither politically desirable nor economically efficient. Can we avoid value choices about who to favour by letting the impersonal mechanism of the market decide?

Actually this proposition – that markets in healthcare are both the fairest and the most efficient means of allocating scarce resources – is not illustrated in any Western healthcare system. Even in healthcare systems which were never overtly socialist, such as that of the USA, a managed market is the reality, a free market largely rhetorical. Who gets treatment is effectively decided by health-insurance plan managers, directors of Health Maintenance Organizations, and officials of companies providing insurance plans or HMO membership to their employee: by the phenomenon of 'managed care'. The decision about whom not to treat is made in the first instance on the basis of who is covered by one of these categories, or who is not a player in the market; the rest form the nearly 50 million Americans with no healthcare insurance. Of course market systems produce terrible health inequalities, particularly on a global level. That is itself an issue of justice, meaning that we cannot avoid questions about justice by letting the market decide.

One important illustration of these inequalities in international health resource allocation is provided by the reports of the Global Health Forum (Global Forum for Health Research, 2004, 2008), which found that 90% of medical research spending was being devoted to conditions that only affect the wealthiest 10% of the world's population. Market factors come in here, too: the 'worried Western well' are a bigger market for the pharmaceutical firms which fund much medical research than the poorer populations of Africa and Asia.

Nevertheless, many medical ethics commentators have argued that markets, whether on a global or national scale, are the only fair and practical way to allocate scarce healthcare resources, particularly organ transplants (Radcliffe Richards, 1998; Harris and Erin, 2002; Savulescu, 2003; Wilkinson, 2003; Cherry, 2005; Healy, 2006). Sometimes these arguments, particularly those focusing on distributive justice, come from unexpected quarters. The African–American legal scholar Michelle Goodwin (Goodwin, 2006) believes that the current prohibition in the USA on payment for any human tissue other than sperm and eggs is unjust to persons of colour. African–Americans have the highest death rates among all Americans on waiting lists for transplant organs. Registrants of colour represented nearly half of those waiting for kidneys in 2003, the majority of them African–Americans. Goodwin argues forcefully that the current system of altruistic donation fails to serve their interests and thus indirectly perpetuates racial injustice.

ACTIVITY: Stop a moment and think about the arguments for and against markets in human organs. Who would gain and who would lose in such a system?

You may have been concerned for the poor in a free-market system which allowed unregulated trade in human organs, since only the financially desperate would presumably want to sell. This concern is indeed borne out by reports of who the sellers actually are in those Third World countries which have become the hub of a trade in kidneys or eggs, such as India (Cohen, 1999). An ethnographic study of kidney sellers in Pakistan (Moazam *et al.*, 2009) found that all but one of the donors regretted their decision and would never advise a relative to sell a kidney, although in many cases their relatives had also been drawn into kidney sale in a widening circle of desperation. They had only done so to clear their debts to landlords or money-lenders, but most of them remained in debt. Altruistic organ donation systems in these countries had been driven out by market systems, meaning that there was still an overall shortage of organs. The author of this report condemns those Western bioethicists who defend organ sales as free, autonomous choices, finding their position simultaneously naïve and cynical. This view is echoed by Western analysts who view the global trade in body parts as profoundly exploitative (Scheper-Hughes, 2002; Dickenson, 2004b, 2005a, 2008; Waldby and Mitchell, 2006; Widdows, 2009).

Advocates of organ markets tend to prefer managed markets with some state intervention, rather than totally free markets. That, they say, better serves the requirements of distributive justice (e.g. Fabre, 2006; Goodwin, 2006; Healy, 2006). A managed market might well run into many of the problems which we encountered in the previous section about deciding on 'worthy' cases for allocation, whittling away at the primary advantage of markets which we identified at the start of this section – that they purport to bypass such issues altogether. But when resource allocation outcomes appear to be the result of market forces rather than deliberate political decisions, they may well appear to remove ethical issues about judgement, responsibility and risk from decision-making.

Since we cannot avoid ethical analysis in resource allocation by appealing to market mechanisms, we must confront it squarely. In the final section of this chapter, we aim to give you some philosophical tools that will better equip you to do so.

Section 5: Philosophical models of resource allocation

In this chapter we have been addressing the question of *distributive justice* in relation to the allocation of scarce healthcare resources. Decisions will have always to be made about how to distribute healthcare: how much ought we to allocate to each region, to each kind of treatment, to primary, secondary or tertiary care and so on. We would want to argue that such distribution inevitably raises important ethical questions for those who have to make these choices. We have, throughout this chapter, looked at a variety of other ways in which healthcare allocation decisions could be made, whether on grounds of medical criteria, social and political criteria, or economic market mechanisms, but in every case it has proven impossible to side-step ethical considerations. In this section we want to address such considerations in relation to distributive justice more directly.

ACTIVITY: Think back for a moment to the example with which we started this chapter, that of distributing pieces of a cake. What did you decide would be the ethical way in which to divide it? On first reflection we might be tempted to allocate the cake equally among those who want it. However, as we suggested earlier, whilst justice requires that we treat equal cases equally, Aristotle also reminds us that it is unjust to treat different cases as if they were the same, and this suggests that a commitment to 'equality' cannot mean that we treat all people the same. We might, for example, decide to allocate the pieces of cake on the grounds of need. If a starving man comes into my house I may decide to forego my share of the cake and give it all to him, even though this might go against the principle of equality. On the other hand, I might decide to give a larger portion to my brother and take a smaller piece myself because he has been working hard all day to collect the ingredients which go into my cake-making and he deserves to be rewarded. Desert, equality and need (see Glossary on the CD) are three possible guiding concepts for the ethical distribution of the cake or of healthcare resources. Can you think of any more? List them here and we will return to them at the end of this section.

John Rawls – justice as fairness

John Rawls has argued in his book *A Theory of Justice* (1971) for a procedural model of justice. What this means is that he attempts to create a method or procedure which, if followed, will lead to a just outcome. He suggests that, in order to allocate what he called primary social goods (such as money and healthcare) in a way which is just, we ought to imagine ourselves making the decision in a hypothetical situation which is characterized by two features. The first feature is that we, as the decision-makers, have to imagine that we have perfect knowledge about the society about which we are making the decision. We would, for example, know all the statistics which were relevant to the decision; we would know the likelihood of success of various treatments, and we would know which age groups are more likely to require certain treatments. In fact, we would have to be capable of knowing all there is to know about the society in question which is of relevance to our decision. The second feature of this imaginary situation would be that we would have absolutely no knowledge at all of our own position in this society. So, for example, we would not know whether we were male or female, a child or elderly, sick or healthy, rich or poor. Rawls calls this imaginary situation the 'veil of ignorance' and suggests that, from behind this veil, it is possible to make an ethical and just decision about the allocation of primary social goods such as healthcare resources.

> **ACTIVITY:** Our first response to this is to ask what would the likely outcome of such a process be and would it be an outcome that we would find ethical? Try this for yourself. Using Rawls's model how would you go about allocating healthcare resources? How would this help us to resolve difficult choices like the one involving Mr K?

Rawls argues persuasively that, in such a position, the rational and just thing to do would be to argue for the equal distribution of resources, except if by distributing resources unequally one could improve upon the situation that would be achieved by the worst-off member of the society in the case of an equal distribution. He calls this the *difference principle*.

What would be the implication of this principle for the distribution of healthcare resources in the cases we have already seen? How would it bear upon the use of age cut-offs in resource allocation?

Norman Daniels – Equality of opportunity

Let us go on now to see how Rawls's model of procedural justice is applied to healthcare by one theorist, Norman Daniels, by reading an extract from a paper by Masja van den Burg and Ruud ter Meulen, which leads us back to our earlier consideration of the relevance of age to the distribution of scarce healthcare resources.

> **Age as a criterion for distributing scarce healthcare resources**
>
> Masja van den Burg and Ruud ter Meulen[2]
>
> Another proposal for age cut-offs has been made by Norman Daniels in his book *Am I My Parents' Keeper?* (1988). According to Daniels the much-discussed competition for resources between the young and the old is misleading insofar as it suggests a conflict between different groups of persons. The issue of distribution should be considered from a diachronic perspective. In fact, it is a matter of individual, prudential decision-making how to distribute resources over the different stages of one's own life. The criterion of age does not differentiate between persons, but between life stages within a person's life. At any particular stage of life, all persons will be treated the same. In this respect the age criterion is different from other criteria such as race, sex or religion.
>
> The starting point for Daniels's theory of distributive justice is the clearly perceived self-interest of the individual. According to Daniels an age-based allocation of scarce healthcare may be justified. However, it should never be put into practice until we have a society in which general principles of justice are realized. A just distribution of social goods requires a 'fair equality of opportunity' for all, not only in regard to healthcare, but also to income and education.
>
> Within Daniels's theory of just healthcare a fair share of healthcare is determined by *what is necessary to maintain a fair equality of opportunity over a lifetime*. The allocation of available healthcare services will then be determined by what a prudent individual would choose. Prudential planning requires neutrality toward the different life stages. For this, Daniels uses the hypothetical contract theory of Rawls and his idea of the 'veil of ignorance'. Behind the veil of ignorance prudential planners do not know their age, health condition and other personal circumstances. In this 'original position' Daniels suggests, it would be prudential for individuals to secure a roughly equal opportunity at each life stage to carry out their plans of life, whatever they may be. It is rational to maximize

the chances of living a normal lifespan. Because their fair share of healthcare will not provide all possible beneficial care for all their health needs, the allocation between the different life stages will be affected by age-related differences in needs (Daniels, 1988).

Like Rawls, Daniels creates a hypothetical situation in which prudential planners are confronted with a scarcity of resources. To simplify the situation they can choose between two distribution schemes. In the first scheme no one over 75 years is offered any high-cost life-extending technology. Persons younger than 75 years will have access to all life-extending treatments. Under this scheme everybody reaches the age of 75 years, and then immediately dies. In the second scheme resources are strictly allocated according to medical need. Only one of the high-cost technologies can be developed and made available to all who need it. This scheme offers a 0.5 probability of living to age 50 and a 0.5 probability of reaching age 100. Life expectancy is identical to the first scheme of distribution.

Prudential planners would prefer the first scheme of distribution. Daniels offers two reasons. Firstly, prudential planners know that the incidence of disease and disability is greater between ages 75 and 100, and so the quality of life is commonly greater under the first scheme than under the second. Secondly, the most important life plans will be completed by the age of 75 years. This makes the 50–75 period more important than the 75–100 period. Daniels underlines that age criteria are only justified if the savings are used for long-term care for the elderly.

ACTIVITY: How does Daniels's use of Rawls's model of justice as fair equality of opportunity compare with your own? What are the implications of the model when assessed using the three concepts we introduced earlier of equality, need and desert?

Daniel Callahan – Setting limits

Daniel Callahan offers a philosophical perspective which is sometimes seen as opposed to that of Rawls in that it is *communitarian* rather than individualistic. Rather than using a principle of equality and rights as the basis of decision-making, communitarians suggest we should base our ethical consideration of questions such as these on the concepts of the natural lifespan, the good society or community, and on the notion of a balance between rights and responsibilities. Read the following section from van den Burg and ter Meulen's paper and try to identify the ways in which this approach differs from the one outlined earlier.

In view of the increasing scarcity of healthcare services, there has been a widely discussed debate about the allocation of these services, first in the USA, but now also in many European countries. Distributing scarce healthcare resources involves many ethical issues. It requires that the goals of medicine are defined and the choices made should reflect major values in society. Besides this, these choices will have considerable consequences for the accessibility to healthcare services.

Since the 1980s, several proposals have been made to re-allocate these services. One of these proposals is to set limits to the elderly in their use of expensive life-extending care. The most debated proposal for such age-based rationing is made by Daniel Callahan in his book *Setting Limits* (1987).

Callahan proposes to set limits on life-extending care for the elderly in exchange for better access to long-term care facilities. According to Callahan, we should set limits to the use of expensive medical technology which extends the lives of elderly people only for a few weeks or months. Instead, this technology should be allocated to the young, in order to increase their chances of reaching old age.

Callahan's proposal should be seen from a communitarian point of view. For communitarians the source of norms and values should be found in society. Criteria for justice are rooted in a moral tradition. In this view modernism and individualism are obstacles to the development of a shared meaning of old age. Our pluralistic society embraces individual liberty and is opposed to a shared notion of the good life which is considered coercive. There are no shared values or even discussion of these values which could give meaning to suffering and decline in life, and the concept of a whole life is absent. Both of these are required, Callahan suggests, in order to give meaning to old age and death.

In Callahan's opinion we need a community-based notion of the meaning of old age. The life cycle and the concept of a whole life are of considerable importance for ageing, dying and death. The meaning and significance of old age have much to do with the role of the elderly in society. In his view, old age is a period of consideration, reflection, disengagement and preparation for death. The elderly are the conservators of the moral tradition; they are able to integrate the past with the present and the future. They have insight in the way in which the generations are connected with each other. In these roles and functions, the elderly have obligations toward the young. The young need the old to develop a meaningful perspective on their lives, as a coherent whole.

The goals of medicine should be defined in this normative framework. The goal of medicine is not the extension of life as such, but the avoidance of premature death and the achievement of a full and natural lifespan. After that point Callahan speaks of a tolerable death: the event of death at that stage in life span when one's possibilities and life goals have on the whole been accomplished and one's moral obligations to those for whom one has responsibility have been discharged. At that point death is understood as a sad but none the less acceptable event. The natural lifespan and tolerable death are thus defined in terms of the fulfilment of a biographic life. When the natural life span has been achieved, medicine should be directed at improving the quality of life and the relief of suffering. This means the control of pain and the active effort to promote physical functioning, mental alertness and emotional stability.

This understanding of old age and death justifies limitations on some forms of medical care for the elderly. Our social obligation to the elderly, he suggests, is to help them live out a natural lifespan. After that point it is legitimate to set limits to life-extending treatments, in favour of life-enhancing care, that is care which tries to improve those physical functions which are needed for normal daily activities. In Callahan's opinion age criteria should be used as part of a national healthcare policy. They should not be considered as medical, but person-centred or biographic criteria.

Callahan's proposal requires a full-scale change in thinking and attitudes. Therefore, he argues that it is time to start a public debate. When consensus on the use of age criteria has been reached, it must be implemented in public policy. Callahan underlines that a policy of age-based rationing can only be morally acceptable within a society that recognizes the positive values of all ages (Callahan, 1987).

ACTIVITY: Communitarians have sometimes been criticized for emphasizing tradition and community at the expense of the rights of individuals. And this can be seen to be expressed most clearly in the concept of the 'good life' or the 'good community', for they leave open the question of who is to decide what would count as the good life. This is particularly important in relation to the question of age cut-offs, for what counts as the good life might be said to vary both with age and between people. It is open to us to reject Callahan's particular conception of the good old age. Stop for a moment and list some of the advantages and disadvantages of the communitarian

approach compared to Rawls and Daniels, before going on to read the next excerpt from the paper.

Now, finally, bearing in mind these different theoretical approaches based on fairness, equality of opportunity and the good life and also the three concepts of need, desert and equality, we would like you to finish this chapter by reading the following report of some empirical research in the Netherlands which involved carrying out interviews with doctors about how they go about making resource allocation decisions. In the light of your consideration of the various perspectives and the issues raised by this chapter, we would like you to use this reading as an exercise. Try to identify the arguments the doctors are using and note them down. When you reach the end of the reading, address each of these arguments in turn and identify their weaknesses and strengths using the arguments and counter-arguments you have explored as you have worked your way through this chapter.

Age as a criterion for distributing scarce healthcare resources (cont.)

Masja van den Burg and Ruud ter Meulen

It is healthcare practitioners who decide upon the distribution of medical care. In a recent study we interviewed 11 Dutch physicians. The main goal of the interviews was to find out how physicians deal with tough choices. Which criteria and arguments influence the process of selection? Special attention was paid to the role of age and the position of the elderly. In the analysis of the interviews, a distinction will be made between the indication and the selection.

Scarcity of resources   First of all, physicians find it difficult to imagine that there will be a scarcity of healthcare resources in the future. If there is a scarcity, they believe that it is created because of budgetary constraints by the government. Many physicians argue that there are enough financial resources in the Netherlands and that the government should enlarge the healthcare budget.

> If it is true that as a consequence of a limitation of resources we cannot do our work any more, we cannot justify this situation towards our patients. And I think that the patients should know that it is not the physician who is responsible for the lack of care, but the politicians. (...) However, if the politicians are going to tell me which patient I have to

refer to the Intensive Care Unit, I will leave the hospital and start working for a pharmaceutical company.

However, other physicians argue that the decision-making would be much easier were the government to make explicit choices and set limits:

If in a situation of scarcity, you have to make a choice between different persons, the government should set the rules for such decisions. The government should make it clear to the voters, that this government has decided that everybody above 90 years does not get a hip replacement. In my opinion I should not have to explain this decision in the treatment room.

In cases where the scarcity is caused by political decisions, the politicians should set the limits for who will get what kind of treatment. As long as the government does not make such choices, most of the physicians will do their best to give every patient the treatment he or she needs. However, this does not apply to heart transplantation, where the scarcity is not the result of political decisions, but of a lack of supply of donor organs.

Age and indication for treatment   On a clinical level, physicians sometimes have to decide between patients. In such situations, age is an important factor for determining the medical appropriateness of medical treatments. In the opinion of the physicians, age is related to the medical condition of the patient and the expected medical benefit. From a medical point of view, the elderly are in a less favourable position. Growing old involves fewer chances of success and more chance of complications. But physicians agree that age alone is not decisive for the medical appropriateness of a treatment. They think it is better to look at the biological age, instead of the chronological age. This is illustrated by the following quotations:

Age does play an important role, but not as an absolute fact. We cannot use a formula: this man has a biological age of 86 years. However, it may be true that an elderly person can't stand a certain treatment any more. So, certain treatments will not be given to older persons. As an example: a 90-year-old person who needs resuscitation, will not get it, because from experience we know that he or she will not survive.

Another physician said about age:

When a colleague proposes to treat an 85-year-old, there will be an intensive discussion, until a consensus is reached. The result can be that the treatment will not be given. Age is an easy and objective substitute for supplementary problems. An 85-year-old with heart problems nearly always has other problems too, which complicates the treatment. So you talk about age, but in fact you mean the whole physical condition of the patient.

Quality of life considerations are taken into account. They are determined by the medical, social, psychological and mental condition of a person. Important aspects are vitality, co-morbidity, the social context and the future perspective of patients. These factors are negatively related to age. In general, elderly patients will not be treated as aggressively as younger patients.

Age and selection for treatment   The principle of beneficence is difficult to realize in a situation of scarcity. Physicians are expected to provide optimal care to patients. Beneficence obliges them to act in accordance with their interests. Scarcity in healthcare may force them to withhold an appropriate treatment, which may cause medical and/or social harm for the patient involved. The reluctance to accept scarcity and the selection of patients is illustrated by the following quotation:

It is important to be clear about the indication and that has nothing to do with scarcity. As a doctor you cannot accept it when a politician or a hospital director says that some kind of appropriate care will not be provided. These people don't know what they are talking about.

Scarcity, due to a lack of money is not accepted. In practice, physicians try to find solutions, or, if that is not possible, create one.

When the shortages in healthcare are due to, for example, a lack of organs, it is hard to steer clear of scarcity. This kind of scarcity is considered to be absolute. Physicians are forced to select patients. Different arguments and values are relevant for the selection procedure. The position of the elderly in the process of selection depends on the weight physicians attach to these values. It is not always clear which selection criteria are acceptable. Is it justified to use utilitarian criteria in order to maximize the medical benefit? Can it be justified to base the decisions with regard to selecting patients on the notion of the natural lifespan? Below, the arguments of the physicians are grouped under the headings equality, efficiency and the natural lifespan.

Equality From the legal point of view, equity and equality are leading principles. Persons who are equal from a medical viewpoint, should be treated equally. The question is whether age can be considered as a medically relevant criterion. Several authors argue that chronological age cannot be considered as a medical criterion (Jahnigen and Binstock, 1991). Therefore, the principle of equality is being violated when physicians distinguish between patients on grounds of their differences in age.

In the interviews with the physicians it appeared that the principle of equality is taken into account. However, this barely influences the medical decision-making with regard to the selection of patients. Physicians think that people who are equal in a relevant sense, must be treated the same. However, in their view age is a medically relevant criterion. Therefore, for them it is justified to distinguish between people of different ages.

I have learned that it is unethical to say that 5 years of life for a 25-year-old has more importance than 5 years for a 75-year-old. In general, for the 75-year-old, it is as important to see his grandchild as it is for the 25-year-old to see his child. But this argument does not take into account that age might be an indicator for concomitant diseases.

Some physicians stated it more explicitly:

You cannot say that when you take age into account in your decision-making, that is a kind of discrimination. There are medical and social arguments that lead you to start a different treatment for a 90-year-old than for a 46-year-old. In that sense, age is not a discriminatory criterion. Age is a medical criterion.

Even when the chance for success is equal for a 25-year-old and for a 75-year-old, the 25-year-old gets priority on the basis of the duration of the benefit:

It is not age, but the situation of the patient, his rate of success, the time that is left. So, the proportion of the investment compared to the benefit. An operation at the age of 75 that results in hospitalization of many months and a benefit of one year longer life at best, is different compared to an operation on a person of 25, because the benefit is much greater in the latter case.

Efficiency Efficiency is promoted by utilitarian arguments. The principle on which utilitarian arguments are based is 'the greatest good for the greatest number'. The objective is to realize maximal health benefits with minimal costs. Potential candidates for a medical treatment are compared to each other; priority will be given to patients who are expected to have the greatest medical benefits.

Patients who statistically have lower chances of success will be excluded. This is illustrated by the following quotation:

I think that you have to choose for the patient who is expected to have the best results. You ought to use such a scarce resource as efficiently as possible.

In most cases, priority will be given to younger patients. The elderly are in a less favourable condition with regard to utilitarian criteria. In general, the rates of success of medical treatments are lower for elderly people. Risk of co-morbidity increases with age and elderly patients normally have diminished physiological reserves. Furthermore, the benefits of life after extensive treatments are lower for the elderly, because of limited life expectancy. Most physicians argue that it is reasonable to apply age criteria for heart transplantation. Some are in favour of flexible age criteria, others believe in strict age criteria. The following quotations are illustrative:

The whole situation is determined by the scarcity, you have to do something. And I believe that doctors use the following principle: how long can a patient profit from a medical treatment? And a younger person has a longer profit than an older person. (. . .) In 90 per cent of the cases age is decisive.

In situations of absolute scarcity, physicians favour the patients with the best chances:

It is a matter of supply and demand. So, in case of absolute scarcity, those persons (. . .) with the best possible medical outcome will be treated first.

Imagine that if two people need at the same time a complex treatment, then you will favour the patient with the fewest supplementary problems, and with the best prognosis after treatment. When I have two ruptured aortic aneurysms, one of 40 years old and one of 70 years old, then the 40-year-old will probably be treated first.

Under normal circumstances physicians do their very best for the individual patient. Beneficence is the leading principle. However, under conditions of absolute scarcity utilitarian arguments are used in medical decision-making. Physicians weigh lives and compare patients. Priority will be given to patients with the best rates of success. The objective is to maximize the medical benefit.

The natural lifespan The notion of the natural lifespan seemed reasonable to some physicians. For them it is important not to forget that, at a certain point, life comes to an end. In their opinion, it is fair to give everybody the chance to grow old. They do not think it is a matter of discrimination if it is decided on nonmedical grounds that a 25-year-old person gets a treatment and a 75-year-old person does not get it. One physician argued that a different treatment on the basis of age is acceptable:

> This is not bad, because discrimination always takes place. I mean you have to distribute the scarce treatments. You can close your eyes and start a lottery, but that does not solve the problem. In such cases I would give priority to a 25-year-old. That looks reasonable to me. If you let people participate in a lottery, you walk away from your responsibility.

This physician thinks that it is more reasonable to give everybody a fair chance to become old than to treat everybody equally. However, this moral notion cannot easily be framed into a rule. Another physician who was in favour of the philosophical argument about 'natural lifespan' argued:

> This is reasonable: the glass may be half empty or the glass may be half full. Of course, for the one person life has just started, for the other there is just a little left. The further you are on the road, the more you are looking back and the less you can look forward. That is all true, but you cannot turn it into a general rule. (. . .) We do not need rules, but we need an ethics which guides our decision-making.

Most of the physicians in this study stuck to their own rule that only medically relevant facts may influence clinical decision-making.

At the end of their article, Masja van den Burg and Ruud ter Meulen comment that:

> Using utilitarian criteria in the selection procedure conflicts with the principles of dignity

and equality. Using utilitarian criteria involves a comparison between human lives and implies that some (longer) lives have more value than other (shorter) lives. Dignity and equality do not allow lives to be weighed against each other. Finally, when utilitarian criteria become the leading principle in the selection procedure, access to healthcare services for some groups of patients may be threatened, especially the elderly. When scarcity increases in future, it can be expected that utilitarian criteria will be used more often and that elderly people will get into an increasingly less favourable position.

> The objections to the application of utilitarian criteria need to be taken seriously. Physicians, who continue to be confronted with scarcity in future, have to be aware of the ethical implications of their choices and decisions. In medical education attention should be paid to the ethical dimensions and aspects of clinical practice. This may contribute to the prevention of being discriminatory against the elderly.

When resource allocation decisions are being made we need to be wary of making the vulnerable worse off than they already are. What the case studies and other materials in this chapter show is that, whilst medical, economic and legal considerations are central to any decision-making process, it is not possible to avoid the pressing ethical and moral questions with which we are confronted as practitioners in an era of limited resources.

Notes

1   Adapted with permission from Berkeley Greenwood (2009), 'Bang for the buck: what purchasers and commissioners think and do'. In *Reproductive Ageing*, ed. S. Bewley, W. Ledger and D. Nikolaou, pp. 303–13. London: Royal College of Obstetricians and Gynaecologists Press.

2   Reproduced with permission from Masja van den Burg and Ruud ter Meulen, 'Age as a criterion for distributing scarce health care resources'. Paper presented at EBEPE workshop.

9 Thinking about ethics: autonomy and patient choice

Introduction

Human rights and the associated emphasis on liberty or freedom belong to a well-established tradition of ethical reasoning. Their origins can perhaps be traced to the recognition by the Stoic philosophers in Ancient Greece of the possibility that the actual laws and conventional practices in a particular community might be seen to be unjust when contrasted with a 'natural law' (Almond, 1993). For this reason the concept of 'universal human rights' which grew out of the 'natural law' tradition has often appealed to those who have felt themselves to be vulnerable or to be oppressed by the powerful. For the appeal to a concept of universal human rights transcending any particular community and its laws makes it possible to call for the upholding of the rights of individuals *against* their community and against such laws, and in recent years the concept of universal human rights has come to play an important role. It helps us to recognize and express the importance of the protection of the weak and vulnerable.

In medicine this has tended to be expressed as the belief that the protection of vulnerable patients and the practice of ethical medicine can best be guaranteed in a context of patient-centred medicine, that is, in medicine which places a very high value on respect for autonomy and patient choice. An emphasis on patient-centredness means that in cases where practitioners wish to override the expressed wishes of a patient, the burden of justification lies with the practitioner.

The demand for this kind of respect for autonomy and patient choice in healthcare practice has increasingly been recognized officially, such as in the Declaration of Helsinki 1964 (as amended by the 59th World Medical Assembly in Seoul 2008):

> Medical research is subject to ethical standards that promote respect for all human subjects and protect their health and rights. Some research

populations are particularly vulnerable and need special protection. These include those who cannot give or refuse consent for themselves and those who may be vulnerable to coercion or undue influence.
> (Declaration of Helsinki, Basic principle 9, 2008)

Few today would dispute the importance of autonomy and of an emphasis on the value of the patient's voice and informed choice to ethical medicine. Recently, however, the call for more patient autonomy has come under challenge from some of the quarters where it might previously have been expected to find a powerful resonance. For example, some of those arguing for the need to protect minority ethnic and cultural rights have asked whether the call for individual rights is compatible with the recognition of a diversity of cultures and of cultural identities, arguing that a more sophisticated concept is required (O'Neill, 1996; Barry, 2002; Hirschmann, 2003; Dickenson, 2004a; Donchin, 2004; Salles, 2004). In this final chapter of the workbook, we look more closely at the methods of medical ethics itself and investigate the extent to which the concepts of 'autonomy' and of 'patient choice' are capable of resolving the types of ethical questions we have been exploring throughout this workbook, as well as the extent to which they need to be either supplemented or perhaps replaced by other approaches.

Section 1: The importance of autonomy in medical ethics

In this chapter we will be exploring the concepts of 'autonomy' and of 'patient choice' in medicine and healthcare more widely. What does it mean to be autonomous? What are the conflicts between autonomy and other values? How ought such conflicts to be resolved? You can begin your consideration of these questions by reading the following account.

The case of Peter Noll

When he was 56 years old, the Swiss law professor and author Peter Noll discovered that he had advanced cancer of the bladder. He was advised to have surgery but chose not to, as he explained in his book *In the Face of Death*:

> Survival chances in bladder cancer are relatively good, especially if the surgery is combined with radiation treatment. How favourable the odds were was a matter of statistics – about 50%. In response to my questions, [the urologist] says that sexual intercourse would no longer be possible since there could be no erection; but there was no other essential limitation – biking, sports in moderate measure, even skiing. Patients who survived the critical first five years all grew accustomed to the curtailed life. When I explained that I would never consent to such an operation under any conditions, he said that he had great respect for such a decision but that I should really get as much information as possible from other doctors as well. Did I want to take the X-rays with me? I said no; the case seemed quite clear to me.
>
> What bothers me is the loss of freedom; having others in charge of you, to be drawn into a medical machine which controls a person and which one cannot fight. Naturally intolerable pain will disturb me too. In order to escape it, one enters the machine that takes away pain and at the same time freedom. And it's precisely this enslavement that I don't want.
>
> I don't want to get sucked into the surgical-urological-radiological machinery because I would lose my liberty bit by bit. With hopes getting more and more reduced my will would be broken and in the end I will end up in the well-known dying chamber, [to] which everybody tends to give a wide berth – the outer office of the cemetery.

Peter Noll died nearly a year after his diagnosis, during which he had lived alone and administered his own pain relief. However he had continued to write, to work and to meet his friends until the last few days of his life.

As a part of his preparation for death Peter Noll planned his own funeral.

ACTIVITY: Peter Noll argues forcefully for patient autonomy. Take a few minutes to consider how far you think the emphasis on autonomy and patient choice should be pursued. What do we do if patients make choices about their treatment about which we feel uneasy or which appear to be at odds with our assessment of their best interests? What if the patient's choices conflict with the other demands we feel upon us as part of our commitment to the practice of ethical medicine? Can you think of any other ethical features of ethical medicine with which patient choice might conflict? Make a list of what you consider to be the key 'principles' of ethical medicine. Start the list with something like 'Place a particular emphasis on the value of the patient's autonomy and choices'. We would like you to keep this list close at hand as you progress through the chapter, adding to it when possible. Once you have completed your list spend a few minutes going through it identifying ways and circumstances in which each of the principles might conflict with 'autonomy and patient choice'.

We would now like you to read the following commentary on the Peter Noll case by Christian Hick, who is a doctor from Germany.

The right to refuse treatment

Christian Hick[1]

Treatment refusal as the realization of a 'free death'
For Aristotle, things in medicine seemed to be clear.

> We deliberate not about ends but about means. For a doctor does not deliberate whether he shall heal, nor an orator whether he shall persuade, nor a statesman whether he shall produce law and order, nor does anyone else deliberate about his end. They assume the end and consider how and by what means it is to be attained.
>
> (Aristotle, *The Nichomachean Ethics III*, p. 3)

But today, on the contrary, we must deliberate not only about means but also about the ends of medicine. The very meaning of health, as the end of medicine, is submitted to our power, as becomes evident in predictive genetic testing. It is questionable, and this is where our consideration of the right to refuse treatment starts, whether medical treatment provides the patient with the health he is expecting, with the experience of personal health, of health adapted to his conception of existence and of a human life.

In his autobiographical book, which takes the form of a diary, Peter Noll records his thoughts from the moment of his being diagnosed with bladder cancer until immediately before his death. The relevance of this day-to-day description of the progression of an incurable disease for the discussion of the 'right to refuse treatment' lies in the motives Peter Noll had for his refusal. In fact, the whole book can be seen to some extent as a long, written, argumentative meditation explaining his refusal, a refusal which might prima facie seem unreasonable.

ACTIVITY: Take a moment at this point to re-read Peter Noll's account of his reasons for refusing treatment. While you do so, try to pick out and note down Noll's own arguments for asserting his right to refuse treatment and any comments you might like to make about these arguments. Then go on with your reading of Hick's commentary below.

Taking the quotations above together with the arguments Noll presents in the rest of his book, the following reasons are those he gives for his refusal of the treatment offered.

Negative reasons
- After the treatment he will need an artificial urine collection device.
- Sexual intercourse will no longer be possible.
- There is a 50–50 chance of a relapse.

Positive reason
- To have certainty about one's death instead of a mere statistical possibility of death or survival.

This 'positive' reason is, for him, the most important one and seems to be, at the same time, the one most easily overlooked by medical professionals who have difficulty imagining themselves in the role of such a patient. The *certitude* of death, even if it should occur earlier, is in general easier to deal with than the *incertitude* which lies in the statistical possibility of healing. Certitude permits planning, active coping and the shaping of one's life; incertitude breeds passivity and might very well spoil the rest of one's lifetime. Noll refuses treatment because he wants to master his own death. This presupposes that dying is not merely an objective, biological process but, as life, a personal affair. In this way Noll discriminates between three different ways of dying:

- Sudden death by accident
- Prolonged dying controlled by the 'medical machinery'
- 'Self-controlled' dying – 'to see death as it comes'.

The positive reason Noll gives for refusing medical treatment lies in the possibilities he sees in a 'self-

controlled' dying, which permits the integration of death into the biographical life of an individual:

> It is a real chance to see death as it comes. First, there is nothing left to be taken into consideration; nobody can take from you more than your life. Second, one can prepare oneself and bring everything to a close.

As a way of clarifying his view on the relation between personal freedom and death, Noll quotes some famous passages from Montaigne's *Essays*, especially chapter XVII of the first book entitled, 'That to study philosophy is to learn to die'.

> The premeditation of death is the premeditation of liberty; he who has learned to die, has unlearned to serve. There is nothing of evil in life, for him who rightly comprehends that the privation of life is no evil: to know how to die, delivers us from all subjection and constraint.

And how should one premeditate death in an intensive care unit, how should one find any link from death in a 'machine' with the preceding part of a free and personal life story? To refuse to be treated seems by this view to be the only way to safeguard a person's liberty and biographical integrity. And in the second book of his essays Montaigne continues, as does Peter Noll in quoting him, as if he had foreseen the problems of modern medicine and the pitfalls of 'healing' – when there is nothing left to heal.

> The common way of healing goes at the expense of life: one is incised, one is cauterised, our members are cut off, food and blood are taken away. One step further and we are definitively healed.

ACTIVITY: What do you think are the strengths and weaknesses of Noll's arguments? Are some of them stronger than others?

When we read through the case we felt that some of the arguments were quite weak. The idea that he was any more certain that he was going to die because he didn't get treatment for his cancer just isn't true. Clearly there is an obvious sense in which we are all certain to die from the moment we are born. What Noll is perhaps reasonably sure about now is that without treatment he is going to die 'sooner' than he would with treatment but even this is not certain. Noll might perhaps have replied that at least by refusing treatment he has kept control of his death, for he has made the decision. But even here, it would have been him who made the decision had he decided to accept treatment.

His argument that he now has certainty about the form of death rather than statistical possibility is again wrong. If he continues to live a 'normal' life for a year (as he did) then during that year there was as much chance as before that he would be killed by a 'sudden accident' or by a heart attack, for example. So certainty is not gained by his choice, nor are statistics avoided. Moreover, the idea of having a self-controlled death and of 'seeing death as it comes' could as easily be reinterpreted as a reason to go on living and to accept the treatment. Certainly the quotations from Montaigne could and perhaps should be interpreted as calls for us to use the awareness of the certainty of the finite nature of our lives as a motivation to enhanced living, not as a reason to choose death, now. If life is indeed enhanced by the anticipation of death, then one ought perhaps to attempt to have more of it rather than less. The most certain way to take control over death and to make it certain would be for Noll to kill himself, and he does not suggest this.

What Noll may in fact have been attempting to avoid was the 'unnatural' death and the 'unnatural' life (one with a colostomy bag and one without sex). For he suggests that medicine and the 'medical machine' are inevitably the enemies of autonomy and that being 'treated' necessarily involves a loss of self, especially at the end of life. What do you think about these claims?

Noll argues that personal autonomy and patient choice ought to be the guiding principles in medical ethics. There is a sense in which the case itself might be seen as extreme, but it usefully brings the concept of autonomy and patient-centred choice into question. For, how can we have patient-centred care if the patient doesn't want care?

The case of Peter Noll (continued)

Peter Noll's friends varied in their responses to his decision to refuse treatment. He wrote,

> The expression of respect seems, to a certain extent, to be a standard response, for I heard it several times afterward. Naturally, it is appropriate to show a patient who chooses metastasis [the spread of the original cancer to other organs] instead of the technological prolongation of death a certain admiration, even though, strictly speaking, he hardly

> deserves it, for he really has only a choice between two evils, and it is almost purely a question of taste as to which he prefers.

> But his friend Ruth informed him that his decision was difficult to accept for several of his friends.

> You see, you're upsetting people with your decision. If someone has cancer, he goes to hospital and has surgery – that's what's normal. But if someone has cancer and goes around cheerfully like you, it gives people the creeps. They are all of a sudden challenged to confront dying and death as a part of life, and that they don't want. Nor are they able to do it as long as they are not in your situation. That is why it is irritating and confusing that you sit here and say 'I have cancer' while refusing to go to the hospital. If you went to the hospital everything would be all right. Then everything would be fine again; people could visit you, bring flowers, and after a certain time say, 'Thank God, he's been released' and again after a certain time, 'Now he's back in', and they'll come again with flowers, but always for shorter periods. But at least they would know where to find you. They would know that you hadn't been run over by a car but have cancer and that you were going to the hospital to have things cut out, all as it is supposed to be. You scandalise them (this isn't the way she expressed it) – you are showing them that death is in our midst and you are acting it out before their very eyes; they suddenly are forced to think of what they have always suppressed. And of course they think only of themselves. Which makes it all the worse. They cannot help imagining what their own fate will be at some future time.

Whilst there is obvious irony in Ruth's comments, it does seem to be important to recognize that decisions like that taken by Peter Noll are always inevitably going to affect people other than the patient him or herself. How would we feel about Peter Noll's decision if he was the single-parent father of dependent children, for example? Should factors such as these make a difference? If not, why not?

We would like you to return now to the conflicts between autonomy and other principles of ethical medicine which you listed at the start of this chapter. In their influential book *Principles of Biomedical Ethics*, Tom

Beauchamp and James Childress identified what have come to be known as the 'four principles of biomedical ethics'. They suggested in that book that ethical problems in medical ethics are best analysed using a framework provided by the principles of 'autonomy', 'beneficence', 'non-maleficence' and 'justice' and this has come to be known as the principlist approach.

> Four prima facie moral principles [can be identified] which seem defensible from a variety of theoretical moral perspectives and can ... help us to bring more order, consistency and understanding to our medico-moral judgements. These principles – respect for autonomy, beneficence, non-maleficence and justice – plus attention to the scope of each of them – may not give us THE ANSWER to a particular medico-moral problem. But they can and do give us a widely acceptable basis for trying to work out our answers more rigorously. If, when confronted with a medico-moral problem, we consider the possible relevance of each of these principles to the particular circumstances then it seems to me that we are at least unlikely to omit any relevant moral concerns.
>
> (Gillon, 1985, p. viii)

ACTIVITY: Below is a very brief account, using extracts from Beauchamp and Childress (1994), of each of these terms. As you read through their account of the four principles we would like you to compare them with the list you made earlier and see how they compare. Do you think that it would be possible to regroup your principles so that they fit easily gathered together under these four headings? If not, what are the problem areas which make this difficult?

The four principles of biomedical ethics

1. Respect for Autonomy

We start with what we take to be essential to personal autonomy, as distinguished from political self-rule: personal rule of the self that is free from both controlling influences by others and from personal limitations that prevent meaningful choice, such as inadequate understanding. The autonomous individual freely acts in accordance with a self-chosen plan. ... A person of diminished autonomy, by contrast, is in at least some respect controlled by others or incapable of deliberating or acting on the basis of his or her desires or plans.

> (Beauchamp and Childress, 1994, p. 121)

2. Non-maleficence

The principle of non-maleficence asserts an obligation not to inflict harm intentionally. It has been closely associated in medical ethics with the maxim 'primum non nocere': 'Above all [or first] do no harm'. ... An obligation of non-maleficence and an obligation of beneficence are both expressed in the Hippocratic oath: 'I will use treatment to help the sick according to my ability and judgement, but I will never use it to injure or wrong them'.

> (Beauchamp and Childress, 1994, p. 189)

3. Beneficence

In ordinary English the term 'beneficence' connotes acts of mercy, kindness and charity. Altruism, love and humanity are also sometimes considered forms of beneficence. We will understand beneficent action even more broadly, so that it includes all forms of action intended to benefit other persons. 'Beneficence' refers to an action done for the benefit of others; 'benevolence' refers to the character trait or virtue of being disposed to act for the benefit of others; and the 'principle of beneficence' refers to a moral obligation to act for the benefit of others. Many acts of beneficence are not obligatory, but a principle of beneficence, in our usage, asserts an obligation to help others further their important and legitimate interests.

> (Beauchamp and Childress, 1994, p. 260)

4. Justice

Beauchamp and Childress present an essentially Aristotelian account of justice:

> Common to all theories of justice is a minimal requirement traditionally attributed to Aristotle: Equals must be treated equally, unequals must be treated unequally. This principle of formal justice sometimes called the 'principle of formal equality' is 'formal' because it states no particular respects in which equals ought to be treated equally and provides no criteria for determining whether two or more individuals are in fact equals. It merely asserts that whatever respects are under consideration as relevant, persons equal in those respects should be treated equally.
>
> (Beauchamp and Childress, 1994, p. 328)

ACTIVITY: How does this list of principles compare with your own? Do you have more or fewer than Beauchamp and Childress? Is it possible to fit your principles under their headings? If not, why not? Do you anticipate any problems with applying these principles to real cases?

One problem, which Beauchamp and Childress recognize is that there will always, in real cases, be conflicts between the four principles, which will need to be resolved in order to make an ethical decision. One way of dealing with this is to arrange the principles in a hierarchy, so that one of the principles always overrides the others. Raanan Gillon is a strong supporter of principlism, and he recommends that respect for autonomy should be considered 'first among equals':

Let me [explain] why I personally believe that emphasis on respect for autonomy is in many circumstances morally desirable and why I personally am inclined to see respect for autonomy as primus inter pares – first among equals – among the four principles. Firstly, autonomy – by which in summary I simply mean deliberated self rule; the ability and tendency to think for oneself, to make decisions for oneself about the way one wishes to lead one's life based on that thinking, and then to enact those decisions – is what makes morality – any sort of morality – possible. For that reason alone autonomy – free will – is morally very precious and ought not merely to be respected, but its development encouraged and nurtured and the character traits or "habits of the heart" that tend to promote its exercise should indeed be regarded and extolled as virtues.

Secondly, beneficence and non-maleficence to other autonomous agents both require respect for the autonomy of those agents. Although there are some general norms of human needs, benefits and harms, people vary in their individual perceptions and evaluations of their own needs, benefits, and harms. Jehovah's Witness attitudes to blood are simply vivid illustrations of this variability. Thus even to attempt to benefit people with as little harm as possible requires, where possible, discovery of what the proposed beneficiary regards as a benefit, regards as a harm, and regards as the most beneficial and least harmful of the available options. Moreover even if the person agrees that one available intervention would be more beneficial than another, he or she may simply wish to reject the beneficial intervention. It may be because of an idiosyncratic basis of assessment of harm – for example, the autonomous belief that a blood transfusion will lead to eternal damnation or some equivalently massive harm. Or it may be a relatively trivial assessment . . .

When it comes to justice, again, I argue that respect for autonomy must play an important role. First comes the problem, true of all our moral values, but perhaps especially acute in the case of justice, of deciding which substantive account of justice we should adopt in different contexts such as those of distributive justice, rights based justice, and legal justice. But for any substantive theory within each of these contexts it seems morally impossible to avoid a place for respect for autonomy. In distributive justice, for example, while a needs based criterion must surely have a central role, so too must respect for autonomy. Why? Both because, as I've just argued, responding to people's needs justly will require respect for those people's autonomous views, including autonomous rejection of offers to meet their needs; and, more importantly, because providing for people's needs requires resources, including other people's resources. Again it seems reasonable to claim that appropriating those resources without at least a political and law making system that, through a democratic process, respects the autonomy of those people would be unjust. But if this is accepted then respect for people's autonomy must be an integral component of any substantive theory of distributive justice just as meeting people's needs must be an integral component. When it comes to rights based justice, an integral component again must be, it is widely acknowledged, respect for people's autonomy rights. And in the context of legal justice (which I interpret as the prima facie moral obligation to respect morally acceptable laws) yet again respect for autonomy must surely play an important role. Why? Because if people are to be morally bound by laws they ought to have some opportunity to autonomously accept or reject being thus bound. Hence the moral need for some sort of democratic law making system that – to the extent possible – respects the autonomy of those governed by the laws it creates. Hence, too, the lack of an even prima facie moral obligation for people to obey laws that are not open to democratic revision (revision compatible with the *four* universal prima facie principles!).

So yes, for all these reasons it seems clear to me that respect for autonomy – in so far as such respect is consistent with respect for the autonomy of all potentially affected – should be seen as an integral component of the other three of the four principles and thus should be regarded as first among equals.

(Gillon, 2003, pp. 310–11)

ACTIVITY: Gillon sees autonomy as the primary principle, which implies that any apparent conflict between principles can be resolved by ensuring – first and foremost – that we respect autonomy. Do you find this argument persuasive? Can you think of any situations when this approach will not give us an answer or at least will not give us a satisfactory answer?

One example that occurred to us concerned the patient who is not – and maybe never has been – autonomous, for example, like a very young child. When working out whether or not (or how) to treat such a patient, we might well use the other principles, particularly beneficence and non-maleficence, as our moral compasses, but it seems wholly artificial to say that any decision we make is informed by the patient's autonomy. Of course, in order to work out when autonomy is important and, indeed, when it has come into conflict with another principle we need first to have some idea of what is meant by 'autonomy'. We will consider this issue in the next section.

Section 2: What is autonomy?

In Section 1, we examined the conflicts between respect for autonomy and other principles and values in ethical medicine. Bearing this in mind, we are now going to look more closely at the concept of autonomy itself. This is a theme which has emerged in several places throughout this workbook as a whole, most notably in the chapter on long-term care, and it seems to lie at the heart of the question of what counts as ethical medicine. What do we mean by autonomy and how do the various interpretations of autonomy relate to medical practice?

We would like to start off by asking you to read the following case study from Finland in the light of your work in the previous section.

The case of Carl

Carl suffers from dementia and for this reason lives in a residential nursing home. During the day, Carl functions well, but towards the evening, and in particular when it is time for him to go to bed, Carl becomes very distressed, irritable and nervous. This manifests itself in a desire to wake up the people in the beds and rooms around him. The staff have tried their best to help Carl to relax and to find ways of avoiding his feelings of nervousness. They have tried letting him stay up for longer and they have tried talking to him and trying to soothe him. But as soon as the 'coast is clear' he leaves his bed and starts waking the others. Recently the staff have used some sedatives, but

---

these too have failed to solve the problem. The night staff find it very difficult to manage and the other residents are clearly suffering. What ought to be done?

At a staff meeting several suggestions were made. One of these was to set up a 'gate' around Carl's bed and another was to 'lure' Carl into taking a sleeping pill.

ACTIVITY: The case of Carl is a much more every-day kind of case than that of Peter Noll. Even so, the problem with which the staff at Carl's home are faced might in some ways be said to be more complex and challenging. What would it mean to 'respect autonomy' in this case? Clearly there are conflicts here between Carl's autonomy and the interests of others. Nevertheless, having made the decision that Carl's behaviour is unacceptable in a residential setting such as this, how can the staff act in such a way as to respect his autonomy? What would be your decision? Give reasons.

In order to get a sense of the variety of different approaches to the concept of autonomy we would now like you to go on to read the following section from a paper by John Coggon,[2] a UK medical lawyer, which introduces three different ways of describing autonomy. While you are doing so, consider what this conception of autonomy would mean both in the case of Carl and in that of Peter Noll. Coggon suggests three possible conceptions of autonomy:

1. *Ideal desire autonomy* – Leads to an action decided upon because it reflects what a person should want, measured by reference to some purportedly universal or objective standard of values.
2. *Best desire autonomy* – Leads to an action decided upon because it reflects a person's overall desire given his own values, even if this runs contrary to his immediate desire.
3. *Current desire autonomy* – Leads to an action decided upon because it reflects a person's immediate inclinations, i.e. what he thinks he wants in a given moment without further reflection.

Let us consider each of these in a little detail.

Ideal desire autonomy is compatible with a Kantian or neo-Kantian conception of autonomy (Kant, 1998). As such, it requires an agent's decision-making to accord with some objective set of ideals.

A good example of a contemporary account of autonomy that would fall under this head is Onora O'Neill's 'principled autonomy' (O'Neill, 2002). This theory holds that whilst it is important that we be in control of our decision-making, we must not try to imagine ourselves in the untenable vacuum that is sometimes implied by individualism. Ideal desire autonomy requires agents to consider their reason for acting, and only to pursue a course of action if it could be made a universal law. That is, if it could be a successful maxim for all agents to follow. Therefore, if a person chooses to act in a way that is incompatible with a universalizable theory, that person is not acting autonomously. Also, ideal desire autonomy might include simple reference to a purportedly objective system of ideals that for some other reason would lead to an agent's being considered 'irrational' were he to ignore it. On this account, obedience of the will does not necessarily equate with acting autonomously: autonomous action requires 'responsible decision-making'.

Best desire autonomy is akin to the conception of autonomy advanced by Harry Frankfurt (1971) and Gerald Dworkin (1988). These commentators famously distinguish 'first-' and 'second-order desires', and hold that being able to act in accordance with second-order desires is what makes a being autonomous. On this account, we find a person to be autonomous if he acts in accordance with his own value system. This will sometimes require him to act against his immediate inclination, but differs from ideal desire autonomy because the values that command an action inhere in the individual. They may be selfish, self-destructive, or subject to some other condition that would make them impossible to hold as a universal. They are, nonetheless, settled – although not necessarily permanent – and an agent recognizes them as his values, and seeks to act in accordance with them.

Current desire autonomy looks close to an agent's 'first-order desires'. It may refer either to a person's impulsive desire, or to a person's desire that is settled and lasting but on which he has not reflected.[3] When we say that someone is acting in accordance with his current desire autonomy, we suggest a level of conscious choice, but one that is not very (if at all) reflective. If it is reflective, it nonetheless succumbs to the call of the moment, even if that may be a matter of contemporary regret for the agent – i.e. even if the agent would not wish to be subject to the desire (Coggon, 2007, pp. 235–6).

ACTIVITY: How would adopting each of these perspectives have affected the practitioners' behaviour in the cases of Carl and of Peter Noll? With which of the three approaches do you have most sympathy? Why?

In the next section we will be going on to explore the various ways in which autonomy and patient choice have been expressed in European law. Then, in Section 4, we shall return to the question of concepts of autonomy by looking at some alternative, contemporary, conceptions of medical ethics which place less emphasis on autonomy.

Section 3: Autonomy: alternative models in European law

In the previous two sections of this chapter, you've encountered some case examples testing the limits of autonomy. In this section, we will be looking at its limitations in law, and conversely at some new initiatives intended to give it greater weight.

Before we do that, however, we need to point out that autonomy is actually a concept from ethics, not law. Autonomy doesn't usually appear in the index of major texts on healthcare law, whereas it notches up more references than any other entry in the index for a classic text in ethics, Beauchamp and Childress's *Principles of Biomedical Ethics*. Perhaps that seems a trivial observation; but the differences go deeper than that. Autonomy may or may not be the ethical value that legal systems are most concerned to protect.

ACTIVITY: Stop here for a moment and think about what ethical values the legal system in your country is most concerned to protect. If you had to name just one such value as dominant in your country's law, what would it be? In particular, would it be autonomy? You may have to confine your answer to one particular example from practice; after all, this is quite a sweeping question. Think, for instance, about the law in your country about consent to treatment. What ethical values lie behind the law?

Although Beauchamp and Childress argue that 'rules requiring consent in medicine and research are rooted in concerns about protecting and enabling autonomous choice by patients and subjects' (Beauchamp and Childress, 1989, p. 67), this is not universally true, even if it holds for the USA. In English law, for example, the legal requirement of consent has quite a different basis, which is more reflective of the value of trust between doctor and patient.

This difference is consistent with the fact that in English law there is no right to *informed* consent, as there is in the USA. In the common law which underpins both systems, treatment without consent is regarded as a civil wrong (the tort of battery). Whereas a doctrine of informed consent has grown up in the USA, particularly since the Second World War, the original requirement for consent, which persists in England, is primarily required as a defence to an alleged tort of battery. The older underlying reasoning has less to do with enabling autonomous choice than with preserving the patient's bodily integrity and the physician's professional integrity, with keeping alive the value of trust in the fiduciary relationship between doctor and patient.

To put it another way, the basis for consent in English law is not the patient's autonomy, but rather the doctor's duty to provide the patient with the information needed (Trew, 1998, p. 280). Despite some pro-autonomy developments in recent years (e.g. *Chester* v *Afshar* [2005] 1 AC 134), the English position has sometimes been seen as doctor-centred, even paternalistic (Faulder, 1985). By contrast, the standard for consent in American law is what the reasonable patient would want to know, not what the reasonable doctor would want to reveal. Furthermore, American law is rooted in constitutional rights to privacy and property, while English law lacks any such constitutional rights and has only recently begun to engage with questions of privacy, following the Human Rights Act 1998. To sum up, fully informed consent is an American doctrine, so to argue backwards from the right to fully informed consent to patient autonomy won't work in England because there is no right to fully informed consent.

More generally, European models concerning autonomy and consent are likely to differ from the dominant American literature on autonomy. The overall theme of this section, then, is that autonomy is not the sole value of any European legal system. Although the bioethics literature, particularly in the USA, was dominated by the concept of autonomy until recently (with a few long-standing exceptions, such as the work of Daniel Callahan), the legal codes under which European practitioners work are not.

But within Europe we can distinguish different levels of emphasis on autonomy. In an article called 'Cross-cultural issues in European bioethics', Donna Dickenson suggests that there are at least three principal models in European healthcare law, each with its own dominant ethical values (Dickenson, 1999b). Rather than a unitary 'Western' cultural and legal framework in which the rights of the individual are paramount and autonomy is the core value, she identifies at least three 'different voices' (following Gilligan, 1982). In one of these systems, patient autonomy is much more important than in the other two, but even there it is not the sole value.

ACTIVITY: As you read the summary of the article below, make entries in the following table.

	Southern Europe	Western Europe	Nordic Europe
Dominant concept			
Dispute solution			
Legal examples			

Dickenson distinguishes these three separate models, building on the philosophical distinction between positive and negative liberties that you have encountered elsewhere in this workbook, particularly in Chapter 5 on mental health (following Berlin, 1969):

- The deontological codes of southern Europe (and Ireland), in which the patient has a *positive duty* to maximize his or her own health and to follow the doctor's instructions, whilst the physician is constrained more by professional norms than by patient rights
- The liberal, rights-based models of Western Europe, in which the patient retains the *negative right* to override medical opinion, even if his or her mental capacity is in doubt
- The social welfarist models of the Nordic countries, which concentrate on *positive rights* and entitlements to universal healthcare provision and entrust dispute resolution to non-elected administrative officials (Dickenson, 1999b, p. 250).

This tripartite division carries over into the three systems' different approaches to conflict resolution: for example, what to do when patients and their doctors disagree about what treatment is best, or whether treatment has been adequately carried out, and at what expense. The Western European rights-based systems afford patients a greater right to override medical opinion and to pursue their own notions of wellbeing, by court action if necessary. By contrast, the deontological systems of southern Europe more typically posit a positive duty to follow the doctor's instructions and to maximize one's own health and wellbeing, sometimes even enshrining such requirements in constitutional provisions. The Nordic social welfarist models generally prefer to resolve disputes in an administrative manner, through an ombudsman or other appointed individuals, although the underlying assumption is that disputes are unlikely to arise if a proper social welfare system is in place.

As Dickenson remarks, 'Of course these three models are caricatures of much more complex realities, but like all models, they have their analytical uses. It is particularly interesting, I think, to disentangle the Western European rights-orientated models from the Nordic administrative one, since the two are often confused' (Dickenson, 1999b, p. 250). It is also interesting to note that the division into three systems is not purely geographical: although Ireland is not part of southern Europe, it has largely rejected the liberal rights-orientated model of autonomy, for example by continuing its constitutional ban on abortion. While Ireland has never experienced Fascist rule – unlike the countries of southern Europe – there is a long-standing absence of pluralism at official levels (though not in the population), according to at least one Irish writer (Dooley, 1997). Here the influence of the Catholic Church is clearly important, but it doesn't explain why the Netherlands, with its substantial Catholic population, has embraced the individualist model. Nor is the role of the Catholic Church the only explanation for rejection of the rights-based, autonomy-centred model in southern Europe. Often politics and history have more to do with it: in Italy, codes of medical ethics date back to the Fascist period, retaining a positive duty in the name of the collectivity to maximize one's own health and to allow the doctor free rein in the exercise of his or her beneficence.

Because Italian doctors are also bound by legislative requirements, for example in article 28 of the Deontological Code of 1995, it would actually be a legal duty of beneficence for the doctor to proceed with treatment of an incompetent person, even if relatives or the patient refused treatment. As the Italian child psychiatrist Carlo Calzone has written, 'in actual clinical practice doctors are given substantive discretion to resolve potential conflicts between the right of patients to be informed and the need to ensure their compliance' (Calzone, 1996). Although there are formal guarantees against enforced treatment in Article 32 of the Italian constitution, Calzone thinks that physicians tend to rely on implicit consent except in surgery, when formal written consent will normally be obtained. While article 4 of the 1995 code calls on doctors to 'respect the rights of the individual', another commentator judges that the paramount values in the Italian deontological codes are the professionalism of physicians and the dignity (rather than the rights) of patients (Lebeer, 1998).

The concept of dignity has been condemned as hopelessly 'woolly' by some writers (Schuklenk and Pacholczyk, 2009). It has also been said, perhaps cynically or perhaps accurately, that dignity is what is allotted as a consolation prize to those who are not in charge. Critics of that persuasion will be naturally more comfortable with the second model in European law, of which the Netherlands is a strong example and the UK a weaker one. This patient's rights perspective is the closest of the three European models to the dominant emphasis in American biomedical literature on autonomy (e.g. Engelhardt, 1986, 1996), But as we've already seen, the law of consent, as one of several possible examples, is very different in English law from the US position.

While the Italian code of professional conduct largely relies on self-regulation by the medical profession, deliberately leaving the doctor 'as free as possible from the strict confines of the law' (Barni, 1991), in the Western European rights-orientated model there is a much greater role for the law as the ultimate enforcement mechanism for patients' rights. One Greek commentator has claimed that his country actually views the patient as in some sense a defective person, incompetent by mere virtue of being a patient (Peonidis, 1996). By contrast, Western European practice increasingly refers to patients as 'service users' and upholds the presumption of adult competence even in extreme cases, such as that of *Re C*.

Of course it might also be said that the terminology of 'service users' is consumerist rhetoric, influenced by the privatization and outsourcing of healthcare, and that the veneer of rights merely adds respectability to a policy which is nothing like as driven by choice and responsiveness to patients' needs as it claims to be (Rowland and Pollock, 2004). How sincere is the patient's rights terminology in those Western European countries ostensibly committed to this model?

As Ron Berghmans reported in his article in Chapter 5, Dutch mental health legislation does attempt to take a strong line on patients' rights. As in the UK, the basic assumption of patient autonomy is not vitiated in Dutch legislation by a finding of mental incapacity. But whereas in the UK a compulsorily detained psychiatric patient cannot refuse treatment for his psychiatric condition – unlike a physical treatment such as amputation, which Mr C was allowed to refuse (*Re C* [1994]) – Dutch law goes further by allowing such a patient to refuse either sort of treatment. The law thus makes no distinction between the rights and treatment decisions of a competent patient and an incompetent patient, which some Dutch commentators find an extreme version of the patients' rights position (Verkerk, 1998). Unlike most southern European countries, which allow the patient's family to override a refusal, Dutch relatives have no power to override the patient's wishes.

Even the Netherlands, however, must be seen in the context of a national, insurance-based system of healthcare provision, in which solidarity with less advantaged members of society is as important a value as autonomy. The notion of social solidarity and communal healthcare leads naturally into the territory of the third model, associated with the Nordic nations. Patients' rights are hollow, in this model, unless they also enjoy the facilities to make those rights real. This outlook is epitomized in the Finnish Act on the Status and Rights of the Patient (Statute no. 785, 1992, which came into force on 1st March 1993), and the earlier Patient Injury Act (1986).

Although the Finnish Act does view autonomy as an important issue, essentially it is seen as secondary to social justice. Once an acceptable level of welfare provision has been attained, autonomy can be added as an additional benefit. The patient's rights are still primarily conceived in the social context, against the background of the mature Nordic welfare state (Lahti, 1996). This outlook is the exact opposite of the American model, in which universal provision has still to be attained – with the so-called 'public option' of government-sponsored healthcare having been dropped from President Obama's proposals in 2010 for healthcare reform – but awareness of patients' rights is high. To put the contrast another way, in the American model negative liberties – freedom *from* arbitrary actions – are foregrounded, whereas the Nordic systems emphasize positive liberties – freedoms *to* enjoy certain healthcare entitlements.

Nor is recourse to the law viewed as a central mechanism for enforcing patients' rights in the Nordic model. As in the southern European systems, self-regulation by the profession is central, but with an added assumption that where that fails, administrative resolution is preferable to litigation.

> In Finland the control over the health care and medical personnel has for a long time focused on the administrative sanctions and ethical self-regulation of the personnel. Criminal trials brought against medical personnel have remained very rare … The interests of the patient as well as of the health and medical care personnel would be better served if the disagreements arising from the patient's care and treatment could be settled as flexible [sic] as possible in each unit of health and medical care.
>
> (Lahti, 1994, p. 210)

In that context it is not so surprising – although odd to anyone from a culture that regards autonomy as something individuals exercise *against authority* – that the source of the recent greater concern for patient autonomy in Finland was a government official, not a grass-roots demand or a court decision in a case brought by a patient. In 1973 the Finnish Parliamentary Ombudsman ruled that patients' rights were protected by article 6 of the Constitution, on personal liberty. If you contrast this 'top-down' holding with the piecemeal 'bottom-up' development of rights through cases brought against the medical profession by patients and their representatives, like *Re C*, you can immediately see the difference from the rights-based model. Here, unlike in the case of informed consent, the Anglo-Saxon nations resemble each other more than either resembles the Nordic group.

Similarly, failure to obtain informed consent is not itself actionable in the Finnish system: only worsening of the patient's condition as a result of that failure. Lahti (1994) describes the case of a dentist who failed to obtain the patient's consent before removing four teeth which could have been filled. When the patient brought a suit against the dentist, the Finnish Supreme Court awarded damages for the lost teeth but conspicuously declined to rule in the patient's favour on the consent issue. 'It should be noticed that a therapeutic measure performed in the absence of the patient's consent is not considered – exceptional cases excluded – punishable as an offence encroaching on life, liberty or bodily integrity, i.e. as a crime in the nature of assault and battery ... In this respect *a patient's right to self-determination is not protected ...*' (Lahti, 1994, p. 213, emphasis added). By contrast, in the US case of *Mohr* v. *Williams*, a woman consented to an operation on her right ear, as the surgeon mistakenly asked her to do, but it was actually the left ear that required surgery. Although the surgery on the left ear was successsful, the woman won an action for battery because she had not actually given informed consent for that operation, only to surgery on the right ear. The benefit to her of the successful operation on the left ear was outweighed, the US court held, by the affront to her autonomy.

Similarly, we might contrast the way in which a young person's right to refuse treatment was taken to court in the UK case of *Re W* [1992], with the provisions in the 1992 Finnish Act. In the Finnish statute the provisions on competence and right to refuse treatment for children and young people are barely spelled out at all, except for the rather vague provision that a competent minor has to be treated 'in mutual understanding'. If there is a failure of mutual understanding, an administrative mechanism is to be used, rather than recourse to the courts in adversarial fashion. The Finnish Act also lacks a formal definition of mental capacity. 'Instead, it seems to be assumed that conflicts can be resolved in the public health care system precisely because it is a public health care system, with the virtues of universality and solidarity built in' (Dickenson, 1999b, p. 254). Raimo Lahti, the act's principal drafter, has described it as a 'soft law' which concentrates more on making practitioners' attitudes more patient-centred than on creating sanctions for infringement of patients' rights (Lahti, 1996).

This aim might sound laudably non-litigious, but some members of the nascent Finnish patients' rights movement are sceptical. They feel that their system should import a more stringent concept of patient autonomy from outside the Nordic nations – from the Netherlands in particular (Sodergard, 1996). Ombudsmen, they argue, are mere officers of the 'system'; unless the liberal notion of separation of powers is preserved, the Finnish patients' rights advocates argue, there can be no real accountability.

ACTIVITY: To what extent do you think Dickenson's analysis of the European legal situation is an accurate reflection of differences of emphasis on ethical values? As Dickenson herself emphasizes strongly, whilst a model of this kind has analytical uses, there is sure to be significant variation 'on the ground'. Can you think of any examples of cases, judgements or situations which do not fit this model?

These three 'ways of doing ethics' are of course somewhat schematic, and the differences are by no means absolute. Arguably they may have lessened since Dickenson's article was written, with the incorporation of European-wide human rights legislation into individual countries' own legal systems. However, that process of homogenization has been consciously resisted by some European countries, such as France, whose long-established national ethics committee strongly defends a model which is communitarian rather than individualist, suspicious of commercialization of the human body, and sensitive to social solidarity (Dickenson, 2005b, 2007).

Clearly there is some movement in each of the three models towards increasing the weight given to autonomy; equally clearly, autonomy is not the sole value in any of them, although it is most central to the second, rights-orientated model typical of Western Europe. This movement is two-way: the concept of autonomy is likely to be changed by its encounter with other, pre-existing values in these three legal systems. Autonomy is not simply being imported unaltered into previously 'primitive' systems; what emerges from these new developments will be something very different from the standard model of instrumental, rational individualism.

Section 4: Autonomy: alternative models in new theories

In Section 3 we saw that no European legal system is as autonomy-conscious as the American system. Autonomy is working its way into systems based on other core values – such as the Finnish one – but it will be incorporated in a very different way, building onto the prior value of universal provision in the Nordic example. These new initiatives in law will produce a new sort of hybrid, a different kind of autonomy, perhaps.

Similarly, new initiatives in *theory* have also challenged the dominance of standard notions of autonomy in medical ethics. There is increasing dissatisfaction with 'the notion, which nowadays is almost obsessive, of respect for the patient's autonomy' (Silva, 1997). But this opposition is not rooted in medical paternalism; it does not seek a return to the 'bad old days' of 'doctor knows best'. Indeed, it can be seen as a logical progression in the notion of autonomy, an extension of it to groups previously excluded – particularly when we look at feminist ethics. These new models seek to refine the notion of autonomy rather than replace it altogether. In this section we will look at two such models and ask what lessons they offer for practice, where a narrow model of autonomy may well be insufficient. They are as follows:

- Narrative/feminist ethics
- Deliberative ethics

We begin with narrative/feminist ethics, in an article by the British philosopher Susan Mendus, 'Out of the doll's house'. You will see that Mendus uses Ibsen's play *A Doll's House* as an extended metaphor and explanatory device. We think this use of literature is important in teaching medical ethics, enriching our responses and moving beyond the exclusively scientific training which most doctors and medical students have had since early adolescence. But it will take a little more unravelling than you may be used to, so we suggest that you read it actively, using the grid below. As you read, please begin filling in this table, a similar activity to that you did for the three different legal systems in Section 3. What we want you to concentrate on is, first, what criticisms the new model offers of the standard autonomy-centred model in principlist medical ethics; what alternative concepts it stresses as equally or more important; and finally, what concepts it retains from the standard model.

	Narrative ethics	Deliberative ethics
Critique of autonomy model		
Alternative concepts to model		
Retained concepts from model		

Out of the doll's house

Susan Mendus[4]

Autonomy is, without doubt, one of the most important concepts (maybe the most important concept) in modern moral and political philosophy. John Rawls (1971), Ronald Dworkin (1977) and Joseph Raz (1986)

(three of the most influential political philosophers of the late twentieth century) all accord a central place to autonomy, and all agree that political arrangements are to be judged in large part by their ability to create the conditions in which people may lead autonomous lives. Autonomy is crucial [in this view] for individual flourishing and, by extension, for a good society. But what exactly is autonomy? Here agreement runs out:

> [T]he term is used in an exceedingly broad fashion. It is used sometimes as an equivalent of liberty, sometimes as equivalent to self-rule or sovereignty, sometimes as identical with freedom of the will. It is equated with dignity, integrity, individuality, independence, responsibility and self-knowledge. It is identified with qualities of self-assertion, with critical reflection, with freedom from obligation, with absence of external causation, with knowledge of one's own interests. It is related to actions, to beliefs, to reasons for acting, to rules, to the will of other persons, to thoughts and to principles. About the only features held constant from one author to another are that autonomy is a feature of persons and that it is a desirable quality to have.
>
> (Christman, 1988)

Autonomy, it seems, is a 'catch all' term, lacking clear definition and deployed primarily for the purposes of evincing approval. Cynically, we might say that nobody knows what it is, but that whatever it is, it is a good thing for individuals to have and for society to promote.

My aim is to question that conclusion. I want to argue that the assumption that autonomy is a desirable quality to have, and the concomitant assumption that political arrangements are to be judged (in some part) by their ability to foster autonomy, overlook an important set of prior considerations. When those considerations are taken into account, autonomy will be seen to be less important to individuals than is usually supposed, and, by extension, to be less central to the construction of social and political policies. In brief, I shall suggest that we should worry less about autonomy than most moral and political philosophers are inclined to do.

First, however, I must say something about what I take autonomy to be. As has already been emphasized, the philosophical literature is replete with diverse and often contradictory accounts. However, one prominent claim, and the one I shall concentrate on here, is that autonomy is a personal ideal according to which individuals are authors of their own lives. To be autonomous is to be able to live out one's plans, projects and aspirations and, in that sense, to 'write the story' of one's own life. Thus Joseph Raz, subscribing to this conception, defines autonomy as follows:

> The ruling idea behind an ideal of personal autonomy is that people should make their own lives. The autonomous person is a (part) author of his own life. The ideal of personal autonomy is the vision of people controlling, to some degree, their own destiny, fashioning it through successive decisions throughout their lives.
>
> (Raz, 1986, p. 369)

ACTIVITY: Does this definition of autonomy fit the case of Peter Noll? Consider this entry in his diary after he learned the diagnosis of bladder cancer:

> What bothers me is the loss of freedom: having others in charge of you, to be drawn into a medical machine which controls a person and which one cannot fight. Naturally, intolerable pain will disturb me too. In order to escape it, one enters the machine that takes away pain and at the same time freedom. And it's precisely the enslavement that I don't want.

We think it probably does: what Peter Noll most feared was that the narrative of his life (and death) would be written not by himself but by what he called 'the medical machine'. Once he consented to the surgery and radiation for his bladder cancer, he felt, the script would be out of his authorship: things would take their own course, and he would be sucked into one procedure after another.

The notion of exercising autonomy as writing one's own script also entails possible conflict with the approved roles, the conventional script; you may recall that Peter Noll's friend Ruth pointed out to him that some of those close to him found it 'irritating and confusing that you sit here and say "I have cancer" while refusing to go to hospital'. By exercising his autonomy in the sense of refusing to read from the socially acceptable script for cancer sufferers, but insisting instead on writing his own narrative, Noll placed himself outside the bounds: people no longer knew where to locate him in the usual story – not just literally.

Now continue with your reading of Susan Mendus.

On this understanding, then, my life is a story and what matters is that I should, so far as possible, write that story myself. Of course, and as Raz is at pains to point out, such authorship can never be complete, nor can it be attained in a social vacuum. Thus, the kinds of stories I can write will always depend, in some part, on the constraints imposed by the circumstances in which I find myself. [However], social and political arrangements are, we might say, justifiable to the extent that they foster and encourage individual autonomy understood as authorship, and they are suspect to the degree that they obstruct the pursuit of that ideal.

One further warning: just as the ideal of autonomy need not imply total and unconstrained freedom of choice, so it need not imply a single object of choice. The autonomous agent will not be required to make a single, once-for-all decision about how his life should go. As Raz expresses it: 'The ideal of personal autonomy is not to be identified with the ideal of giving one's life a unity … The autonomous life may consist of diverse and heterogeneous pursuits. And a person who frequently changes his tastes can be as autonomous as one who never shakes off his adolescent preferences' (Raz, 1986, pp. 370–1).

Autonomy, then, understood as authorship, is consistent with limitation on choices, and distinct from any requirement that a life shall have a unity. The story of my life, we might say, will have a setting, and it may well be a story with diverse strands rather than a single 'plot'. It is, nevertheless, an autonomous life to the extent that I am able to mould and fashion it for myself.

In what follows, I want to argue that autonomy, so understood, is less important than is commonly believed. My aim is to show that by giving centrality to the concept of autonomy, moral and political philosophers neglect what is of most significance to many people (particularly to women), that they simultaneously misrepresent the nature of personal relationships, and that, in consequence, they advocate social and political arrangements which are false to the realities of life.

I shall try to substantiate these claims via the examination of a single dramatic case: the case of Nora in Ibsen's play 'The Doll's House'. My claim will be that we should not understand Nora as lacking in autonomy. There is an alternative account of her predicament, one which identifies it as problematic not because she is unable to *write* the story of her own life, but because, and in ways to be explained, she is unable to *read* the story of her own life.

In Ibsen's play the two central characters are Torvald Helmer and his wife, Nora. Torvald is a successful businessman who, as the play opens, is on the verge of promotion to a high-ranking position in the local bank, which will bring with it wealth and respect from the local community. However, his success and status have been hard-won, and during the early years of his marriage to Nora, he suffered serious ill-health. At that time, and unknown to him, Nora borrowed money to pay for his medical treatment. Because women were not allowed to borrow money without a male guarantor, she forged her father's signature on the official loan documents. As the play progresses it becomes increasingly likely that her misdeed will be exposed, Torvald's career in the bank will be threatened, and his reputation as a pillar of the community will be destroyed. In the final scene, Torvald does indeed discover what Nora has done. She hopes that when he discovers this, he will realize how much she has loved him and how much she has been prepared to do for him. To her horror, he receives the news as proof that he has been married to a forger, a liar and a cheat. His wife is not an innocent and guileless 'doll'. Rather, she is a common criminal.

The case of Nora, as the title of the play makes clear, is the case of a woman who is treated as a 'doll', more generally as a child, incapable of making decisions for herself, incapable of understanding, much less handling, financial matters. It is a picture endorsed as appropriate by the society in which she lives. It is a picture which portrays what is 'suitable' for a married woman in a society such as hers. The final traumatic scene, in which Nora realizes that this is the picture endorsed by her husband and her society, is the focus of most critical discussion.

The autonomy of individuals is, we might say, acknowledged by allowing them a voice in the determination of the rules which are to govern their society. Social institutions are just if they are such that autonomous agents could and would agree to them. However, as a woman, Nora has had no voice in this 'initial conversation' which determines the rules of justice that prevail in her society. In this respect she has been denied autonomy. Where autonomy is understood as authorship, Nora has been denied a voice in writing the rules. Additionally, and yet more worryingly, she has been denied the language in which to express her disagreement with those rules, once they have been decided upon.

What I wish to concentrate on is the quite general assumption that denying individual autonomy is suspect, together with the connected assumption that autonomy is a matter of authorship. It is also part of my aim to provide an alternative model of autonomy, or, more correctly, a model of what makes life valuable which depends much less heavily on autonomy or authorship.

In *After Virtue* Alasdair MacIntyre writes:

> Man is in his actions and practice, as well as in his fictions, essentially a story-telling animal. He is not essentially, but becomes through his history, a teller of stories that aspire to truth. But the key question for men is not about their own authorship; I can only answer the question 'What am I to do?' if I can answer the prior question, 'Of what story or stories do I find myself a part?'
>
> (MacIntyre, 1981, p. 216)

ACTIVITY: Stop here for a moment and think about how this might apply to medical ethics and to clinical practice. What is the importance of the question, 'Of what story or stories do I find myself a part?' One answer might be that it is only by understanding how the patient understands the story of his or her life and illness that doctors and nurses can communicate effectively with patients. But the converse is also true: the patient is caught up in the narrative of medicine. In our age this is a story about overcoming illness through the heroic discoveries of modern science and the application of wonder technologies. (In this script Peter Noll refused to play a part.) Now continue with your reading of Mendus.

In what follows I want to take MacIntyre's central claim (that I can only answer the question 'What am I to do?' if I can answer the prior question 'Of what story or stories do I find myself a part?') and apply it in the case of Nora. I shall argue that Nora's predicament is not essentially that of a woman who is unable to *write* the story of her life. Rather, it is the predicament of a woman who has systematically *misread* the story of her life. More generally, and following MacIntyre, I shall argue that successful reading is primary and successful writing only secondary. To that extent, modern emphasis on autonomy is partial and potentially distorting of our understanding of what makes life valuable and what makes political and social institutions legitimate.

First, Nora misreads the relationship between the laws of society and personal attachments. In other words, she misreads the world in which she finds herself. Secondly, and connectedly, she misreads her relationship with Torvald, and finally, she misreads herself.

Nora's misreading of her society is seen in her astonishment that the law can forbid an act which is undertaken from love. Although she knows that she has broken the law in forging her father's signature, she nevertheless believes that her act is justifiable because it was done to help her husband. Although of course Nora understands that she has acted illegally, she cannot believe that she has acted morally badly. If the law says she has, then the law is wrong. Here, then, we have a sense in which Nora misreads the world. She is mistaken about the status of law relative to personal loyalties, and when she discovers what that status is, she is appalled.

Moreover her misreading of the world brings with it a misunderstanding of her relationship with Torvald, and indeed a misreading of Torvald himself. For her discovery that law takes priority over personal relationships is also a discovery that *for Torvald* law stands above personal relationships. Thus, when faced with a choice between obedience to the law and loyalty to Nora, he chooses the law, saying: 'Nora, I'd gladly work night and day for you, and endure poverty and sorrow for your sake. But no man would sacrifice *his honour* for the one he loves.' (To which she replies, 'Thousands of women have.') Here we find another way in which Nora has misread her life: not only has she been mistaken about the relative priority of law and personal attachment, she has also been mistaken about their relative priority in Torvald's eyes, and as a consequence she has been mistaken about Torvald himself. She had imagined that he would sacrifice everything, including honour, for her, as she would sacrifice everything for him. In this she is wrong, and her mistake now leads her to conclude that for eight years she has been married to a stranger.

Thirdly, and most poignantly, in the final scene Nora is brought to a realization that she has misread herself. It follows from her misreading of the relationship between law and personal attachment, and the misreading of the relationship between Torvald and herself (he is exposed as a man who cares more about honour in the eyes of the world than about his own wife) that Nora's own life, her hopes, her plans, her aspirations and her actions have all been a deceit. She concludes, 'I thought I had, but really I have never been happy.' The final remark reveals the extent to which Nora's predicament is more a function of her misreading of the world and her place in it, than it is a function of her inability to write the story of her life. In fact, though in a rather perverse sense, she *has* written the story of her life. She has attained the things she set out to attain – has helped her husband, brought up her children, earned money and in general 'moulded' her life and theirs. What is tragic in her situation is not that she has lacked autonomy, but

rather that she has exercised autonomy in a world she has systematically misunderstood.

The discussion of Nora suggests that the ideal of autonomy does not merely make claims about what makes a life valuable for the person who leads it. It is also an ideal which has implications for the ways in which we relate to one another. Thus the claim that what matters most is that 'I mould and fashion my life' implies a clear distinction between myself and others; *my* life and *my* projects are to be distinguished from the projects of other people. Of course, other people may contribute to my projects, but it is *my* projects to which they are contributing. Conversely, of course, other people can constitute a threat to my pursuit of my projects.

What we have here, I suggest, is an account of what makes an individual life worthwhile which implies something rather worrying about the relationship which will hold between the autonomous person and others. What it implies . . . is that a society premised on the value of autonomy will be, at root, a society of strangers – a society which will have difficulty accommodating 'constitutive' relationships such as those of friendship and love. For it is precisely in such relationships that a clear distinction between my projects and those of another person is at least plausible.

Thus, when Nora refers to Torvald as a stranger, there are two ways in which her statement can be interpreted: he is a stranger because he is not what she has always believed him to be, and he is also a stranger because, by giving priority to law over personal loyalty, he indicates that the demands of strangers (lawmakers) are more important than his attachment to his own wife. Faced with a choice between the impersonal laws of society and the needs of his wife, he chooses law, and thus in a quite literal sense 'estranges' Nora. Her demands matter less to him than the demands of strangers. More specifically, by refusing to give up his 'honour' for her, he indicates that *his* life and *his* projects are still and always distinct from hers. And in this sense, too, they are strangers to one another.

There are, I think, some very general conclusions to be drawn from these considerations, and the conclusions have implications for our practical dealings with others. First, if we aspire to encourage and develop autonomy, then we must be aware that autonomy is not simply an individual ideal. It is an ideal which has implications for how we relate to others. Put bluntly, a world of autonomous individuals will be, more or less, a world of strangers.

Second, and connectedly, the ideal of autonomy cannot be one which merely enables each person to live whatever life he or she chooses: if autonomy implies something about the ways in which we can relate to others, then some kind of relationships will be deformed by the attempt to render them compatible with autonomy. Nora's understanding of marriage is an example of just this.

Finally, and most importantly, the ideal of autonomy presupposes a background of values, and where an individual misunderstands that background, it is not the case that she is damaged by being denied autonomy. She is mocked because her life is based on a deception. Therefore if we are to write the story of our lives, we must first read the context of our lives. We can only answer the question 'What am I to do?' if we can answer the prior question 'Of what story or stories do I find myself a part?' And we must read our own stories accurately.

ACTIVITY: Please go back to the summary table and fill in the narrative/feminist ethics section. What critiques of autonomy does Mendus suggest? What alternative concepts does she offer?

The dominant principlist school in medical ethics focuses primarily on actions, on particular decisions, on medical dilemmas. In an account like that of Joseph Raz, the autonomous agent's life is not a unity; rather, it is a series of possible diverse decisions. This concentration on life as a string of separate action choices has had several consequences which critics view as undesirable:

- The dilemmas have generally tended to be the 'big issues' like abortion and euthanasia. This does not adequately convey the tenor of ordinary practice, which is much more about routine cases that may not even be immediately recognizable as ethical dilemmas; at most they may just look like practical questions. So what sustains clinicians in their everyday work is much more like something that could be called the 'narrative dimension of medicine'. That's also akin to what has sustained us as authors in the writing of this book. Although we did begin this chapter with the unusual case of Peter Noll, we followed it with the much more everyday example of Carl. Our approach in this book has been informed by our belief that everyday cases matter to practitioners, and that they are also consistent with an experiential approach, to which we are very sympathetic.
- In a dilemma-focused approach, the four principles become – at worst – a mechanical formula for busy clinicians: simply apply autonomy, beneficence, non-maleficence and justice to the situation and a 'solution' emerges. This is of course a parody, even a travesty to advocates of the principles, but narrative ethicists warn us to resist the temptation for superficial thinking which the approach presents. Again, we have tried to resist that temptation in writing this book: rather than presenting a checklist of principles to be applied in a 'top-down' fashion to the various topics we cover, we have tried to encourage you as the reader to deepen your own thinking by working from the 'bottom up' through a case-based analysis.

- The same principles are to be applied to every situation, in every culture and country. This is insensitive to different institutional structures, to multiculturalism and to the nuances of relationships – in all of which autonomy is not necessarily the be-all and end-all. People don't make their own lives, particularly not the sick and vulnerable people clinicians encounter in daily practice. In Mendus's terms, prioritizing autonomy means failure to read the situation in which you find yourself: insistence on imposing another script instead.
- It also posits a model in which other people are a threat to 'my' project. Translated to the healthcare context, the autonomy approach is too conflictual. It leads us to expect conflict in the doctor–patient relationship, when doctors stand in the way of patients' autonomy, and that could turn out to be a self-fulfilling prophecy. Although Mendus does not touch explicitly on the doctor–patient relationship, she does say that 'some kinds of relationships will be deformed by the attempt to render them compatible with autonomy'. Is the doctor–patient relationship one of them? Or does even admitting that it might be return us to blatant medical paternalism?
- As MacIntyre says, the approach which concentrates on the right action is in fact self-defeating unless it asks questions about the entire narrative. But the key question for men is not about their own authorship; I can only answer the question 'What am I to do?' if I can answer the prior question, 'Of what story or stories do I find myself a part?"

Developing this last point, Michael Parker suggests that bioethics itself tends to tell one of two different stories about us: either an individualistic one, where we are all individuals first and foremost, or a communitarian one, where we are essentially part of a community. Parker thinks there is something worthwhile in both of these accounts, which he seeks to combine in a deliberative approach to bioethics. Like narrative ethics, a deliberative approach to ethics is also sensitive to embeddedness in relationships. Like feminist ethics in particular, it does not necessarily seek to jettison the concept of autonomy altogether, but rather to broaden and deepen it: 'Autonomy, the root of ethics ... has an essential dialogical dimension which must not be forgotten' (Silva, 1997, p. 16). You can explore this approach in the final reading in this section, by Parker, and while you read remember to complete the remaining boxes on your grid.

A deliberative approach to bioethics

Michael Parker[5]

A 'rivalry of care' case   In their book, *The Patient in the Family*, Hilde and James Lindemann Nelson describe the case of a man whose daughter is suffering from kidney failure (Lindemann Nelson and Lindemann Nelson, 1995). She is spending six hours, three times a week on a dialysis machine and the effects of this are becoming increasingly hard for her and her family to bear. She has already had one kidney transplant, which her body rejected, and her doctors are unsure whether a second would work but are willing to try if they can find a suitable donor. After some tests the paediatrician privately tells the father that he is compatible and therefore a suitable donor.

It may seem inconceivable that a father would refuse to donate his kidney to his daughter under such circumstances. Yet he does refuse and justifies his decision both on the grounds that the success of the transplant is uncertain and also on the basis of his concerns about the implications of the operation itself for him and his family. He is frightened and worried about what would happen to him and his other children if his remaining kidney were to fail. But he is ashamed to feel this way and cannot bear to refuse openly so he asks the paediatrician to tell the family that he is in fact not compatible. However, whilst having some sympathy, she says she cannot lie for him and, after a silence, the father says, 'OK then I'll do it. If they knew that I was compatible but wouldn't donate my kidney, it would wreck the family'.

But why should this decision wreck the family, ask the Lindemann Nelsons? Does a father have a special

obligation to donate his kidney to his daughter? What is it about families and the values that underpin them which leads to the expectation that parents will sacrifice themselves for their children (and in particular for the child who is ill)? What is it about modern *patient-centred medicine* that intensifies such expectations?

The case is used by the Lindemann Nelsons because they believe it suggests that there is a conflict in healthcare between two sets of values: those individualistic values which underlie patient-centred medicine and the communitarian (community-based) values which sustain families and communities. They argue that modern medicine's overriding focus on the benefit of the individual patient has distorted the ways in which family members interact with one another and in particular with those who are sick. They argue that at times of stress families often adopt the individualistic values of the medical world and this leads them unintentionally to trample on the values and concerns that sustain families. It is with this tension, they suggest, that the father wrestles in the case described.

ACTIVITY: The Lindemann Nelsons think that patient-centred medicine has had a damaging effect on the values which sustain families and communities. To what extent do you agree? If you do agree, do you think that this is a price worth paying?

In the next section Parker contrasts two different approaches to ethics, each of which starts, he claims, from a different view of the person. As you read this section try to pick out the characteristics of the person in each model

Who am I?   The claim that there are important tensions between the values of patient-centred medicine and those which sustain families and communities reflects an ongoing and important contemporary debate in bioethics (and in ethics more widely) between what have been called 'individualistic' approaches and those which have come to be known as 'communitarian' (Parker, 1999) The conflict is one that is characterized by Michael Sandel and other communitarians as one between two conceptions of what it is to be a moral subject (Sandel, 1982).

The communitarian analysis of the case offered by the Lindemann Nelsons urges the father to seek a resolution of his moral problem in an answer to the question 'who am I?', where his identity is to be seen as informed by his membership of a community (in this case, a family) rather than through an analysis of rights (Lindemann Nelson and Lindemann Nelson,

1995) or a 'balancing' of principles (Beauchamp and Childress, 1994). For, as Kukathas and Petit suggest,

> [For communitarians] the end of moral reasoning is not judgement but understanding and self-discovery. I ask, not 'what should I be, what sort of life should I lead?' but 'Who am I?' [And] to ask this question is to concern oneself first and foremost with the character of the community which constitutes one's identity.
>
> (Kukathas and Petit, 1990)

Sandel too, argues that,

> I [should] ask, as I deliberate, not only what I really want but who I really am, and this last question takes me beyond attention to desires alone to reflect on my identity itself.
>
> (Sandel, 1982, p. 180)

At the heart of this communitarian approach to the moral which urges us to emphasize the values which sustain families and communities over those of autonomy and patient choice, is the ontological claim that the moral world consists of fundamentally and essentially 'socially embedded' beings who draw their identities, and their moral values, from their constitutive attachments to a 'community'.

Interestingly, Sandel argues that the individualist too, whose approach it is which is rejected by the Lindemann Nelsons and other communitarians, agrees that the question of who I am is at the core of moral deliberation (Sandel, 1982). In contrast to the communitarian, however, the individualist is said to conceive of the moral subject in terms of the autonomy and the free choice of the individual 'free chooser', rather than in terms of a being constituted by his or her embeddedness in a constellation of social and communal values, and this leads to an approach to bioethics which emphasizes the values of autonomy and patient choice over those of community and family.

The individualist argues that the value of such freedom is independently derivable by virtue of the fact that it is a necessary condition of the very possibility of the moral, and hence of the very possibility of a constellation of values at all, and it is this which means that autonomy ought to 'trump' other values (Dworkin, 1977). As Sandel explains,

> For justice to be primary, certain things must be true of us. We must be creatures of a certain kind, related to human circumstance in a certain way. In particular, we must stand to our circumstance always at a certain

distance, conditioned to be sure, but part of us always antecedent to any conditions. Only in this way can we view ourselves as subjects as well as objects of experience, as agents and not just instruments of the purposes we pursue.
>
> (Sandel, 1982, p. 11)

The basis of an emphasis on autonomy is thus not the ends we choose but the capacity of us to choose them, and such capacity depends upon the free and independent nature of the subject. As Kant argues, in response to the question of what makes the moral possible,

> It is nothing else than personality, i.e., the freedom and independence from the mechanism of nature regarded as a capacity of a being which is subject to special laws (pure practical laws given by its own reason).
>
> (Kant, 1956 [1788])

Sandel's claim, then, is that both the individualist and the communitarian seek an explanation of the moral in an answer to the question of what it means to be a moral subject, each rejecting the other on the grounds that it is incapable of providing such an explanation. I shall be going on to argue in the rest of this paper, however, that each of these conceptions must themselves be rejected and that this rejection of both individualism and community has important and far-reaching implications for the practice of bioethics, some of which I shall tease out in the final section.

ACTIVITY: Parker identifies two different conceptions of the moral subject or of the moral person – the individualistic and the communitarian. Choose the model with which you have most sympathy and then try to identify two arguments for why this ought to be rejected and two for why it ought to be supported.

In the section which follows, Parker goes on to provide reasons for rejecting both of the models in favour of a third, discursive approach.

Three reasons for rejecting the liberal individual moral subject   It seems to me that the communitarian is right to reject the liberal individualist model as conceived in this way and the grounds for such a rejection can, I want to argue, be grouped under three headings.

The first of these grounds might best be collected under the heading, 'the impossibility of moral understanding,' and draws together arguments from both philosophy and psychology, which suggest that the individualist account of morality must be rejected because it is not possible to provide an explanation of the development of moral understanding from an individualistic epistemological perspective. For, the very possibility of moral understanding and moral language, it is claimed, is dependent upon the social dimension of human experience. Ludwig Wittgenstein's 'private language argument' is one powerful argument to this effect, in which Wittgenstein argues that the very possibility of meaning and hence language depends upon the existence of standards of established social practice (Wittgenstein, 1974, n 150–200). But this is not the only argument to this effect. Alasdair MacIntyre in *After Virtue* argues that,

> In so far as persons must be understood as partly individuated by their membership of traditions, the history of their lives will be embedded in the larger narrative of a historically and socially extended argument about the good life for human beings
>
> (MacIntyre, 1981)

The second group of arguments are those which claim, against the individualist, that the having of moral problems and moral identity at all depends on the fact that we are all socially embedded. That is, it is claimed, we are all inevitably located in social, intersubjective networks from which we draw our identity and that the liberal conception of the subject as divorced from such networks inevitably comes at a price. For, as Michael Sandel writes,

> To imagine a person incapable of constitutive attachments such as these is not to conceive an ideally free and rational agent, but to imagine a person wholly without character, without moral depth.
>
> (Sandel, 1982, p. 179)

Perhaps the strongest proponent of this type of argument is Charles Taylor, who argues that to be a self at all is to be an essentially moral being located within what he calls evaluative frameworks and that such frameworks are inevitably linguistic and hence social.

> This is the sense in which one cannot be a self on one's own. I am a self only in relation to a certain interlocutor: in one way in relation to those conversation partners who are essential to my achieving self-definition; in another in relation to those who are now crucial to my continuing grasp of languages

of self-understanding – and , of course, these classes may overlap. A self exists only within what I call 'webs of interlocution'.

> (Taylor, 1989, p. 36)

The third groups of arguments are those which attempt to describe the unacceptable social consequences of individualism. Communitarians sometimes argue that historically the over-emphasis on rights in liberal democracies has had unacceptable consequences both for societies and individuals (i.e. the breakdown of traditional structures such as the family) and for this reason should be rejected (Etzioni, 1993).

Whilst I have my doubts about the strength of the third group of arguments in a world in which perhaps the most striking moral challenge is the oppression of individuals by communities, the combination of these arguments taken together means that if communitarians are right it seems to me to call for the rejection of what I have called elsewhere 'overly individualistic' approaches to ethics (Parker, 1999).

Three reasons for rejecting the communitarian 'embedded moral subject' The communitarian argument for the 'socially embedded subject' must itself be rejected, however, for three sets of reasons which, again for reasons of space, I shall simply state here.

Firstly, the explanation of morality in terms of the 'socially embedded self' and of 'constitutive attachments' means that communitarianism is incapable of recognizing *the moral status of the individual*. Feminists, for example, have argued that whilst communitarianism is very good at describing the benefits of community, it says very little about the damage caused by families and communities and says nothing for those at the periphery of societies, for whom we expect moral theory to have special concern. Taken to its logical conclusion, communitarianism seems capable of justifying the oppression of minorities and of the weak by the majority, of the novel by the traditional (Parker, 1996). And whilst we might agree with the communitarians that overly individualistic approaches to ethics must be rejected, we would surely not want to reject with it that which is valuable about the individualistic approaches: namely a recognition of the moral status of the individual. For this would be to throw out the baby with the bathwater.

Secondly and following from the above, the communitarian approach is, it is argued, incapable of providing an explanation of social change or of the need for the critical moral reflection, creativity and criticism necessary for the change and development of communities. Another way of saying this is to say that communitarianism is incapable of providing an account of how the individual can come to have an effect upon the society within which they live and upon their constitutive values and relationships (Mendus, 1992; Parker, 1995b).

Thirdly, Jürgen Habermas has argued that it is not in fact possible to identify the shared values required by communitarians (Habermas, 1993). The breakdown of shared values and traditions identified by communitarians brings into question the viability of the communitarian project itself. For, when we look around us there appear few if any candidates for the shared values upon which a communitarian New World might be built. We live in a world characterized by diversity, in which candidates for the role of paradigmatic communities are revealed to be as often the sites of conflict and violence as of mutual support (Campbell, 1995); a world in which it is not possible to identify the kind of shared values or traditions upon which a communitarian morality might be founded.

ACTIVITY: Do you think that Parker's argument withstands scrutiny? You may find it helpful to write out the main stages of his argument, so as to assess each step.

As you read the next section, in which Parker attempts to elaborate a deliberative approach to medical ethics, consider how this approach might deal with the cases you have encountered in this chapter.

A resolution? The deliberative moral subject   Both the individualist and communitarian models of the moral subject (and of the person) in ethics must be rejected. But where does this leave us? If we wish to elaborate a coherent moral theory and, if appeal is no longer possible either to the kind of detached, individual, rational decision-making called for by the liberal individualist or to communitarian shared values and traditions as the basis of ethical decision-making in healthcare, how are we to approach the making of ethical decisions of the kind confronting the father at the beginning of this paper? What seems clear is that any coherent explanation of the moral will have to be one capable of capturing the insights of both communitarianism and individualism whilst avoiding their weaknesses and pitfalls, and what this means is that it must be capable of capturing both the value of the individual voice and the moral status of the individual and at the same time of recognizing the intersubjective and social context of morality and the value of social relationships and their various manifestations.

It is worth pausing here for a moment to reflect upon the interdependent nature of the relationship between the two sets of arguments I have identified for the rejection of individualism and of communitarianism. For it is an important feature of each of these arguments that such rejection is in each case put in terms of the necessity of the other to any coherent account of the moral. The argument that individualism must be rejected, for example, is based on the claim that recognition of the role of the social is a necessary element of any coherent explanation of morality. The argument for the rejection of overly social accounts on the other hand, is phrased in terms of the necessity of a recognition of the role of the individual.

My point in juxtaposing the arguments in this way is to suggest that both the social and the individual are together necessary and it is their combination that makes a coherent account of the moral possible. I want further to argue that these features of our moral world are jointly and together only explicable in terms of the actual relations between people in the intersubjective contexts which constitute their everyday lives with others. For it is only here, in the intersubjective relations between people, that the community meets the individual and vice versa. It is here that morality is elaborated and here that the maintenance and the transformation of social practice occur. This is to suggest following Harre and Gillett (1994) and Shotter (1993) and other discursive psychologists that the primary social reality is neither the individual nor the community but people in conversation. To quote Alasdair MacIntyre from *After Virtue*,

> Conversation, understood widely enough, is the form of human transactions in general.
> (MacIntyre, 1981)

This must indeed be the case, I suggest, for the reasons above and because it is through such 'conversations' that we are both introduced into the world of human affairs and negotiate our identity and our moral concerns. It is also here that we discover the ethical voice with which we reflect upon, deliberate and change the nature of our relations to our community and other people. From this deliberative perspective, it seems to me, it is possible to begin to recognize the particular value, and indeed the necessity, of the engagement of human beings in deliberation about the moral features of their own lives. And of the nature of their relations with those around them, with those who constitute their communities. For the development of much that is of value in what it is to be human is made possible by such relationships. Hence, within a moral framework of this kind is it possible to capture, as neither individualists nor communitarians are able, both the value of communal life and the moral significance of the individual ethical voice. It is to claim that it is neither the freedom of the abstracted individual nor the emphasis of community values which ought to be given a special place in the constellation of values but the interrelationship between the two. It is also to claim that deliberation is the developmental fundamental of human experience and that it is this that makes the moral possible (Parker, 1995b).

Implications for bioethics   What then are the implications of this deliberative approach for bioethics? It seems to me that there are several key features of an approach such as this and I shall attempt to outline these very briefly in conclusion.

(i) The value of deliberation with others   Firstly, to adopt this perspective is to argue, as I have already suggested, that the deliberative search for moral meaning is at the core of what it is to be human in a world with others. This is to locate morality and the search for moral meaning very firmly at the centre of human life. To adopt this perspective therefore is to recognize the particular value of the engagement of human beings in the attempt to 'make moral sense' of their lives and the nature of their relation with those around them. This is necessarily a social process but it is also necessarily part of what it is to be and to become autonomous. It is also by these means to recognize as neither individualists nor communitarians are able, both the value of communal life and the moral significance of the individual ethical voice. Whilst placing an emphasis on the social therefore, this approach nevertheless has the advantage of providing, as communitarianism does not, space for a critique of accepted or traditional values on the basis of a respect for the discursive nature of human experience. For whilst such recognition is capable of capturing our social embeddedness it is also capable of recognizing that individuals need both to be protected from, and to have a voice in, their community.

To assert the value of deliberation is in many respects to follow Alasdair MacIntyre, who argues for a conception of the moral life as one which is constituted by engagement in a conversation with history and tradition in an attempt to establish the narrative unity of one's life. It is also to align oneself with Charles Taylor's claim that the identity of the self is inextricably linked to its sense of the significance, and meaning of the situations it encounters in life and this is to see, as does Ronald Dworkin, life as a series of 'challenges' which must be addressed (Dworkin,

1988) The good life is at least to some extent one in which we are engaged in the attempt to make sense of the challenges with which we are confronted.

(ii) Subsidiarity and participation   Secondly, it follows from the emphasis on the value of 'making sense' that ethical decisions are best made and in fact might only be capable of being made by those most closely involved, and this is to suggest that the process of making ethical decisions ought to adhere to a principle of 'subsidiarity'. Nevertheless, such an approach is also and perhaps primarily one which emphasizes the participation of all those who have a legitimate interest, and this means that the requirement that decisions be made by those most likely to be affected needs to be balanced against a responsibility to ensure that all who have a legitimate interest are involved. This is to suggest that decision-making in bioethics will need to take a range of different forms, from the establishing of public consensus conferences about ethical issues of widespread public or even global concern, to conversations among doctors, patients and families or within families themselves about the ethical questions raised by a particular case or treatment option, and in some cases, perhaps even most, this will mean that decisions will be made by the patient alone, or in collaboration with his or her doctor.

However, whilst taking a variety of forms, such fora would have to share a commitment to recognition of the fundamental value of deliberative involvement and hence would have to place an emphasis on both participation and subsidiarity.

(iii) Openness and truthfulness in ethical decision-making processes   Thirdly, and briefly, the emphases on the values of 'making sense', 'participation' and 'subsidiarity' all imply a requirement both for the openness of the processes of decision-making and for truthfulness in the decision-making forum. This is clearly crucial to any deliberative approach to ethics, and whilst it might be argued that such an emphasis on truthfulness might be captured by the first principle which argues for the engagement in a genuine attempt to 'make sense', it seems to me that having it as a separate principle highlights the formal elements of the deliberative ethical space within which 'making sense' is possible (Habermas, 1993).

(iv) A decentralised bioethics   Finally, and perhaps most importantly, this is an argument for the democratisation and decentralisation of ethics (see Parker, 2007a). For, whilst the philosophical analysis of ethical problems and ethical theory and the elaboration of biomedical principles can be useful in creating a

framework for the discussion of ethical problems, the resolution of such problems in an ethical way involves the creation and maintenance of ethical fora of the kind I have described, in which those who have a legitimate interest in a case can engage jointly in the process deliberation. This is to argue for a genuinely participatory, democratic and discursive bioethics, and such a perspective has, I suggest, profound and radical political implications both for the medical profession and beyond.

We began this chapter by reflecting on the key roles played by the concept of 'autonomy' in contemporary understandings of the ethical dimensions of medical practice and in particular in the ways it informs an increasing emphasis on the centrality of 'patient choice' in notions of good medical practice. We also provided examples of the ways in which these concepts have been integrated into healthcare policymaking.

In this chapter we have explored the limits of these concepts and commitments. We have investigated competing definitions of autonomy and their implications, explored the different and to some extent competing ways in which autonomy is enshrined in European law, and finally, critically reflected on two alternative conceptions of ethics and their implications for the ways in which autonomy and respect for patient choice might be understood. Despite the differences and tensions between these approaches and between them and the 'autonomy' approach with which we began this chapter, there remains in common between them a view that something like emphasis on and support for 'autonomy and patient choice' in the context of day-to-day healthcare practice, whether this is engaged with through narrative or through deliberation, seems to offer the best chance of protecting the vulnerable in healthcare. As this chapter has progressed, however, we have begun to see that the question of how this is to be enacted effectively in practice demands an increasingly sophisticated understanding of the ethical dimensions of medicine and of medical practice more widely than that which sees ethical practice too narrowly as patient-centredness. As the chapter, and indeed the book, draw to a close, we are left not only with the question of what should be done, but also of 'method' in ethics: that is, what the implications of different models of ethics are not only for what we think should be done, but also for how we are to understand the 'problem'.

We leave you with a final case, from Sweden, and a challenging question. Please read through this case with this question in mind: How would this case be approached from each of the 'patient-centredness', 'narrative' and 'deliberative' perspectives, and what are the ethical implications of thinking about ethics and this case from these different, but overlapping perspectives?

The case of Olle

Olle is 84 years old and suffers from Parkinson's disease. In addition to this he has poor vision and hearing. Olle has lived in a residential home for several years but he is not happy there. One particular source of discontent is his love of good food and consequent dissatisfaction with the meals provided at the home.

The problem for the staff and for other residents, however, is that Olle has an electric wheelchair which he drives around in, occasionally going too fast to be safe. The other residents have complained about this, saying that they find it frightening, and the atmosphere in the home has become tense and irritable as a consequence. Some of the staff and some of the other residents feel that Olle should have his electric wheelchair replaced with an ordinary one because he is a danger to the safety of others.

But this would mean that Olle would become dependent upon the staff for mobility as he is not able to propel himself in a manual wheelchair. The electric chair provides him with freedom.

References and Notes

1. Reproduced with permission from Christian Hick, 'The right to refuse treatment'. Paper presented at EBEPE workshop in Turku.

2. With permission from John Coggon (2007), 'Varied and principled understandings of autonomy in English law: justifiable inconsistency or blinkered moralism?' *Health Care Analysis*, 15(3), 235–55.

3. My thanks to Professor Søren Holm for pointing out this distinction to me.

4. Reproduced with permission from Susan Mendus, 'Out of the doll's house'. Paper presented at EBEPE workshop in Turku.

5. Adapted with permission from Michael Parker, 'A deliberative approach to bioethics'. Paper presented at EBEPE workshop.

Appendix 1: Study guide for teachers

Each of the chapters in this workbook is intended to be a flexible educational resource, and we would encourage both learners and teachers to use the materials in a way which best suits their requirements. In some cases this might mean working through an entire chapter, but more often it might mean using a case study and the related activities as an educational resource to be used in conjunction with other materials. The chapters and the activities within them are intended to be used in a variety of ways at different points in the medical or nursing curriculum or for post-qualifying training; they are equally suitable for use as distance learning materials for self-study.

We aim to present a kind of medical ethics and a way of teaching it which we believe doctors and nurses will find highly relevant to their everyday practice. Although we sometimes refer to the 'big' cases and issues, as evidence of legal positions, for example, we concentrate on 'everyday ethics' by beginning each chapter with a very ordinary and typical sort of case. So we answer the question '*why* study medical ethics?' by beginning from examples which will resonate with practitioners, we hope. The headline topics are important, demonstrating that the issues of medical ethics are of widespread interest to the population as a whole – of which healthcare practitioners are of course a part. We do not ignore them, but we do not begin from them, as many texts and courses in medical ethics have done. Nor do we start from abstract 'principles' such as 'autonomy', 'beneficence', or whatever, and then work down to cases, in a deductive fashion. Instead we begin empirically from typical cases and, importantly, from the narratives which practitioners construct around them. They write those stories in different ways according to what professional part they play in them, according to their disciplinary background.

Using a case study

Here is an example of the sorts of cases we use, and of the interactive, experiential way we ask you to look at

them. Like almost all the others in this workbook, it is a real-life case which has been heavily anonymized to protect patient confidentiality. After the case you will find an activity with comments; again, this is a typical structure in the chapters, designed to enhance interactive learning. The typical activity in these chapters is not merely a 'quiz' on factual aspects of the case; here, it requires you to do some thinking about the arguments for and against the proposition that although this is an everyday sort of case, it is not about ethics, but rather simply a matter of good and bad patient management. This sort of activity is common to the workbook as a whole, deriving from our aim of encouraging 'reflective practice'. We would encourage you to enter your reflections on these activities in a learning journal. You might also wish to compare your reactions with those of colleagues; indeed, in a more formal teaching or training setting, the activities are a good focus of groupwork, and a possible means of formative or summative assessment. But they, and the cases on which they centre, can also be read and analysed by individuals working on their own. Later in this guide, we will give some suggestions on different approaches to reading the cases, particularly for those working alone. But first, you should read the case without any such 'coaching'.

The case of Mr P

Mr P, who is 64 years old, has pre-senile dementia of the Alzheimer's type. His condition is deteriorating rapidly, and for the past four months he has lived in a nursing home. Now he is confined to a wheelchair and cannot feed himself. His wife Susan comes to visit him every day, bringing a home-cooked evening meal. The nursing home's guidelines for good practice encourage relatives' involvement, and Mr P does seem pleased to see Susan when she first arrives. But although Mr P has a hot meal at lunch time in the nursing home, Susan thinks he also needs 'a proper

---

meal' in the evening, rather than the sandwiches and cakes provided at the home. Mr P appears to resist Susan's attempts to feed him, tossing and turning in his wheelchair. She in turn has taken to 'playing a little game': holding his nose, so that when he opens his mouth for air, she can spoon-feed him. This seems to make Mr P very agitated, and he is often hard to calm after Susan's visits.

The nursing home staff have asked Susan not to feed Mr P, but this has led to worsening relations. They feel that Mr P is clearly indicating that he does not want to be forcibly fed. Susan, very hurt by this comment, insists that she is handling Mr P in a playful but caring fashion, and that she has to do something about Mr P's weight loss, which she blames on inadequate nutrition in the home. 'If you can't even feed him properly, what else are you doing wrong? He's not getting any better, you know.' The nursing staff themselves are divided, some feeling that Susan is trying to help, and others that she is in denial about her husband's impending death. The doctors at the nursing home, however, are unanimous. They see no reason to allow Susan to continue feeding Mr P, as it is contrary to his medical best interests and indeed risks asphyxiation. The manager of the home agrees with the doctors: this unnecessary trouble is upsetting the smooth running of the home, and should be stopped.

ACTIVITY: First, consider the response that this case has nothing to do with medical ethics, that it is simply a matter of patient management. What are the arguments for and against that view? Second, make a list of the ethical issues which you feel this case evokes. In doing so, try to think of what issues would be identified by (a) the nurses on both sides of the question, (b) the doctors, (c) Susan, (d) the home manager and, interestingly, (e) Mr P in his pre-senile condition.

Let us look first at the viewpoint which insists that this case is just an illustration of bad management, and that it does not raise any difficult ethical dilemmas: it is clear what should be done. Arguably, the problem could have been avoided by not allowing Susan to feed Mr P in the first place. There is no medical need, and Mr P's weight loss is due to his condition, which Susan apparently cannot accept. Perhaps her behaviour is due to her denial about his impending death, in that view. Alternatively, the bad practice is seen as lying in poor communication. Better communication might have prevented the breakdown in relations

between Susan and the nursing home staff. But the difficulty here is about what should have been communicated, not just how it should have been communicated. If the nursing home staff were obliged to tell Susan that she was not permitted to feed Mr P, it is hard to see how conflict could have been avoided altogether, no matter how tactfully it was done.

These sorts of interpretations are commonly heard, but what is less often realized is that this 'anti-ethics' position itself rests on a value or ethical base. Not allowing Susan to feed Mr P, because it is not in his medical best interests, or because it upsets the routine of the home, is a *paternalistic* stance. It implies that 'doctor (or nurse, or manager) knows best'. The home has in fact not taken that stance; the staff have allowed Susan to feed Mr P. Implicitly, they are accepting a different ethical stance, one which gives weight to non-medical factors. It is a more consultative, *egalitarian* position, which accords some rights to the patient's relatives (or alternatively, for competent patients, to patients themselves). This dynamic between *paternalism* and *rights* has been the wellspring of much of modern medical ethics over the past 40 years. So this very ordinary case – much more everyday than most of the questions raised in medical ethics during the past four decades, which originally concentrated more heavily on death and dying, abortion and other 'big' topics – seems to us to prove that no, you can't avoid 'doing ethics' in everyday practice. Ethics, in our view, is also about institutional structures and power relations, not just about individual choices, and when seen in that light, it is difficult for practitioners to avoid.

What about the second question? That is, the ethical issues which would be identified in different professional 'narratives'. We have already suggested one set of issues, around rights and paternalism. Others might include:

- Consent to treatment, particularly for incapacitated patients.
- The prior question of whether feeding is treatment.
- Communication of a terminal diagnosis to the patient's relatives.
- How actively we should treat patients at the end of life.
- The formulation of hospital and nursing home internal guidelines and consultation between different categories of staff.
- Resource issues, such as the amount of staff time devoted to calming Mr P after Susan's visits.

- Nurse advocacy: what does it mean to be the patient's advocate in this case?
- Best interests of the patient: are they purely medical? Or does Mr P derive some emotional benefit from Susan's visits?

You may also have identified other questions. So this abbreviated, ordinary case raises a wide range of ethical questions (and 'meta-ethical' ones, about whether something is an ethical matter in the first place). It is worth noting at this point that you might therefore wish to use this textbook either in the way in which it is presented – i.e. by using a particular chapter when teaching on issues pertaining to that particular topic – or as a broader resource, for 'dipping into' in order to illustrate the particular issue on which you are teaching (like consent, say) with appropriate cases and commentaries. We would encourage both approaches. The topics and cases we have selected should raise issues of relevance wherever you are practising (or teaching) and, indeed, whichever curriculum you are following – be it a country-specific document like the UK's 'core content' of learning for medical ethics and law, pioneered by retired obstetrician Gordon Stirrat and colleagues (Stirrat *et al.*, 2010), or wider educational initiatives, such as those promoted by UNESCO (ten Have, 2008).

Howsoever one might choose to use the workbook, once we have identified the sorts of ethical questions which arise in such cases as Mr P's, we need to know where to go from there. It is not enough simply to say that an ethical issue has been raised; we need to know how to get a better purchase on the ethical question. Many people believe that there are no absolute answers to ethical questions, and that each person's point of view is equally valid. This can lead to a crippling form of *moral relativism*. In clinical practice, teams need to make decisions; clinical and ethics research committees need to decide on guidelines. On what basis can this possibly be done if everyone's opinion is equally good? (Perhaps this, coupled with a view of ethics as abstract and difficult philosophy, is one reason why people are sometime reluctant to identify a question as a matter of ethical debate; it will be impossible to get agreement once that concession has been made.) And in terms of ethics education, the dilemma is equally compelling. Doesn't teaching ethics either imply forcing a particular viewpoint on people, or throwing up one's hands in despair and conceding that it's all a matter of opinion? We have tried to avoid either course in these chapters. In the next section, we

present a view of ethics as communicative activity which underpins our approach and which we feel forestalls total relativism. Again, we present the substance and the method of the chapters together in the next chapter; you will be asked to read part of an article by the German ethicist Dieter Birnbacher, arguing for the view of ethics not as grand, impenetrable theory but as communicative activity. This illustrates both the ways in which the chapters typically proceed – from case examples to guided reading exercises based on papers – and the 'philosophy' behind the chapters.

Using a reading exercise

Each of the chapters in the workbook starts off with a set of interactive, experiential activities structured around real, everyday cases and commentaries upon those cases by practitioners from Europe, the USA and Australia. In addition to this, the chapters also include guided reading exercises based around papers written by expert commentators, who may be practitioners, lawyers, philosophers, patients, economists or social policy analysts.

As an example of how we do this we have included a short extract from a paper below by Dieter Birnbacher, in which he discusses the role of medical ethics and how it ought to be taught. We have included this paper in the study guide because this appendix is largely concerned with just this question. The papers included in the other chapters, such as that on resource allocation, are much more clinically and case-based. In the other chapters we generally introduce the question of, say, resource allocation, by means of an everyday case, such as the one in the previous section. (Sometimes we do this through the text alone, but in three chapters – on reproductive ethics, genetics and research ethics – the cases are presented through branching video scenarios on the accompanying CD-ROM.) Often we then lead into a reading exercise, in which we ask the student to read the paper in the light of the issues raised by the case. The activities and the questions we ask are designed to encourage the student to question the thesis which the paper presents. In this case, for example, whilst we largely agree with Birnbacher that ethics ought to be practically based, we would encourage the student to reflect on this question for him or herself.

To see how this would work, we would now like you to read the following short extract from the paper, which is concerned with a conflict between two quite different approaches to medical ethics. As you do so we would like you to reflect on the case of Mr P with which we began this study guide. How would you go about analysing the case from each of the two perspectives Birnbacher introduces? Are the two approaches necessarily in conflict or might they be complementary in some respects? What would an ethics as practice look like? To what extent do you think students of medical ethics require a sense of ethics as theory in order to make an ethics of practice possible?

Teaching clinical medical ethics

Dieter Birnbacher

Which aims and functions of medical ethics are achievable by means of an exchange between the views of patients and doctors? Is this kind of exchange a genuine and constitutive part of medical ethics, or is it an exercise in which concepts, principles and norms of medical ethics are simply applied?

The answer depends on how medical ethics is conceived. A conception of ethics as theory has tended to predominate in the tradition of philosophy. Its task was the theoretical clarification of moral concepts, the study of moral arguments and the development of a maximally coherent and well-founded set of moral principles. Ethics in this sense was academic work done in writing books, giving lectures and holding seminars.

Even since the times of the Sophists and of Socrates, however, there has also existed a rival conception of ethics according to which ethics is practice rather than theory, more analogous to art than to science. According to this conception ethics (and philosophy generally) is an activity rather than a doctrine, where 'activity' means an essentially communicative activity of problem identification, deliberation and problem-solving. Though making use of methods similar to those of theoretical ethics and requiring similar skills (in fact, some more), this kind of doing ethics is quite different in its performance aspects. Ethics as theory is mainly monologue, ethics as practice mainly dialogue. Ethics as theory deals mainly with intellectual problems and intra-disciplinary controversies, whereas ethics as practice deals mainly with real-life problems and extra-disciplinary controversies. Ethics as theory deals mainly with potential cases, ethics as practice mainly with real cases. Taken as ideal types, ethics as theory is done in the ivory tower, ethics as practice in the marketplace.

ACTIVITY: Stop here for a moment and consider the case of Mr P with which we began this

study guide. When you read the case earlier, we asked you to consider the question of the extent to which cases like this are matters of patient management rather than of ethics. We also asked you to list the ethical issues which you felt the case posed. What are the relative advantages and disadvantages of the two approaches, that is, 'ethics as theory' and 'ethics as practice' in the process of case analysis of this kind?

Now continue with your reading of Birnbacher.

The idea of medical ethics as a truly practical discipline derives from the Socratic idea that ethics (and philosophy generally) is an activity, and an activity that is in principle open to everyone prepared to subject himself to the discipline of controlled dialogue. Correspondingly, the role of the professional ethicist radically changes. Far from functioning as a teacher of ethical wisdom, his role is rather that of a catalyst, moderator and mediator. His task is to see to it that the ethical dialogue keeps its aims firmly in view and is not led astray by extraneous motives, without himself prejudging or manipulating its results.

ACTIVITY: Try to make a list of the kinds of aims you think an ethicist should have in view in such a dialogue. What precisely is his or her role vis-à-vis the other participants?

Dieter Birnbacher answers this question as follows. As you read through his list compare it with your own, adding any of those that are missing to your list.

(1) A definition of the problem. It must be clear what the problem is. The ethicist can support the group in fixing the object of the debate.
(2) Articulation of views. The ethicist can give help, where needed, in making these views explicit and giving them adequate expression.
(3) Arguing for one's views. 'Arguing' does not mean, of course, rigorous philosophical reasoning. It should be open to all kinds of relevant inner and outer experiences.
(4) An effort to understand the others' views and arguments. This is the task for which the help of the ethicist is probably most needed. He should insist that the reasons others have for their views are not only taken notice of but understood in depth, taking into account their cognitive and

emotional background: Which normative principles are presupposed by these views? On which kind of experience do they depend? Which commitments and attitudes do they manifest? How far are they guided by external (legal, institutional, financial) constraints?

(5) The potential revision of views in the light of step 4. Confrontation with conflicting views of others may lead to a rethinking of reactions and positions, or to a weakening of claims to absolute truth.

(6) Finding common ground, consensus formation. Ethics is, among other things, the endeavour to solve practical problems in a way acceptable to all sides. The ethical standpoint is the 'view from nowhere' (Nagel, 1986) in which the partiality of all particular viewpoints is transcended but in which all particular viewpoints are somehow taken account of. The ethicist may be helpful as a mediator, paving the way to consensus.

Ethics education for practitioners

The structure of the chapters varies slightly, depending on the topic they address. In some, after a reading exercise of this kind, readers might be asked to look at another case, perhaps one which involves the law more directly. In others they might be asked to read another paper or perhaps a commentary on the case by a practitioner, or they might be asked to relate the issues raised to their own practice. In the three chapters already mentioned, readers are asked to return to the video scenarios on the CD-ROM: analysing a new case, drawing if they wish on additional resources such as the glossary, or adding to the learning log they will already have constructed as part of the guided exercises.

Nevertheless, despite their differences the chapters adopt a consistent and coherent overall educational and theoretical approach. The topics themselves might be said to each relate in a different way to a single theme, which might be expressed as a concern with the nature of relationships as the focus of ethical problems in medical practice. Each of the chapters can be seen to some extent as testing the relationship between practitioners and patients and their families in a variety of ways, illustrating and analysing the various difficulties which arise as a result.

This study guide has told you something about our view of the 'why, how and what' of ethics education; in self-reflexive fashion, it has also illustrated that view by having you do a bit of ethics learning in our preferred experiential, activity-based format. You will have seen that our style uses case material as a base. We think the case-based approach has several advantages:

- It cuts across disciplinary and cultural boundaries. Everyone can 'relate' in some sense to an actual case, even if they come from very distinct religious or cultural traditions which dictate different principles of ethical conduct. Similarly, different healthcare disciplines have increasingly evolved their own forms of healthcare ethics: nursing ethics, for example, sees its concerns and approach as quite distinct from those of medical ethics proper. But in a case-based approach, the different slants of different disciplines can be explicitly built in.
- It requires little previous knowledge of ethics and reassures students who think of philosophy as abstruse and difficult.
- It encourages students to think of comparable cases of their own, and thus to generalize what they have learned from one case to another, comparing similarities and differences.
- In the broader context, it allows students to learn from practice in other countries.

But before you begin work on the workbook itself, you may wonder how to approach these cases. Cases, like any other narrative, are constructed by their authors; the facts do not just speak for themselves. Although the Mr P case study comes from a true account, it is a selective account, it also had to be anonymized, and thus 'fictionalized' to some extent. It is always worth asking just how 'realistic' is this case? What has been left out?

From the reader's point of view, it is also true that cases do not necessarily just speak for themselves. So before ending this study guide, we want to present two possible approaches to reading the case studies. You may choose either (or neither!), but it may be helpful to have different frameworks of analysis before you start. Even if you decide to use these frameworks, however, it is important not to do so mechanically. It is important to be sensitive to the nuances of the actual case, rather than trying to fit it into a straitjacket of a framework.

In a text written primarily for medical students, Alan Johnson develops what he calls 'pathways in medical ethics'. These are decision trees which require a choice at several stages among possible responses.

For example, the first thing to ask about a clinical situation, in Johnson's framework for ethical analysis, is whether it is a question of ethics at all. The first part of the tree therefore reads: 'Clinical situation: is it:

(1) Technical?
(2) Ethical?
(3) A matter of professional etiquette?
(4) An emotional question?'

Perhaps you can see some problems with this framework already: it assumes 'only one of the above', but a situation could easily manifest all four components. In particular, we have our doubts about the distinction between 'ethical' and 'emotional'. It implies that ethics is divorced from emotion, but this represents an increasingly outdated and out-of-touch view of philosophical reasoning (Blum, 1980; Lloyd, 1993; Lindemann Nelson and Lindemann Nelson, 1995). However, let us continue with Johnson's framework.

If the situation is viewed as 'ethical', Johnson suggests you should subdivide the components of the case next. He limits the components to four again, assuming that any question can be typified as being about one of the following:

(1) Aims of medical care in this situation
(2) Value questions (e.g. about quality of life)
(3) Autonomy (the capacity to determine one's own actions)
(4) Truth, confidentiality and promise-keeping.

The next stage is to enunciate the general and specific moral principles which apply, including law and professional codes. If these principles are in conflict, what should be the outcome? Through another series of choices, Johnson eventually suggests applying the standard of *best consequences*. This implies a particular philosophical slant, generally termed consequentialist or utilitarian. It is worth noting, then, that Johnson's framework is not value-free; indeed, no framework is. If cases do not speak for themselves, neither do the analytical frameworks for analysing cases.

An alternative method of case analysis is offered by David Seedhouse and Lisetta Lovett in their *Practical Medical Ethics* (1992). This is the 'ethical grid', which suggests that in any clinical case the doctor should take account of each of the following:

(1) The principles behind health work (defined as respecting persons equally, creating autonomy, respecting autonomy and/or serving needs first).
(2) The duties of a doctor (defined as minimizing harm, doing the most positive good, telling the truth and/or keeping promises).
(3) The general nature of the outcome to be achieved (defined as the most beneficial outcome to society, the most beneficial outcome for the patient, the most beneficial outcome for the practitioner, and/or the most beneficial outcome for a particular group).
(4) The pertinent practical features of the situation (such as the law, the wishes of others, resources available, the effectiveness and efficiency of action, the risks, codes of practice, the degree of certainty of the evidence on which action is taken, and disputed facts).

At each level, some aspects will be relevant and others will not; however, all four levels of the grid are always relevant.

As Seedhouse and Lovett write,

> In one sense the Grid is merely a reminder that there are at least four separate levels at which to think, and that within these levels there are several different ways of deciding on strategy. As the Grid is used it soon becomes apparent that it is not the Grid that is working – but the doctor. To say 'I am using the Ethical Grid' is simply to say 'I am engaged in moral reasoning'.
> (Seedhouse and Lovett, 1992, p. 19)

Whether or not you choose to use 'pathways' or 'the ethical grid', or some other approach, this point holds. It is not the mechanism for analysing cases and clinical situations that is doing the work: it is you. We hope that this workbook will provide you with the necessary motivation, interest and support to help you to think critically and constructively about medical ethics.

Appendix 2: Using keywords to explore this book

In this appendix we have mapped *The Cambridge Medical Ethics Workbook* against the most commonly used keywords scheme in medical ethics: the Kennedy Institute of Bioethics classification (otherwise known as the National Reference Center for Bioethics Literature Library Classification Scheme).

For some chapters in this book, such as Chapters 1 (Death and dying: decisions at the end of life) and 2 (Reproduction: decisions at the start of life), there are copious and obvious Kennedy keywords, whereas other chapters appear at first to be less well matched to the scheme. Chapters 6 (Long-term care: autonomy, ageing and dependence) and 7 (Children and young people: conflicting responsibilities) are both major topics to us, whereas neither occupies more than a sub-sub-heading in the Kennedy Institute classification. This difference in emphasis should not, of course, be taken to imply that Chapters 1 and 2 are richer or more 'heavyweight' than Chapters 6 and 7. As it turns out, the list of keywords for Chapter 6 is no shorter than that for Chapters 1 or 2, because in the course of dealing with everyday ethical issues that arise in the care of the elderly, we cover major topics such as truth-telling, disclosure and conflicting ethical principles. Chapter 7 actually garnered the longest list of cross-references of any topic, including confidentiality, right to refuse treatment, and availability of genetic testing, abortion counselling or HIV testing to minors. In the end, then, the classification system did prove productive and appropriate for these chapters, despite initial appearances.

Other Kennedy Institute keywords, such as 1.3 'Applied and professional ethics' or 2 'Bioethics', can be taken as applying to the entire book and so have not been listed separately for each chapter. By contrast, some topics treated in this book do not occur at all in the Kennedy scheme, or have at best a very approximate match. An example is the role of commercial interests and the commodification of the body as they impinge on medical care and research – which has a growing literature in bioethics and biolaw but does not occur as

such in the Kennedy list. The nearest matches, which we have listed under Chapter 3 on Genetics: information, access and ownership, are 9.7, 'Drugs and drug industry' and 15.8 'Genetic patents'. Another example, from the same chapter, is the development of genetic databases and biobanks, for which there is no match at all.

Overall, however, even when the match is less than perfect, we felt it was important to provide you with a widely accepted keywords map to help you orient yourself as you work through the book. It will also allow you to search for further readings by number headings in the online National Reference Center for Bioethics Literature Library: http://bioethics.georgetown.edu/databases/searchtips.htm

We hope that you will find this appendix useful.

Chapter 1: Death and dying: decisions at the end of life

4.1.2 Theory and practice of the health professions: medicine
4.1.3 Theory and practice of the health professions: nursing
4.4 Quality/value of life/personhood
5.3 Social control of science/technology
6 Codes of practice/statements on professional ethics
8 Patient relationships: 8.2 Truth disclosure, 8.3 Informed consent
9.5 Healthcare for specific diseases/groups: 9.5.3 Mentally disabled persons, 9.5.7 Newborns and minors
20 Death and dying: all categories *except* 20.6 (capital punishment)

Chapter 2: Reproduction: decisions at the start of life

5.3 Social control of science/technology
8.4 Patient relationships: confidentiality

9.5 Healthcare for specific diseases/groups: 9.5.5 Women, 9.5.7 Embryos and fetuses
10 Sexuality/Gender
11 Contraception
12 Abortion
14 Reproduction/Reproductive technologies
15.2 Genetic counselling/Prenatal diagnosis

Chapter 3: Genetics: information, access and ownership

4.2 Concept of health
5 Science, technology and society: 5.1 General, 5.2 Technology/risk assessment, 5.3 Social control of science/technology
6 Codes of/position statements on professional ethics
7.3 Professional/professional relationship
8 Patient relationships: 8.2 Truth disclosure, 8.3 Informed consent, 8.4 Confidentiality
9.5. Healthcare for specific diseases/groups: 9.5.4 Minorities, 9.5.7 Minors
9.7 Drugs and drug industry
15 Genetics, molecular biology and microbiology: 15.2 Genetic counselling/prenatal diagnosis, 15.3 Genetic screening/testing, 15.5 Eugenics, 15.8 Genetic patents, 15.11 Genetics and human ancestry
21.7 International/political dimensions of biology and medicine: cultural pluralism

Chapter 4: Medical research: participation and protection

1.3 Applied and professional ethics: 1.3.5 Government/criminal justice, 1.3.6 International affairs, 1.3.9 Scientific research
2.2 History of health ethics/bioethics
5 Science/technology and society: 5.2 Technology/risk assessment, 5.3 Social control of science/technology
6 Codes of/position statements on professional ethics
7.4 Professional misconduct
8 Patient relationships: 8.2 Truth disclosure, 8.3 Informed consent
9 Healthcare for specific diseases/groups: 9.5.6 HIV infection and AIDS
15.5 Eugenics

18 Human experimentation: all categories *except* 15.4 Behavioural research and 15.7 Stem cell research
21.2 International/political dimensions of biology and medicine: war
21.7 International/political dimensions of biology and medicine: cultural pluralism

Chapter 5: Mental health: consent, competence and caring

1.1 Philosophical ethics
4 Philosophies of medicine and health, *especially* 4.3 Concept of mental health
6 Codes of/position statements on professional ethics
8.3 Informed consent
9.5.3 Healthcare for specific diseases/groups: mentally disabled persons
9.5.7 Healthcare for specific diseases/groups: minors
9.7 Drugs and drug industry
17 The neurosciences and mental health therapies
20.7 Suicide/assisted suicide

Chapter 6: Long-term care: autonomy, ageing and dependence

1.1 Philosophical ethics
4.1 Theory and practice of the health professions: 4.1.2 Medicine, 4.1.3 Nursing
4.3 Philosophies of medicine and health: quality/value of life/personhood
8.2 Patient relationships: Truth disclosure
8.3 Patient relationships: Informed consent, *especially* 8.3.3 Third-party consent/incompetents and 8.3.4 Right to refuse treatment
8.4 Confidentiality
9.5.2 Healthcare for specific diseases/groups: aged
10 Sexuality/gender
17.3 The neurosciences and mental health therapies: behaviour modification

Chapter 7: Children and young people: conflicting responsibilities

1.1 Philosophical ethics
2.4 Bioethics: commissions/councils
4.1.2 Theory and practice of the health professions: medicine
8.3.2 Parental consent/minors

Chapter 8: Resource allocation: justice, markets and rationing

Chapter 9: Thinking about ethics: autonomy and patient choice

Adapted from the National Reference Center for Bioethics Literature document: http://bioethics.georgetown.edu/databases/searchtips.htm, last updated May 2009, accessed November 2009.

Bibliography

Abel, E. K. and Browner, C. B. (1998). Selective compliance with biomedical authority and the uses of experiential knowledge. In *Pragmatic Women and Body Politics*, ed. M. Lock and P. Kaufert, pp. 310–26. Cambridge: Cambridge University Press.

Adshead, G. and Dickenson, D. (1993). Why do doctors and nurses disagree? In *Death, Dying and Bereavement*, ed. D. Dickenson and M. Johnson, pp. 162–8. London: Open University and Sage.

Agich, G. (1990). Reassessing autonomy in long-term care. *Hastings Center Report*, **20**(6), 12–17.

Agich, G. (1993). *Autonomy in Long-term Care*. New York, NY: Oxford University Press.

Aiken, W. and LaFollette, H. (eds) (1980). *Whose Child? Children's Rights, Parental Authority and State Power*. Totowa, NJ: Rowan and Littlefield.

Airedale NHS Trust v. Bland (1993) 2 WLR 816.

Alderson, P. (1990). *Choosing for Children*. Oxford: Oxford University Press.

Alderson, P. (1992). In the genes or in the stars? Children's competence to consent. *Journal of Medical Ethics*, **18**, 119–24.

Alderson, P. (1994). *Children's Consent to Surgery*. Buckingham: Open University Press.

Allen, C. (1995). Helping with deliberate self-harm: some practical guidelines. *Journal of Mental Health*, **4**, 243–50.

Allmark, P. (1995). Can there be an ethics of care? *Journal of Medical Ethics*, **21**, 19–24.

Almond, B. (1991). Education and liberty. *Journal of Philosophy of Education*, **25**(2), 193–202.

Almond, B. (1993). Rights. In *Companion to Ethics*, ed. P. Singer, pp. 259–69. Oxford: Blackwell.

American Fertility Society (1990). Surrogate mothers. In *Surrogate Motherhood: Politics and Privacy*, ed. L. Gostin, pp. 259–69. Bloomington, IN: University of Indiana Press.

American Psychiatric Association (1983). Guidelines for legislation on the psychiatric hospitalisation of adults. *American Journal of Psychiatry*, **140**, 622–79.

American Psychiatric Association (1990). Task Force Report. *The Practice of Electroconvulsive Therapy: Recommendations for Treatment, Training and Privileging*. Washington, DC: American Psychiatric Association.

American Psychiatric Association, American Psychiatric Nurses Association, and the National Association of Psychiatric Health Systems (2003). *Learning from Each Other: Success Stories and Ideas for Reducing Restraint/Seclusion in Behavioral Health*. Washington, DC: American Psychiatric Association.

American Psychiatric Association (1994). *Diagnostic and Statistical Manual. Version IV*. Washington, DC: American Psychiatric Press.

Andrews, K., Murphy, L., Munday, R. and Littlewood, C. (1996). Misdiagnosis of the vegetative state: retrospective study in a rehabilitation unit. *British Medical Journal*, **313**(7048), 13–16.

Andrews, L. B. (2002). Genes and patent policy – rethinking intellectual rights. *Nature Reviews Genetics*, **3**, 803–8.

Andrews, L. B. (2005). Harnessing the benefits of biobanks. *Journal of Law, Medicine and Ethics*, **33**(1), 22–30.

Andrews, L. B. and Nelkin, D. (2001). *Body Bazaar: The Market for Human Tissue in the Biotechnology Age*. New York, NY: Crown.

Angell, M. (1996). Euthanasia in the Netherlands – good news or bad? *New England Journal of Medicine*, **335**(22), 1678–8.

Angell, M. (2000). Is academic medicine for sale? *New England Journal of Medicine*, **342**, 1516–18.

Archard, D. (1993). *Children, Rights and Childhood*. London: Routledge.

Archer, L. (2002). Commentary on genetics and insurance, at TEMPE (Teaching Ethics: Materials for Practitioner Education) workshop, Milan, 2001. In *Ethics and Genetics: A Workbook for Practitioners and Students*, ed. G. de Wert *et al.* Oxford: Berghahn Books.

Aristotle (1908/2002). *The Works of Aristotle*, trans. W. D. Ross. 1908, Clarendon Press, reprint 2002. Oxford: Oxford University Press.

Aristotle (1908). *The Nicomachean Ethics*, trans. W. D. Ross. Oxford: Oxford University Press.

Ashcroft, R. E., Chadwick, D. W., Clark, S. R. L. *et al.* (1997). Implications of sociocultural contexts for ethics of clinical trials. *Health Technology Assessment*, **1**(9), 1.67. DOI 10.3310/hta1090/www, hta.ac.uk/927.

Attanucci, J. (1988). In whose terms: a new perspective on self, role and relationship. In *Mapping the Moral Domain*, ed. C. Gilligan *et al.* Cambridge, MA: Harvard University Press.

Bailey, S. (2002). Decision-making in health care: limitations of the substituted judgement principle. *Nursing Ethics*, **9**(5), 483–93.

Barlow, D. (2009). Evidence-based and cost-effective fertility investigation and treatment of older women: moving beyond NICE. In *Reproductive Ageing*, ed. S. Bewley, W. Ledger and D. Nikolaou, pp. 293–301. London: Royal College of Obstetricians and Gynaecologists Press.

Barnett, A. and Smith, H. (2006). Cruel cost of the human egg trade. *Observer*, 30 April, pp. 6–7.

Barni, M. (1991). La medicine legale e le ethiche esterna alla legge. *Rivista Italiana di Medicine Legale*, **13**, 375–80.

Barry, B. (2002) *Culture and Equality*. Cambridge, MA: Harvard University Press.

Bauby, J.-D. (1997). *The Diving Bell and the Butterfly*. New York, NY: Alfred A. Knopf.

Baylis, F. and Sherwin, S. (2000). Judgements of noncompliance in pregnancy. In *Ethical Issues in Maternal–Fetal Medicine*, ed. D. L. Dickenson. Cambridge: Cambridge University Press.

Beauchamp, R. (2009). Scientists flag concern about Africa's place in worldwide genomic research developments. *Bionews*, 9 June

Beauchamp, T. L. and Childress, J. F. (1989). *Principles of Biomedical Ethics*, 3rd edn. Oxford: Oxford University Press.

Beauchamp, T. L. and Childress, J. F. (1994). *Principles of Biomedical Ethics*, 4th edn. Oxford: Oxford University Press.

Beauchamp, T. and Childress, J. (2009). *Principles of Biomedical Ethics*, 6th edn. New York, NY: Oxford University Press.

Beecher, H. (1966). Ethics and clinical research. *New England Journal of Medicine*, **274**(24), 1354–60.

Bell, D. (1993). *Communitarianism and its Critics*. Oxford: Clarendon Press.

Benatar, S. R. (2004). Linking moral progress to medical progress: new opportunities for the Declaration of Helsinki. *World Medical Journal*, **50**, 11–13.

Benhabib, L. (1997). Ethical issues in child psychiatry in the Algerian community in France. Paper represented at the Seventh European Biomedical Ethics Practitioner Education (EBEPE) Workshop, Maastricht, 21–22 March.

Benjamin, M. (2001). Between subway and spaceship: practical ethics at the outset of the twenty-first century. *Hastings Center Report*, **31**(4), 24–31.

Bennett, R. and Harris, J. (2002). Are there lives not worth living? When is it morally wrong to reproduce? In *Ethical Issues in Maternal–Fetal Medicine*, ed. D. L. Dickenson. Cambridge: Cambridge University Press.

Benson, P. (1994). Free agency and self worth. *Journal of Philosophy*, **91**(12), 650.

Berghmans, R. (1992). *Om bestwil. Paternalisme in de psychiatrie* [For the patient's good. Paternalism in psychiatry]. Amsterdam: Thesis Publishers.

Berghmans, R. (1994). Zelfbinding in de psychiatrie. Ethische aspecten. [Self-binding in psychiatry. Ethical aspects]. *Tijdschrift voor Psychiatrie*, **36**(9), 625–38.

Berghmans, R. (1996). The Netherlands. In *Informed Consent in Psychiatry. European Perspectives of Ethics, Law and Clinical Practice*, ed. H-G. Koch, S. Reiter-Theil and H. Helmchen, pp. 197–229. Baden-Baden: Nomos Verlagsgesellschaft.

Berghmans, R. (1997a). Physician-assisted death, the moral integrity of medicine and the slippery slope. Paper presented at the Seventh European Biomedical Ethics Practitioner Education (EBEPE) Workshop, Maastricht, 21–22 March.

Berghmans, R. (1997b). Protection of the rights of the mentally ill in the Netherlands. Paper presented at the Tenth European Biomedical Ethics Practitioner Education (EBEPE) Conference, Turku, Finland, June.

Berlin, I. (1969). Two concepts of liberty. In *Four Essays on Liberty*. Oxford: Oxford University Press.

Beyleveld, D. and Brownsword, R. (2001). *Human Dignity in Bioethics and Biolaw*. Oxford: Oxford University Press.

Biggs, H. (2001). *Euthanasia, Death with Dignity and the Law*. Oxford: Hart Publishing.

Biller-Andorno, N., Lie, R. K. and ter Meulen, R. (2002). Evidence-based medicine as an instrument for rational health policy. *Health Care Analysis*, **10**, 261–75.

Birke, L., Himmelweit, S. and Vines, G. (1990). *Tomorrow's Child: Reproductive Technologies in the 90s*. London: Virago.

Black, D. (1991). Psychotropic drugs for problem children. *British Medical Journal*, **302**, 190–1.

Blank, R. and Merrick, J. S. (1995). *Human Reproduction, Emerging Technologies, and Conflicting Rights*. Washington, DC: Congressional Quarterly.

Blasszauer, B. (1993). Ethical issues in institutional care. Paper for the May Conference of the Project Care for the Elderly: Goals and Priorities, Maastricht, 7–8 May.

Bloch, S. and Chodoff, P. (1993). *Psychiatric Ethics*, 2nd edn. Oxford: Oxford University Press.

Blum, L. (1980). *Friendship, Altruism and Morality*. London: Routledge and Kegan Paul.

Blum, L. (1988). Gilligan and Kohlberg: implications for moral theory. *Ethics*, **98**, 472–91.

Blustein, J. (1982). *Parents and Children: The Ethics of the Family*. Oxford: Oxford University Press.

Bok, S. (1989). *Secrets: On the Ethics of Concealment and Revelation*. New York, NY: Vintage Books.

Bolam v Friern Hospital Management Committee [1957] 1 WLR 582.

Borry, P., Fryns, J.-P., Schotsmans, P. and Dierickx, K. (2006). Carrier testing in minors: a systematic review of guidelines and position papers. *European Journal of Human Genetics*, **14**, 133–8.

Borry, P., Stultiens, L., Goffin, T., Nys, H. and Dierickx, K. (2008). Minors and informed consent in carrier testing: a survey of European clinical geneticists. *Journal of Medical Ethics*, **34**, 370–4.

Borst-Eilers, E (1990). Leeftijd als criterium. In *Grenzen aan de Zorg. Zorgen aan de Grens*, ed. J. K. M. Gevers and H. J. Hubben, pp. 66–72. Alphen aan de Rijn: Tjeenk Willink.

Borthwick, C. (1995). The proof of the vegetable: a commentary on medical futility. *Journal of Medical Ethics*, **21**, 205–8.

Bosanquet, N. (1998). The case for investing in quality health services for older people. Paper delivered to British Geriatric Society, October 1998.

Bouman, N. (1997). Ethical issues in child psychiatric consultations and liaison in paediatrics. Paper presented at the Eighth European Biomedical Ethics Practitioner Education (EBEPE) Workshop, Rome, 7–8 March.

Bowlby, J. (1988). *A Secure Base: Clinical Applications of Attachment Theory*. London: Routledge.

Boyle, J. (1996). *Shamans, Software and Spleens*. Cambridge, MA: Harvard University Press.

Bracalenti, R. and Mordini, E. (1997). The role of psychiatric and psychological support at the end of life. Paper presented at the Seventh European Biomedical Ethics Practitioner Education (EBEPE) Workshop, Maastricht, 21–22 March.

Bradshaw, A. (2009). Measuring nursing care and compassion: the McDonaldised nurse? *Journal of Medical Ethics*, **35**, 465–8.

Breggin, P. (1991). *Toxic Psychiatry, Drugs and Electroconvulsive Therapy: The Truth and the Better Alternatives*. New York, NY: St. Martin's Press.

Breslau, N., Davis, G. C., Andreski, P., Peterson, E. and Schultz, L. (1997). Sex differences in posttraumatic stress disorder. *Archives of General Psychiatry*, **54**, 1044–8.

Bristol Crisis Service for Women (1995). *Women and Self-injury: A Survey of 76 Women. A Report on Women's Experience of Self-injury and their Views on Service Provision*. London: Mental Health Foundation.

British Broadcasting Corporation (1995). Open University course K260 (*Death and Dying*). Radio programme.

British Medical Association (1995). *Medical Ethics Today*. London: BMA.

British Medical Association (1998). *Human Genetics: Choice and Responsibility*. Oxford: Oxford University Press.

British Medical Association, Resuscitation Council (UK) and Royal College of Nursing (2007). *Decisions Relating to Cardiopulmonary Resuscitation*. London: British Medical Association.

Brock, D. (1993). A proposal for the use of advance directives in the treatment of incompetent mentally ill persons. *Bioethics*, **7**, 244–56.

Brody, H. (1997). Medical futility: a useful concept? In *Medical Futility and the Evaluation of Life-sustaining Interventions*, ed. M. B. Zucker and H. D. Zucker, pp. 1–14. Cambridge: Cambridge University Press.

Brooks, J. D. and King, M. L. (2008). *Geneticizing Disease: Implications for Racial Health Disparities*. Washington, DC: Center for American Progress.

Brown, D. (1994). Self-development through subjective interaction: a fresh look at ego training in action. In *The Psyche and the Social World*, ed. D. Brown and L. Zinkin, pp. 80–98. London: Routledge.

Brown, G. and Harris, T. (1978). *The Social Origins of Depression*. London: Tavistock.

Brown, L. and Gilligan, C. (1992). *Meeting at the Crossroads: Women's Psychology and Girls' Development*. Cambridge, MA: Harvard University Press.

Brownsword, R. (2006). Biobank governance: property, privacy and consent. In *Ethics and Law of Intellectual Property*, ed. C. Lenk, N. Hoppe and R. Andorno. Aldershot: Ashgate.

Buchanan, A. and Brock, D. (1989). *Deciding for Others: The Ethics of Surrogate Decision Making*. Cambridge: Cambridge University Press.

Button, E. (1992). *Rural Housing for Youth*. London: Centrepoint.

Calabresi, G. and Bobbitt, P. (1978). *Tragic Choices*. New York, NY: Norton.

Callahan, D. (1987). *Setting Limits. Medical Goals in an Ageing Society*. New York, NY: Simon and Schuster.

Callahan, D. (1990). *What Kind of Life: The Limits of Medical Progress*. New York, NY: Simon and Schuster.

Callahan, J. (ed.). (1995). *Reproduction, Ethics and the Law: Feminist Perspectives*. Indiana: Indiana University Press.

Calzone, C. (1996). Consent or compliance? From informed consent to the right to informed guidance. Paper presented at the Sixth European Biomedical Ethics Practitioner Education (EBEPE) Workshop, Naantali, Finland, 6–7 September.

Calzone, C. and D'Andrea, M. S. (1996). New offspring in a family with a handicapped child. Paper presented at the

First European Biomedical Ethics Practitioner Education (EBEPE) Workshop, Rome, May.

Campbell, A. V. (1998). Euthanasia and the principle of justice. In *Euthanasia and the Churches*, ed. R. Gill, pp. 83–97. London: Cassell.

Campbell, A. V., Gillet, G. and Jones, G. (1997). *Medical Ethics*, 4th edn. Oxford: Oxford University Press.

Campbell, B. (1995). *The London Independent*, 16 March.

Caplan, A. (2009). Apples, oranges and comas. www.blog.bioethics.net, 7 December.

Capron, A. M. (1995). Baby Ryan and virtual futility. *Hastings Center Report*, **25**(2), 20–1.

Carlson, R. V., Boyd, K. M. and Webb, D. J. (2004). The revision of the Declaration of Helsinki: past, present and future. *British Journal of Clinical Pharmacology*, **57**, 695–713.

Carlson, R. V., van Ginneken, N. H., Pettigrew. L. M. *et al.* (2007). The three official language versions of the Declaration of Helsinki: what's lost in translation? *Journal of Medical Ethics*, **33**, 545–8.

Carr, V., Dorrington, C., Schrader, G. and Wale, J. (1983). The use of ECT for mania in childhood bipolar disorder. *British Journal of Psychiatry*, **143**, 411–15.

Carse, A. L (1991). The 'voice of care': implications for bioethical education. *Journal of Medicine and Philosophy*, **16**, 5–28.

Casey, R. J. and Berman, J. S. (1985). The outcome of psychotherapy with children. *Psychological Bulletin*, **98**, 388–400.

Chadwick, R. (1987). *Ethics, Reproduction and Genetic Control*. London: Routledge.

Chadwick, R. (1999a). Are genes us? Gene therapy and personal identity. In *The Moral Status of Persons: Perspectives on Bioethics*, ed. G. K. Becker, pp. 183–94. Amsterdam: Editions Rodopi.

Chadwick, R. (1999b). The Icelandic database – do modern times need modern sagas? *British Medical Journal*, **319**(7207), 441–4.

Chadwick, R. (2009). Introduction. Reproductive autonomy – a special issue. *Bioethics*, **23**.

Charmaz, K. (1987). Struggle for a self: identity levels of the chronically ill. In *Research in the Sociology of Health Care*, ed. J. Roth and P. Conrad, Vol. 6, pp. 283–321. Greenwich, CT: J.A.I. Press.

Cheon-Lee, E. and Amstey, M. A. (1998). Compliance with Centers for Disease Control and Prevention, antenatal culture protocol for preventing Group B streptococcal neonatal sepsis. *American Journal of Obstetrics and Gynaecology*, **179**, 77–9.

Cherry, M. (2005). *Kidney for Sale by Donor: Human Organs, Transplantation and the Market*. Washington, DC: Georgetown University Press.

Chesley, L. C., Annitto, J. E. and Cosgrove, R. A. (2000). The remote prognosis of eclamptic women. *American Journal of Obstetrics and Gynecology*, **182**(1 pt 1), 247.

Chester v *Afshar* [2005] 1 AC 134.

The Children Act (1989). London: HMSO.

Choices in Healthcare (1992). Report by the Government Committee on Choices in Healthcare, the Netherlands. Rijswijk: Ministry of Welfare, Health and Cultural Affairs.

Christman, J. (1988). Constructing the inner citadel: recent work on the concept of autonomy. *Ethics*, **99**, 109–24.

Christman, J. (1991). Liberalism and individual positive liberty. *Ethics*, **101**(2), 355.

Cicero (1951). *On Moral Duties. The Basic works of Cicero*, ed. M. Hadas, p. 47. New York, NY: Modern Library.

CIOMS/WHO (1993). *International Ethical Guidelines for Biomedical Research involving Human Subjects*. Geneva: CIOMS/WHO.

Clark, P. G. (1989). Canadian health-care policy and the elderly: will rationing rhetoric become reality in an ageing society? *Canadian Journal of Community Mental Health*, **8**, 132–40.

Clarke, A. (1994). *Genetic Counselling: Practice and Principles*. London: Routledge.

Clarke, A. (2007) Should families own genetic information? No. *British Medical Journal*, **335**, 23–4.

Clinical Genetics Society (1994). The genetic testing of children: report of a working party. *Journal of Medical Genetics*, **31**, 785–97.

Coggon, J. (2007). Varied and principled understandings of autonomy in English law: justifiable inconsistency or blinkered moralism? *Health Care Analysis*, **15**(3), 235–55.

Cohen, L. (1999). Where it hurts: Indian material for an ethics of organ transplantation. *Daedalus*, **128**, 136–65.

Consensus statement by teachers of medical ethics and law in UK medical schools (1998). *Journal of Medical Ethics*, **24**(3), 188–92.

Council of Europe Steering Committee on Bioethics (1999). *The Icelandic Act on a Health Sector Database and Council of Europe Conventions*. Strasbourg: Ministry of Health and Social Security (CDBI-CO-GT2(99)7 1999).

Council of Europe (1981). *Convention for the Protection of Individuals with regard to Automatic Processing of Personal Data*. Strasbourg: Council of Europe.

Council of Europe (1997a). Convention for the Protection of Human Rights and Dignity of the Human Being with regard to the Application of Biology and Medicine: Convention on Human Rights and Biomedicine (Oviedo 4 April 1997). *European Treaty Series* **164**.

Council of Europe (1997b). *Recommendation on the Protection of Medical Data*. Strasbourg: Council of Europe (No R(97)5).

Council of Europe (1997c). *Recommendation Concerning the Protection of Personal Data Collected and Processed for Statistical Purposes*. Strasbourg: Council of Europe (No R(97)18).

Crawford, R. (1980). Healthism and medicalization of everyday life. *International Journal of Health Services*, **10**, 365–88.

Crenier, A. (1996). Child abuse and professional secrecy: doctors and the law. Paper presented at the First European Biomedical Ethics Practitioner Education (EBEPE) Workshop, Rome, 25 May.

Crisp, R. and Slote, M. (eds.). (1996). *How Should One Live? Essays on the Virtues*. Oxford: Clarendon Press.

Crisp, R. (ed). (1997). *Virtue Ethics*. Oxford: Oxford University Press.

Cullity, G. (1995). Moral free-riding. *Philosophy and Public Affairs*, **24**(1), 3–34.

Culver, C. M. and Gert, B. (1982). *Philosophy in Medicine*. Oxford: Oxford University Press.

Dalla Vorgia, P. (1997). Car driving and insight: commentary on the case of Mr A from a Greek viewpoint. Paper presented at the Tenth European Biomedical Ethics Practitioner Education (EBEPE) Workshop, Maastricht, May.

Daniels, C. (1993). *At Women's Expense: State Power and the Politics of Fetal Rights*. Cambridge, MA: Harvard University Press.

Daniels, K. R., Ericsson, H. L. and Burn, J. P. (1998). The views of semen donors regarding the Swedish Insemination Act 1984. *Medical Law International*, **3**(2, 3), 117–34.

Daniels, N. (1988). *Am I My Parents' Keeper? An Essay on Justice between the Young and the Old*. New York, NY: Oxford University Press.

Danish Council of Ethics (1998). *Conditions for Psychiatric Patients – A Report*. Copenhagen: Danish Council of Ethics.

Davies, J. (ed). (1993). *The Family: Is it just Another Lifestyle Choice?* London: Institute of Economic Affairs.

Davis, A. (2002). Living with dignity. *The Observer*, 10 November.

Davison, J. M. (1994). Pregnancy in renal allograft recipients: problems, prognosis and practicalities. *Baillière's Clinical Obstetrics and Gynaecology*, **8**, 501–25.

Dawes, R. M. (1986). Representative thinking in clinical judgement. *Clinical Psychology Review*, **6**, 425–41.

Dawson, A. (2005). The determination of "best interests" in relation to childhood vaccinations. *Bioethics*, **19**, 188–205.

de Beauvoir, S. (1972). *The Coming of Age*, trans. P. O'Brien, p. 28. New York, NY: G. P. Putnam's Sons.

deCODE genetics. www.database.is (Accessed 14 May 1999.)

Dees, M., Vernooij-Dassen, M., Dekkers, W. and Van Weel, C. (2009). Unbearable suffering of patients with a request for euthanasia or physician-assisted suicide: an integrative review. *Psycho-Oncology*, DOI: 10.1002/pon.1612.

de Graeve, D. and Adriaenssen, I. (2001). The use of economic evaluation in healthcare allocation. In *The Cambridge Medical Ethics Workbook: Case Studies, Commentaries and Activities*, ed. M. Parker and D. Dickenson, pp. 251–6. Cambridge: Cambridge University Press.

De Haan, J. (2002). The ethics of euthanasia: advocates' perspectives. *Bioethics*, **16**(2), 154–72.

Dennis, N. (1993). *Rising Crime and the Dismembered Family*. London: Institute of Economic Affairs.

De Roy, P. G. (2004). Helsinki and the Declaration of Helsinki. *World Medical Journal*, **50**, 9–11.

Devereux, J., Jones, D. P. H. and Dickenson, D. L. (1993). Can children withhold consent to treatment? *British Medical Journal*, **306**, 1459–61.

Devinsky, O. and Duchowny, M. S. (1983). Seizures after convulsive therapy; a retrospective case survey. *Neurology*, **33**(7), 921–5.

Dickenson, D. (1991). *Moral Luck in Medical Ethics and Practical Politics*. Aldershot: Avebury.

Dickenson, D. (1994). Children's informed consent to treatment: is the law an ass? *Journal of Medical Ethics*, **20**, 205–6.

Dickenson, D. (1995). Is efficiency ethical? Resource issues in healthcare. In *Introducing Applied Ethics*, ed. B. Almond, pp. 229–46. Oxford: Blackwell.

Dickenson, D. (1997). *Property, Women and Politics: Subjects or Objects?* Cambridge: Polity Press.

Dickenson, D. (1998). Consent in children. *Current Opinion in Psychiatry*, **11**, 4.

Dickenson, D. (1999a). Can children consent to be tested for adult-onset genetic disorders? *British Medical Journal*, **318**, 1003–5.

Dickenson, D. (1999b). Cross-cultural issues in European bioethics. *Bioethics*, **3**(3), 249–55.

Dickenson, D. (2000). Are medical ethicists out of touch? Practitioner attitudes in the US and UK towards decisions at the end of life. *Journal of Medical Ethics*, **26**, 254–60.

Dickenson, D. (ed.) (2002). *Ethical Issues in Maternal–Fetal Medicine*. Cambridge: Cambridge University Press.

Dickenson, D. (2003). *Risk and Luck in Medical Ethics.* Cambridge: Polity Press.

Dickenson, D. (2004a). What feminism can teach global ethics. In *Linking Visions: Feminist Bioethics, Human Rights and the Developing World*, ed. R. Tong, A. Donchin and S. Dodds, pp. 15–30. Lanham, MD: Rowman & Littlefield.

Dickenson, D. (2004b). Consent, commodification and benefit-sharing in genetic research. *Developing World Bioethics*, **4**(2), 126–41.

Dickenson, D. (2005a). Global ethics and human tissue. *Genomics, Society and Policy*, **1**, 41–53.

Dickenson, D. (2005b). The new French resistance: commodification rejected? *Medical Law International*, **7**(1), 41–64.

Dickenson, D. (2007). *Property in the Body: Feminist Perspectives.* Cambridge: Cambridge University Press.

Dickenson, D. (2008). *Body Shopping: The Economy Fuelled by Flesh and Blood.* Oxford: Oneworld.

Dickenson, D. and Fulford, K. W. M. (2000). *In Two Minds: A Casebook of Psychiatric Ethics.* Oxford: Oxford University Press.

Dickenson, D. and Jones, D. (1995). True wishes: the philosophy and developmental psychology of children's informed consent. *Philosophy, Psychiatry and Psychology*, **2**, 287–305.

Dickenson, D. and Vineis, P. (2002). Evidence-based medicine and quality of care. *Health Care Analysis*, **10**, 243–59.

Dingwall, A., Eekelaar, J. and Murray, T. (1983). *The Protection of Children.* Oxford: Blackwell.

Donchin, A. (2004). Integrating bioethics and human rights: toward a global feminist approach. In *Linking Visions: Feminist Bioethics, Human Rights and the Developing World*, ed. R. Tong, A. Donchin and S. Dodds, pp. 31–56. Lanham, MD: Rowman & Littlefield.

Donchin, A. (2009). Toward gender-sensitive reproduction policies. *Bioethics*, **23**(1). http://www3. interscience.wiley.com/journal.121560926/issue

Dooley, D. (1997). *Autonomy, feminism and vulnerable patients.* Paper presented at the Tenth European Biomedical Ethics Practitioner Education (EBEPE) Conference, Turku, Finland, June.

Doyal, L. (2006). Dignity in dying should include the legalisation of non-voluntary euthanasia. *Clinical Ethics*, **1**, 31–56.

Drummond, M., Stoddart, G. and Torrance, G. (1987). *Methods for the Economic Evaluation of Healthcare Programmes.* Oxford: Oxford University Press.

Dubler, N. N. (2005). Conflict and consensus at the end of life. In *Improving End of Life Care: Why Has It Been So Difficult? Hastings Center Report Special Report*, **35**(6), s19–25.

Durlak, J. A., Fuhrman, T. and Lampman, C. (1991). Effectiveness of cognitive-behavioural therapy for maladapting children: a meta-analysis. *Psychological Bulletin*, **110**, 204–14.

Dworkin, G. (1988). *The Theory and Practice of Autonomy.* Cambridge: Cambridge University Press.

Dworkin, R. (1977). *Taking Rights Seriously.* London: Duckworth.

Dworkin, R. (1986). Autonomy and the demented self. *The Milbank Quarterly*, **64** (Suppl. II), 4–16.

Dworkin, R. (1990). The foundations of liberal equality. In *The Tanner Lectures on Human Values*, ed. G. Petersen. Saltlake City, UT: University of Utah Press.

Dworkin, R. (1993). *Life's Dominion: An Argument about Abortion, Euthanasia, and Individual Freedom.* London: Harper Collins.

Dworkin, R. (2000). *Sovereign Virtue: The Theory and Practice of Equality.* Cambridge, MA: Harvard University Press.

Dyer, C. (2002). Pretty's legal battle for dignity in death. *The Guardian*, 13 May.

Eastman, N. and Peay, J. (1998). Bournewood: an indefensible gap in mental health law. *British Medical Journal*, **317**, 94–5.

Edwards, R. (1997). *Ethics of Psychiatry.* New York: Prometheus Books.

Eich, H., Reiter, L. and Reiter-Theil, S. (1996). Bioethical problems related to psychiatric and psychotherapeutic treatment of children. Paper presented at the First European Biomedical Ethics Practitioner Education (EBEPE) Workshop, Rome, 25 May.

Eisenberg, L. (1971). Principles of drug therapy in child psychiatry with special reference to stimulant drugs. *American Journal of Orthopsychiatry*, **41**, 371–9.

Elgesem, D. (1996). Paper given at conference of the European Biomedical Ethics Practitioner Education Project, Turku.

Elias, N. (1971). *Sociologie en geschiedene en andere essays.* Amsterdam: Van Gennep.

Elliott, C. and Abadie, R. (2008). Exploiting a research underclass in Phase I clinical trials. *New England Journal of Medicine*, **358**, 2316–17.

Elliston, S. (2007). *The Best Interests of the Child in Healthcare.* London: Routledge-Cavendish.

El-Sharif, A. (1992). *Link: Cause for Concern.* London: Granada (video).

Emanuel, E. J. & Emanuel, L. L. (1992). Four models of the physician-patient relationship. *Journal of the American Medical Association*, **267**, 2221–6.

Engelhardt, H. T (1986). *The Foundations of Bioethics.* Oxford: Oxford University Press.

English, V., Sheather, J., Sommerville, A. and Chrispin, E. (2009). Ethics briefings. *Journal of Medical Ethics*, **35**, 335–6.

Es, J. C. van. and Hagen, J. H. (1987). Kostenstijging in de gezondheidszorg, externe en interne factoren. In *Verdeling van schaarse middelen in de gezondheidszorg*, ed. A. W. Muschenga, and J. N. D. de Neeling, pp. 69–84. Amsterdam: VU Uitgeverij.

Etzioni, A. (1993). *The Spirit of Community*. London: Fontana.

European Parliament (1995). *Directive on the Protection of Individuals with Regard to the Processing of Personal Data*. Brussels: European Parliament (Directive 95/46/EC.).

Evans, D. and Evans, M. (1996). *A Decent Proposal: Ethical Review of Clinical Research*. Chichester: Wiley.

Evans, M. I., Littman, L., Richter, R. *et al.* (1997). Selective reduction for multifetal pregnancy: early opinions revisited. *Journal of Reproductive Medicine*, **42**, 771.

Ex parte Hincks (1980). (*R. v. Secretary of State for Social Services, West Midlands RHA and Birmingham AHA (Teaching), ex parte Hincks*), 1 BMLR 93, 97.

F. v. West Berkshire Health Authority (1989). 2 All ER 545.

Fabre, C. (2006). *Whose Body Is It Anyway? Justice and the Integrity of the Person*. Oxford: Oxford University Press.

Faden, R. and Beauchamp, T. (1986). *A History and Theory of Informed Consent*. Oxford: Oxford University Press.

Fairbairn, G. and Mead, D. (1990). Ethics and the loss of innocence. *Paediatric Nursing*, **2**(5), 22–3.

Faulder, C. (1985). *Whose Body Is It?* London: Virago.

Feinberg, J. (1970). *Doing and Deserving*. Princeton, NJ: Princeton University Press.

Feinberg, J. (1996). *The Moral Limits of the Criminal Law. Volume III: Harm to Self*. New York, NY: Oxford University Press.

Feinstein, A. R. (1990). On white coat effects and the electronic monitoring of compliance. *Archives of Internal Medicine*, **150**, 1377–8.

Finnish Act on the Status and Right of the Patient (1992). (Statute no.785, enacted 1993.)

Flanagan, O. and Rorty, A. (ed.) (1990). *Identity, Character, and Morality: Essays in Moral Psychology*. Cambridge, MA: MIT Press.

Flew, A. (1979). *A Dictionary of Philosophy*. London: Pan Macmillan.

Fogarty, M. (1998, October). Bring down that Berlin wall. Editorial in *Health and Aging*.

Forbes, K. (1998). Response to 'Euthanasia and the principle of justice'. In *Euthanasia and the Churches*, ed. R. Gill, pp. 98–103. London: Cassell.

Frankel, M. S. (2003). Inheritable genetic modification and a brave new world – did Huxley have it wrong? *Hastings Center Report*, **33**, 31–6.

Frankfurt, H. (1971). Freedom of the will and the concept of a person. *Journal of Philosophy*, **68**, 5–20.

Franklin, S. and Roberts, C. (2006). *Born and Made: An Ethnography of Preimplantation Genetic Diagnosis*. Princeton, NJ: Princeton University Press.

Franklyn, B. (1995). *The Handbook of Children's Rights*. London: Routledge.

French, P., Uehling, T. E. and Wettstein, H. K. (ed.) (1988). *Midwest Studies in Philosophy. Volume 13: Ethical Theory – Character and Virtue*. Notre Dame: University of Notre Dame Press.

Friedman Ross, I. (1999). *Children, Families and Healthcare Decision Making*. Oxford: Oxford University Press.

Fryer, D. (1994). Commentary on 'Community psychologists and politics' by David Smail. *Journal of Community and Applied Social Psychology*, **4**, 11–14.

Fulford, K. W. M. and Hope, T. (1994). Psychiatric ethics: a bioethical ugly duckling? In *Principles of Healthcare Ethics*, ed. R. Gillon. Chichester: Wiley.

Fulford, K. W. M. and Howse, K. (1993). Ethics of research with psychiatric patients: principles, problems and the primary responsibilities of researchers. *Journal of Medical Ethics*, **19**, 85–91.

Garfield, S. L. (1980). *Psychotherapy: An Eclectic Approach*. New York, NY: John Wiley.

Garrard, E. and Wilkinson, S. (2005). Passive euthanasia. *Journal of Medical Ethics*, **31**, 64–8.

Gastmans, C. and Milisen, K. (2006). Use of physical restraint in nursing homes: clinical–ethical considerations. *Journal of Medical Ethics*, **32**, 148–52.

Gater, R. and Goldberg, D. (1991). Pathways to psychiatric care in South Manchester. *British Journal of Psychiatry*, **159**, 90–6.

General Medical Council (1993). *Tomorrow's Doctors*. London: General Medical Council.

General Medical Council (1995). *Duties of a Doctor*. London: General Medical Council.

General Medical Council (2002). *Withholding and Withdrawing Life-prolonging Treatments: Good Practice in Decision-making*. London: General Medical Council.

General Medical Council (2007). *0–18 years: Guidance for all Doctors*. London: General Medical Council.

General Medical Council (2008). *Consent: Patients and Doctors Making Decisions Together*. London: General Medical Council.

General Medical Council (2009). *Confidentiality: Reporting Concerns about Patients to the DVLA or the DVA*. London: General Medical Council.

Gevers, S. (1995). Physician-assisted suicide: new developments in the Netherlands. *Bioethics*, **9**(3/4), 309–12.

Gillick v. *W. Norfolk and Wisbech AHA* (1985) 3 All ER 402.

Gilligan, C. (1982). *In a Different Voice: Psychological Theory and Women's Development.* Cambridge, MA: Harvard University Press.

Gillon, R. (1985). *Philosophical Medical Ethics.* New York, NY: John Wiley.

Gillon, R. (1997). Editorial: futility and medical ethics. *Journal of Medical Ethics*, **23**(6), 339–40.

Gillon, R. (2003). Ethics needs principles – four can encompass the rest – and respect for autonomy should be 'first among equals'. *Journal of Medical Ethics*, **29**, 307–12.

Gindro, S. (1994). Luci ed ombre sul progetto di uomo. In *L'Adolescenza: gli anni difficili*, ed. R. Bracalenti. Napoli: A. Guida Editore.

Global Forum for Health Research (2004). *10/90 Report on Health Research 2003–2004.* Geneva: Global Forum for Health Research.

Global Forum for Health Research (2008). *Equitable Access: Research Challenges for Health in Developing Countries.* Geneva: Global Forum for Health Research.

Glover, J. (1977). *Causing Death and Saving Lives.* Harmondsworth: Penguin.

Glover, J. (2005). *Choosing Children: The Ethical Dilemmas of Genetic Intervention.* Oxford: Oxford University Press.

Goodwin, M. (2006). *Black Markets: The Supply and Demand of Body Parts.* Cambridge: Cambridge University Press.

Goudriaan, R. (1984). *Collectieve uitgaven en demografische ontwikkeling 1970–2030.* Rijswijk: Sociaal en Cultureel Planbureau.

Graham, P. (1981). Ethics and child psychiatry. In *Psychiatric Ethics*, ed. S. Bloch and P. Chodoff, pp. 235–54. Oxford: Oxford University Press.

Greely, H. and King, M. C. (1999). *Letter to the government of Iceland.* www.mannvernd.is (Accessed 14 May 1999.)

Greenwood, B. (2009). Bang for the buck: what purchasers and commissioners think and do. In *Reproductive Ageing*, ed. S. Bewley, W. Ledger and D. Nikolaou, pp. 303–13. London: Royal College of Obstetricians and Gynaecologists Press.

Gremmen, I., Widdershoven, G., Beekman, A., Zuijderhoudt, R. and Sevenhuijsen, S. (2008). Ulysses arrangements in psychiatry: a matter of good care? *Journal of Medical Ethics*, **34**, 77–80.

Griffiths, J. (1995). Assisted suicide in the Netherlands: the Chabot case. *The Modern Law Review*, **58**, 232–48.

Griffiths, J., Blood, A. and Weyers, H. (1998). *Euthanasia and Law in the Netherlands.* Amsterdam: Amsterdam University Press.

Grodin, M. and Glantz, L. (ed.). (1994). *Children as Research Subjects: Science, Ethics and Law.* New York, NY: Oxford University Press.

Groenewoud, J. H., Van der Maas, P. J. and Van der Wal, G. (1997). Physician-assisted death in psychiatric practice in the Netherlands. *New England Journal of Medicine*, **336**(25), 1795–801.

Grubb, A. (1996). Commentary on *Re Y. Medical Law Review*, 204–7.

Grubb, A. (1998). Who decides? Legislating for the incapacitated adult. *European Journal of Health Law*, **5**, 231–40.

Gunn, M. (2009). Hospital treatment for incapacitated adults. *Medical Law Review*, **17**(2), 274–81.

Guttmacher, L. B. and Create, P. (1988). Electroconvulsive therapy in one child and three adolescents. *Journal of Clinical Psychiatry*, **49**(1), 20–3.

Haan, M., Rice, D., Satariano, W. and Selby, J. (ed.) (1991). Living longer and doing worse? Present and future trends in the health of the elderly. *Journal of Ageing and Health*, 3(Special Issue), 133–307.

Habermas, J. (1980). *Theorie des kommunikativen Handelns.* Frankfurt am Main: Suhrkamp.

Habermas, J. (1993). *Justification and Application: Remarks on Discourse Ethics.* Oxford: Polity.

Hagestad, O. (1991). The ageing society as a context of family life. In *Ageing and Ethics*, ed. N. Jecker, pp. 123–46. Clifton, NJ: Humana Press.

Hagger, L. (1997). The role of the Human Fertilisation and Embryology Authority. *Medical Law International*, **3**(1), 1–22.

Halliday, R. (1997). Medical futility and the social context. *Journal of Medical Ethics*, **23**, 148–53.

Hamm, D. (2007). Divorced couple battle for "custody" of their frozen embryos. *Bionews*, **410**, 5 June.

Hammon, K. R. (1998). Multifetal pregnancy reduction. *Journal of Obstetric, Gynecological and Neonatal Nursing*, **27**(3), 338–9.

Hanks, G. W. and Twycross, R. G. 1984. Letter: Pain, the physiological antagonist of opioid analgesics. *Lancet*, 30 June, 1477–8.

Hannuniemi, A. (1996). *The status of minors in healthcare and social care in Finland.* Paper presented at Seminar in Medicine and Law, University of Tartu, Estonia, 6–7 December.

Harre, R. and Gillett, G. (1994). *The Discursive Mind.* London: Sage.

Harris, J. (1982). The political status of children. In *Contemporary Political Philosophy*, ed. K. Graham. Cambridge: Cambridge University Press.

Harris, J. (1985). *The Value of Life: an Introduction to Medical Ethics.* London: Routledge and Kegan Paul.

Harris, J. (1987). QALYfying the value of life. *Journal of Medical Ethics*, **13**, 117–23.

Harris, J. (1993). *Wonderwoman and Superman: The Ethics of Human Biotechnology*. Oxford: Oxford University Press.

Harris, J. (1999a). *Embryonic Stem Cell Research*. Paper given at the Conference on Ethics and the Transformation of Medicine, University College, Oxford, 17–18 September.

Harris, J. (1999b). *Stem Cells and Genetic Manipulation*. Paper delivered at the Conference on Ethics and the Transformation of Medicine, University College, Oxford, 17–18 September.

Harris, J. (2003). Consent and end of life decisions. *Journal of Medical Ethics*, **29**, 10–15.

Harris, J. (2005). Scientific research is a moral duty. *Journal of Medical Ethics*, **31**, 242–8.

Harris, J. (2007). *Enhancing Evolution: The Ethical Case for Making Better People*. Princeton, NJ: Princeton University Press.

Harris, J. and Erin, C. (2002). An ethically defensible market in human organs. *British Medical Journal*, **323**, 114–15.

Harrison, C., Kenny, N. P., Sidarous, M. and Rowell, M. (1997). Bioethics for clinicians: involving children in medical decisions. *Canadian Medical Association Journal*, **156**, 825–8.

Hartogh, G. den (1994). Leeftijdsdiscriminatie bestaat dat? Over leeftijdsgrenzen in de gezondheidszorg. *Tijdschrift voor Gezondheidsrecht*, **3**, 134–49.

Hartouni, V. (1997). *Cultural Conceptions: On Reproductive Technologies and the Remaking of Life*. Minneapolis, MN: University of Minnesota.

Hattab, J. Y. (1996). Ethical issues in child psychiatry and psychotherapy: conflicts between children, families and practitioners. Paper presented at the First European Biomedical Ethics Practitioner Education (EBEPE) Workshop, Rome, 25 May.

Hawks, D. (1994). Commentary on 'Community psychology and politics'. *Journal of Community and Applied Social Psychology*, **4**, 27–8.

Hawton, K., Fagg, J., Simkin, S., Bale, E. and Bond, A. (1997). Trends in deliberate self-harm in Oxford, 1985–1995: implications for clinical services and the prevention of suicide. *British Journal of Psychiatry*, **171**, 556–60.

Hawton, K., Zahl, D. and Weatherall, R. (2003). Suicide following deliberate self-harm: long-term follow-up of patients who presented to a general hospital. *British Journal of Psychiatry*, **182**, 537–42.

Healy, K. (2006). *Last Best Gifts: Altruism and the Market for Human Organs*. Chicago, IL: University of Chicago Press.

Helfgott, A. W., Taylor-Burton, J., Garcini, F. J. *et al.* (1998). Compliance with universal precautions: knowledge and behavior of residents and students in a Department of Obstetrics and Gynecology. *Infectious Diseases in Obstetrics and Gynecology*, **6**, 123–8.

Heller, J-M. (1997). La defense des mineurs en justice, approche ethicojuridique. Paper presented at the Twelfth European Biomedical Ethics Practitioner Education (EBEPE) Workshop, Rome, October.

Hendin, H. (1995). Assisted suicide, euthanasia, and suicide prevention: the implications of the Dutch experience. *Suicide and Life-Threatening Behavior*, **25**, 193–204.

Herring, J. (2008) *Medical Law and Ethics*, 2nd edn. Oxford: Oxford University Press.

Hewitt, D. (2004). Assisting self-harm: some legal considerations. In *New Approaches to Preventing Suicide: A Manual for Practitioners*, ed. D. Duffy and T. Ryan, pp. 148–66. London: Jessica Kingsley Publishers.

Hilberman, M., Kutner, J., Parsons, D. and Murphy, D. J. (1997). Marginally effective medical care: ethical analysis of issues in cardiopulmonary resuscitation. *Journal of Medical Ethics*, **23**, 361–7.

Hillier, S. G. (2009). The science of ovarian ageing: how might knowledge be translated into practice? In *Reproductive Ageing*, ed. S. Bewley, W. Ledger and D. Nikolaou, pp. 75–88. London: Royal College of Obstetricians and Gynaecologists Press.

Hirschmann, N. J. (2003). *The Subject of Liberty: Toward a Feminist Theory of Freedom*. Princeton, NJ: Princeton University Press.

HL v *UK* 45508/99 [2004] ECHR 471.

Hollander, C. F. and Becker, H. A. (eds) (1987). *Growing Old in the Future. Scenarios on Health and Ageing 1984–2000*. Dordrecht: Nijhoff.

Holm, S. (2008). Pharmacogenetics, race and global injustice. *Developing World Bioethics*, **8**(2), 82–8.

Holmes, J. and Lindley, R. (1991). *The Values of Psychotherapy*. Oxford: Oxford University Press.

Holt, J. (1974). *Escape from Childhood*. Harmondsworth: Penguin.

Hope, R. A. (1996). Paper delivered at the Fourth European Biomedical Ethics Practitioner Education (EBEPE) Workshop, Maastricht.

Hope, R. A. (1997). Restraints and the elderly: abuse, enforcement and aggression. Paper presented at the Tenth European Biomedical Ethics Practitioner Education (EBEPE) Workshop, Maastricht, May.

Hope, T. (1995). Editorial: Evidence-based medicine and ethics. *Journal of Medical Ethics* **21**, 259–60.

Hope, T. and Oppenheimer, C. (1996). Ethics and the psychiatry of old-age. In *The Oxford Textbook of Old Age Psychiatry*, ed. R. Jacoby and C. Oppenheimer. Oxford: Oxford University Press.

Hope, T., Lockwood, G. and Lockwood, M. (1995). The interests of the potential child. *British Medical Journal*, **310**, 1455–7.

House of Lords Select Committee (1994). *Report of the Select Committee on Medical Ethics, HL Paper 21*. London: HMSO.

Human, D. and Fluss, S. S. (2001). *The World Medical Association's Declaration of Helsinki: Historical and Contemporary Perspectives*. www.wma.net/ethicsunit/pdf/bibliography.pdf.

Human Genetics Commission (2002). *Inside Information: Balancing Interests in the Use of Personal Genetic Data*. London: Human Genetics Commission.

Human Genome Organization Ethics Committee (1996). Statement on the principled conduct of genetic research. *Genome Digest*, May, 2–3.

Hurka, T. (1992). Virtue as loving the good. In *The Good Life and the Human Good*, ed. E. F. Paul, F. D. Miller and J. Paul. Cambridge: Cambridge University Press.

Hursthouse, R. (1995). Applying virtue ethics. In *Virtues and Reasons: Philippa Foot and Moral Theory – Essays in Honour of Philippa Foot*, ed. R. Hursthouse, G. Lawrence and W. Quinn, pp. 57–75. Oxford: Clarendon Press.

Husak, D. N. (1992). *Drugs and Rights*. Cambridge: Cambridge University Press.

Hutson, S. and Liddiard, M. (1994). *Youth Homelessness: The Construction of a Social Issue*. London: Macmillan.

Huxtable, R. (2000). *Re M (Medical Treatment: Consent)*: Time to remove the 'flak jacket'? *Child and Family Law Quarterly*, 12(1), 83–8.

Huxtable, R. (2004). *Re C (A Child) (Immunisation: Parental Rights)* [2003] EWCA Civ 114. *Journal of Social Welfare and Family Law*, 26(1), 69–77.

Huxtable, R. (2007). *Euthanasia, Ethics and the Law: From Conflict to Compromise*. London: Routledge-Cavendish.

Huxtable, R. (2008). Whatever you want? Beyond the patient in medical law. *Health Care Analysis*, 16(3), 288–301.

Huxtable, R. (2009). The suicide tourist trap: compromise across boundaries. *Journal of Bioethical Inquiry* 6(3), 327–36.

Huxtable, R. and Forbes, K. (2004). Glass *v* UK: maternal instinct vs. medical opinion. *Child and Family Law Quarterly*, 16(3), 339–54.

Huxtable, R. and Möller, M. (2007). "Setting a principled boundary"? Euthanasia as a response to 'life fatigue'. *Bioethics*, 21(3), 117–26.

Ibsen, H. (1992). *A Doll's House*. New York, NY: Dover Publications.

Iglesias, T. (1990). *IFV and Justice: Moral, Social and Legal Issues Related to Human In Vitro Fertilisation*. London: The Linacre Centre.

Jahnigen, D. and Binstock, R. H. (1991). Economic and clinical realities: healthcare for elderly people. In *Too Old for Health Care? Controversies in Medicine, Law, Economics and Ethics*, ed. R. H. Binstock and S. G. Post, pp. 13–43. Baltimore, MD: Johns Hopkins University Press.

Jansen, L. A. and Sulmasy, D. P. (2002). Sedation, alimentation, hydration, and equivocation: careful conversations about care at the end of life. *Annals of Internal Medicine*, 136, 845–9.

Janssen, A. (2002). The new regulation of voluntary euthanasia and medically assisted suicide in the Netherlands. *International Journal of Law, Policy and the Family*, 16, 260–9.

Jinnet-Sack, S. (1993). Autonomy in the company of others. In *Choices and Decisions in Healthcare*, ed. A. Grubb, pp. 97–136. Chichester: John Wiley.

Jones, J. (1994). *Young People in and out of the Housing Market*. Working Papers 1–5. Edinburgh: Centre for Educational Sociology at the University of Edinburgh and Scottish Council for the Single Homeless.

Jonsen, A. R., Veatch, R. and Walters, L. (ed.) (1998). *Source Book in Bioethics*, pp. 1–5. Washington, DC: Georgetown University Press.

Josselson, R. (1988). The embedded self – I and thou revisited. In *Self, Ego and Identity: Integrative Approaches*, ed. D. K. Lapsley and F. Clark Power, pp. 91–106. New York, NY: Springer Verlag.

Jouvenel, H. de (1989). *Europe's Ageing Population. Trends and Challenges to 2025*. Guildford: Butterworths.

Jungers, P., Forget, D., Henry-Amar, M. *et al.* (1986). Chronic kidney disease and pregnancy. In *Advances in Nephrology Year Book*, ed. J. Grunfeld, M. Maxwell, J. Bach *et al.*, Vol. 15, pp. 103–41. Linn, MO: Mosby Inc.

Kaimowitz v Michigan Department of Mental Health [1973] 42 USLW 2063.

Kaivosoja, M. (1996). Compelled to help: a study of the impact of the Mental Health Act on coercive treatment of minors, 1991–1993 (in Finnish). *Sosiaali-ja terveysministerion julkaisuja, 2*. Helsinki.

Kane, R. and Caplan, A. (1990). *Everyday Ethics*. New York, NY: Springer.

Kant, I. (1909). Foundations of the metaphysics of morals. In *Kant's Critique of Practical Reason and other Works on the Theory of Ethics, 6th edn*, trans. T. K. Abbott. London: Longmans Green.

Kant, I. (1956). *Critique of Pure Reason*, trans. L. W. Beck. Indianapolis, IN: Bobbs–Merrill.

Kant, I. (1998). *Groundwork of the Metaphysics of Morals*, ed. M. Gregor. Cambridge: Cambridge University Press.

Kaplan, D. (1994). Prenatal screening and diagnosis: the impact on persons with disabilities. In *Women and Prenatal Testing: Facing the Challenges of Genetic Technology*, ed. K. L. Rothenberg and E. J. Thomson, pp. 49–61. Columbus, OH: State University Press.

Kazdin, A. E. (1988). *Child Psychotherapy: Developing and Identifying Effective Treatments.* New York, NY: Pergamon.

Kazdin, A. E. (1994). Psychotherapy for children and adolescents. In *Handbook of Psychotherapy and Behaviour Change,* 4th edn, ed. A. E. Bergin and S. L. Garfield, New York, NY: John Wiley.

Keenan, K. and Shaw, D. (1997). Developmental and social influences on young girls' early problem behaviour. *Psychological Bulletin,* **121**, 95–113.

Kennedy, I. and Grubb, A. (1994). *Medical Law: Text with Materials,* 2nd edn. Guildford: Butterworths.

Kennedy, I. and Grubb A. (1998). Research and experimentation. In *Principles of Medical Law,* pp. 714–46. Oxford: Oxford University Press.

Keown, J. (1997). *Comments on Berghmans* given at the Seventh European Biomedical Ethics Practitioner Education (EBEPE) Workshop, Maastricht, 21–22 March.

Keown, J. (2002). *Euthanasia, Ethics and Public Policy: An Argument against Legalisation.* Cambridge: Cambridge University Press.

Kiloh, L. G. (1983). Non-pharmacological biological treatments of psychiatric patients. *Australian and New Zealand Journal of Psychiatry,* **17**(3), 215–22.

Kirkevold, O. and Engedal, K. (2005). Concealment of drugs in food and beverages in nursing homes: cross-sectional study. *British Medical Journal,* **330**, 20.

Krugman, S., Giles, J. P. and Jacobs, A. M. (1960). Studies on an attenuated measles-virus vaccine. *New England Journal of Medicine,* **263**, 174–7.

Kruschwitz, R. and Roberts, R. C. (eds) (1987). *The Virtues: Contemporary Essays on Moral Character.* Belmont, CA: Wadsworth.

Kuhse, H. (1991). Euthanasia. In *Companion to Ethics,* ed. P. Singer. Oxford: Blackwell.

Kuhse, H. and Singer, P. (eds) (1998). *A Companion to Bioethics.* Oxford: Blackwell.

Kukathas, C. and Petit, P. (1990). *Rawls: A Theory of Justice and its Critics.* Cambridge: Polity.

L v. *Bournewood* (See *Regina* v. *Bournewood*).

Lahti, R. (1994). Towards a comprehensive legislation governing the rights of patients: the Finnish experience. In *Patient's Rights – Informed Consent, Access and Equality,* ed. L. Westerhall and C. Phillips. Stockholm: Nerenius and Santerus Publishers.

Lahti, R. (1996). *The Finnish Act on the Status and Rights of Patients.* Paper presented at the Sixth European Biomedical Ethics Practitioner Education (EBEPE) Workshop, Naantali, Finland, September.

Lamb, D. (1998). *Down the Slippery Slope: Arguing in Applied Ethics.* London: Croom Helm.

Latham, M. (1998). Regulating the new reproductive technologies: a cross-Channel comparison. *Medical Law International,* **3**(2, 3), 89–116.

Launis, V. (1996). Moral issues concerning children's legal status in Finland in relation to psychiatric treatment. Paper presented at the First European Biomedical Ethics Practitioner Education (EBEPE) Workshop, Rome, 25 May.

Laurie, G. (2004). *(Intellectual) Property: Let's think about Staking a Claim to our own Research Samples.* Edinburgh: Arts and Humanities Research Board Centre, University of Edinburgh.

Lebeer, G. (1998). Name of paper presented at the Second UNESCO Conference on Medical Ethics and Medical Law, Copenhagen, June.

Ledger, W. (2006). The burden of multiple pregnancies after IVF treatment. *Bionews,* 5 June.

Lee, R. G. and Morgan, D. (2001). *Human Fertilisation and Embryology: Regulating the Reproductive Revolution.* London: Blackstone Press.

Leenen, H. J. J. (1988). *Handboek gezondheidsrecht. Rechten van mensen in de gezondheidszorg.* [Handbook healthcare law. Rights of people in health care]. Alphen aan den Rijn: Samsom.

Leenen, H. J. J. (1994). Dutch Supreme Court about assistance to suicide in the case of severe mental suffering. *European Journal of Health Law,* **1**, 377–9.

Levacic, R. (1991). Markets: an introduction. In *Markets, Hierarchies and Networks: The Co-ordination of Social Life,* ed. G. Thompson, J. Frances, R. Levacic and J. Mitchell, pp. 21–3. London: Sage.

Levitt, M. and Weldon, S. (2005). A well placed trust? Public perceptions of the governance of genetic databases. *Critical Public Health,* **15**, 311–21.

Lewis, P. (2007). *Assisted Dying and Legal Change.* Oxford: Oxford University Press.

Lewontin R. C. (1999). A human population for sale. *New York Times,* 23 January.

Lexchin, J., Bero, L. A., Djulbegovic, B. and Clark, O. (2003). Pharmaceutical industry sponsorship and research outcome and quality: systematic review. *British Medical Journal,* **326**, 1167–70.

Lindemann Nelson, H. and Lindemann Nelson, J. (1995). *The Patient in the Family.* London: Routledge.

Lindheimer, M. D. and Katz, A. I. (1992). Pregnancy in the renal transplant patient. *American Journal of Kidney Disease,* **19**, 173.

Lippman, A. (1992), Mother matters: a fresh look at prenatal genetic screening. *Issues in Reproductive and Genetic Engineering,* **5**, 141–54.

Lloyd, G. (1993). *The Man of Reason: 'Male and Female' in Western Philosophy,* 2nd edn. London: Routledge.

Lockwood, G. M. (2000) A case study in IVF: problems of paternalism and autonomy in a 'high-risk pregnancy'. In *Ethical Issues in Maternal–Fetal Medicine*, ed. D. L. Dickenson, pp. 161–6. Cambridge: Cambridge University Press.

Lockwood, G. M., Ledger, W. L. and Barlow, D. H. (1995). Successful pregnancy outcome in a renal transplant patient following in-vitro fertilization. *Human Reproduction*, **10**, 1528–30.

Lopez, I. (1998). An ethnography of the medicalization of Puerto Rican women's reproduction. In *Pragmatic Women and Body Politics*, ed. M. Lock and P. Kaufert. Cambridge: Cambridge University Press.

Lucassen, A. (2007). 'Should families own genetic information? Yes'. *British Medical Journal*, **335**, 22–3.

Lurie, P., and Wolfe, S. (1997). Unethical trials of interventions to reduce perinatal transmission of the human immunodeficiency virus in developing countries. *New England Journal of Medicine*, **337**, 853–6.

Lutzen, K. and Nordin, C. (1994). Modifying autonomy: a concept grounded in nurses' experience of moral decision making in psychiatric practice. *Journal of Medical Ethics*, **20**, 101–7.

MacIntyre, A. (1981). *After Virtue: A Study in Moral Theory*, pp. 190–203. Notre Dame: University of Notre Dame Press.

MacIntyre, A. (1984). *After Virtue: A Study in Moral Theory*, 2nd edn. Notre Dame: University of Notre Dame Press.

MacIntyre, A. (1997). *A Short History of Ethics*. London: Routledge.

MacLean, A. (2008). Keyholders and flak jackets: the method in the madness of mixed metaphors. *Clinical Ethics*, **3**, 121–6.

Macklin, R. (1994). *Surrogates and Other Mothers: The Debates over Assisted Reproduction*. Philadelphia, PA: Temple University Press.

Macklin, R. (2004). *Double Standards in Medical Research in Developing Countries*. Cambridge: Cambridge Univeresity Press.

Magno, G. (1996). The rights of minors in international conventions. Paper presented at the First European Biomedical Ethics Practitioner Education (EBEPE) Workshop, Rome, 25 May.

Makanjuola, J. D. and Oyerogba, K. O. (1987). Management of depressive illness in a Nigerian neuropsychiatric hospital. *Acta Psychiatrica Scandinavia*, **76**(5), 486–9.

Manninen, B. A. (2006). A case for justified non-voluntary active euthanasia: exploring the ethics of the Groningen Protocol. *Journal of Medical Ethics*, **32**, 643–51.

Mannvernd (1999). *Icelanders for Ethics in Science and Medicine*. www.mannvernd.is (Accessed 14 May 1999.)

Marrs, R. P. (ed.) (1993). *Assisted Reproductive Technologies*. Oxford: Blackwell Scientific Publications.

Marteau, T. and Richards, M. (1996). *The Troubled Helix: Social and Psychological Implications of the New Human Genetics*. Cambridge: Cambridge University Press.

Matthiasson, A-C., and Hemberg, M. (1997). Intimacy: meeting needs and respecting privacy. Paper presented at the Tenth European Biomedical Ethics Practitioner Education (EBEPE) Workshop, Maastricht, May.

Mause, de L. (1995). *The History of Childhood*. New York, NY: Jason Aronson Publishers.

Mawby, R. I. and Walklate, S. (1994). *Critical Victimology: International Perspectives*. London: Sage.

McGoey, L. and Jackson, E. (2009). Seroxat and the suppression of clinical trial data: regulatory failure and the uses of legal ambiguity. *Journal of Medical Ethics*, **35**, 107–12.

McKie, J., Singer, P., Kuhse, H. and Richardson, J. (1998). *The Allocation of Healthcare Resources*. Brookfield, VT: Dartmouth Publishing Co.

McNeil, P. (1992). *The Ethics and Politics of Human Experimentation*. Cambridge: Cambridge University Press.

Medical Ethics Advisor (1993). 9(12), December.

Mendus, S. (1992). Strangers and brothers: liberalism, socialism and the concept of autonomy. In *Liberalism, Citizenship and Autonomy*, ed. D. Milligan and W. Watts-Miller. Aldershot: Avebury.

Merck's Manual of the Materia Medica (1899). New York, NY: Merck and Co. Reprinted in *The Merck Manual* (1999). New Jersey: Merck Research Laboratories.

Meulen, R. H. J. ter (1995a). Solidarity with the elderly and the allocation of resources. In *A World Growing Old. The Coming Healthcare Challenges*, ed. D. Callahan, R. H. J. ter Meulen and E. Topinkova, pp. 73–84. Washington, DC: Georgetown University Press.

Meulen, R. H. J. ter (1995b). Limiting solidarity in the Netherlands. A two-tier system under way? *Journal of Medicine and Philosophy*, **20**, 607–16.

Meulen, R. H. J. ter (1996). Care for dependent elderly persons and respect for autonomy. Paper presented at the Fifth European Biomedical Ethics Practitioner Education (EBEPE) Workshop, Maastricht, the Netherlands, June.

Mgbeoji, I. (2007). *Talking Past each Other: Genetic Testing and Indigenous Populations*. American Institute of Biological Sciences. www.ActionBioscience.org (Accessed 1 February 2008.)

Michalowski, S. (2003). *Medical Confidentiality and Crime*. Aldershot: Ashgate.

Midgley, M. (1991). Rights talk will not sort out child abuse. *Journal of Applied Philosophy*, **8** (1), 103–14.

Mill, J. S. (1993). *Utilitarianism, On Liberty, Considerations on Representative Government*. London: Everyman.

Miller, D. L. (1986). Justice. In *The Blackwell Encyclopaedia of Political Thought*, ed. D. Miller, J. Coleman and A. Ryan, pp. 260–3. Oxford: Basil Blackwell.

Miller, R. (1991). The ethics of involuntary commitment to mental health treatment. In *Psychiatric Ethics, 2nd edn*, ed. S. Bloch and P. Chodoff, pp. 265–89. Oxford: Oxford University Press.

Miller, R. B. (2003). *Children, Ethics and Modern Medicine*. Bloomington, IN: Indiana University Press.

Ministry of Health (Iceland) (1998a). *Bill on a Health Sector Database*. Reykjavik: Ministry of Health.

Ministry of Health (Iceland) (1998b). *Act on a Health Sector Database*. Reykjavik: Ministry of Health (No. 139/1998).

Mircea, E. (1979). *Histoire de croyances et des idžes religieuses*. Paris: Payot.

Mitchell, G R. and Happe, K. (2005). Defining the subject of consent in DNA research. *Journal of Medical Humanities*, **21**, 41–53.

Mitchell, J. J., Capua, A., Clow, C. and Scriver, C. R. (1996). Twenty-year outcome analysis of genetic screening programs for Tay Sachs and beta-thalassemia disease carriers in high schools. *American Journal of Human Genetics*, **39**, 793–8.

Moazam, F., Zaman, R. M. and Jafarey, A. (2009). Conversations with kidney vendors in Pakistan: an ethnographic study. *Hastings Center Report* **39**, 793–8.

Mohr v. *Williams*, 104 N.W. 12, 15–16 (Minn., 1905).

Momeyer, R. (1995). Does physician-assisted suicide violate the integrity of medicine? *Journal of Medicine and Philosophy*, **20**, 13–24.

Montgomery, J. (1997). *Health Care Law*. Oxford: Oxford University Press.

Mordini, E. (1997). Mandatory hospitalisation in mental health. Paper presented at the AGM of the European Association of Centres of Medical Ethics, Coimbra, 25 October.

Mullen, P. E. (1990). The long-term influence of childhood sexual abuse in the mental health of victims. *Journal of Forensic Psychiatry*, **1**, 13–14.

Mullen, P. M. (1991). Which internal market? The NHS White Paper and internal markets. In *Markets, Hierarchies and Networks: The Co-ordination of Social Life*, ed. G. Thompson, J. Frances, R. Levacic and J. Mitchell, pp. 21–30. London: Sage.

Muller, M. (1996). *Death on Request. Aspects of Euthanasia and Physician-assisted Suicide with Special Regard to Dutch Nursing Homes*. Amsterdam: Thesis Publishers.

Murch, S. (2003). Correspondence: separating inflammation from speculation in autism. *Lancet*, **362**, 1498–9.

Murray, J. E., Reid, D. E., Harrison, J. H. *et al.* (1963). Successful pregnancies after human renal transplantation. *New England Journal of Medicine*, **269**, 341–3.

Murray, T. (1996). *The Worth of a Child*. Berkeley, CA: University of California Press.

Naaborg, J. (1991). *Benodigde en beschikbare middelen, een groeiend porbleem voor de zorgverlening*. Rapport in opdracht voor de Commissie Keuzen in de Zorg. Hoek van Holland.

Nagel, T. (1986). *The View from Nowhere*. Oxford: Oxford University Press.

Nelkin, D. (1994). *Dangerous Diagnostics: The Social Power of Biological Information*. Chicago, IL: University of Chicago Press.

Nelkin, D. and Lindee, M. S. (1995). *The DNA Mystique: The Gene as a Cultural Icon*. New York, NY: W. H. Freeman.

Nelson, R. M. (1997). Ethics in the intensive care unit: creating an ethical environment. *Critical Care Clinics*, **3**, 691–701.

Neuberger, J. (1992). *Ethics and Healthcare: The Role of Research Ethics Committees in the UK*. London: King's Fund.

Niakas, D. (1997). Commentary on the case of Mr K. Paper submitted to the Ninth European Biomedical Ethics Practitioner Education (EBEPE) Workshop, Maastricht, April.

Noddings, N. (1984). *Caring: a Feminine Approach to Ethics and Moral Education*. Berkeley: University of California Press.

Noll, P. (1989). *In the Face of Death*. London: Viking Penguin.

Nuffield Council on Bioethics (2001). *Consultation on Behavioural Genetics*. London: Nuffield Council on Bioethics.

Nuffield Council on Bioethics (2005). *The Ethics of Research Related to Healthcare in Developing Countries – A Follow-Up Discussion Paper*. London: Nuffield Council on Bioethics.

Nuffield Council on Bioethics (2009). *Dementia: Ethical Issues*. London: Nuffield Council on Bioethics.

Nuremberg Code (1947). In: G. J. Annas, and M. A. Grodin (eds.) (1992) *The Nazi Doctors and the Nuremberg Code*, New York, NY: Oxford University Press.

Nys, H. (1999). Physician involvement in a patient's death: a continental perspective. *Medical Law Review*, **7**, 208–46.

O'Neill, O. (1996). *Towards Justice and Virtue: A Constructive Account of Practical Reasoning*. Cambridge: Cambridge University Press.

O'Neill, O. (2002). *Autonomy and Trust in Bioethics*. Cambridge: Cambridge University Press.

O'Neill, O. and Ruddick, W. (eds) (1979). *Having Children: Philosophical and Legal Reflections on Parenthood.* Oxford: Oxford University Press.

Overall, C. (2000). New reproductive technologies and practices: benefits or liabilities for children? In *Ethical Issues in Maternal–Fetal Medicine,* ed. D. L. Dickenson. Cambridge: Cambridge University Press.

Panksepp, J., Fuchs, T., Garcia, V. A. and Lesiak, A. (2007). Does any aspect of mind survive brain damage that typically leads to a persistent vegetative state? Ethical considerations. *Philosophy, Ethics, and Humanities in Medicine,* **2**, 32.

Parfit, D. (1984). *Reasons and Persons.* Oxford: Clarendon Press.

Paris, J. and Reardon, P. (1992). Physician refusal of requests for futile or ineffective intervention. *Cambridge Quarterly of Healthcare Ethics,* **2**, 127–34.

Parker, G., Roy, K., Hadzi-Pavlovic, D. and Pedic, F. (1992). Psychotic (delusional). depression: a meta-analysis of physical treatments. *Journal of Affective Disorders,* **24**(1), 17–24.

Parker, M. (1995a). Children who run: ethics and homelessness. In *Introducing Applied Ethics,* ed. B. Almond, pp. 58–70. Oxford: Blackwell.

Parker, M. (1995b). *The Growth of Understanding.* Aldershot: Avebury.

Parker, M. (1996). *Communitarianism and its Problems.* Cogito, November.

Parker, M. (ed.) (1999). *Ethics and Community in the Healthcare Professions.* London: Routledge.

Parker, M. (2007a). Deliberative bioethics. In *Principles of Health Care Ethics,* ed. R. Ashcroft, A. Dawson, H. Draper and J. McMillan, pp. 185–91. Chichester: Wiley.

Parker, M. (2007b). The best possible child. *Journal of Medical Ethics,* **33**, 279–83.

Parker, M. and Lucassen, A. M. (2004). Genetic information – a joint account? *British Medical Journal,* **329**, 165–7.

Parker, M. G. (1997). Commentary on the case of Mr K. Paper submitted to the Ninth European Biomedical Ethics Practitioner Education (EBEPE) Workshop, Maastricht, April.

Pattison, S. (2001). Dealing with uncertainty. *British Medical Journal,* **323**, 840.

Paul, M. (1997). Children from the age of 5 should be presumed competent. *British Medical Journal,* **314** (7092), 1480.

Pearce, J. (1994). Consent to treatment during childhood: the assessment of competence and avoidance of conflict. *British Journal of Psychiatry,* **165**, 713–16.

Pearce, J. (1996). Ethical issues in child psychiatry and child psychotherapy: conflicts between the child, parents and

practitioners. Paper presented at the First European Biomedical Ethics Practitioner Education (EBEPE) Workshop, Rome, 25 May.

Pellegrino, E. D. (1992). Doctors must not kill. *Journal of Clinical Ethics,* **3**, 95.

Pellegrino, E. D. (1994). The four principles and the doctor–patient relationship: the need for a better linkage. In *Principles of Health Care Ethics,* ed. R. Gillon, pp. 353–65. Chichester: Wiley.

Pence, G. (1984). Recent work on the virtues. *American Philosophical Quarterly,* **21**, 281–97.

Pence, G. (1991). Virtue theory. In *A Companion to Ethics,* ed. P. Singer. Oxford: Blackwell.

Pennings, G. and de Vroey, M. (2006). Subsidized in-vitro fertilization and the effect on the number of egg sharers. *Reproductive Biomedicine Online,* **13**, 8–10.

Peonidis, F. (1996). A moral assessment of patients' rights in Greece. Paper presented at the Sixth European Biomedical Ethics Practitioner Education (EBEPE) Workshop, Naantali, Finland, September.

Perrett, R. W. (1996). Killing, letting die and the bare difference argument. *Bioethics,* **10**(2), 131–9.

Perry, J. E., Churchill, L. R. and Kirshner, H. S. (2005). The Terri Schiavo case: legal, ethical, and medical perspectives. *Annals of Internal Medicine,* **143**, 744–8.

Persaud, R. D. and Meus, C. (1994). The psychopathology of authority and its loss: the effect on a ward of losing a consultant psychiatrist. *British Journal of Medical Psychology,* **67**, 1–11.

Pincoffs, E. (1986). *Quandaries and Virtues.* Lawrence, KS: University Press of Kansas.

Polack, C. (2001). Is a tattoo the answer? *British Medical Journal,* **323**, 1063.

Psychiatric Bulletin (1990). *Guidelines for Research Ethics Committees on Psychiatric Research Involving Human Subjects.* London: Royal College of Psychiatrists.

Purdy, L. M. (1994). Why children shouldn't have equal rights. *International Journal of Children's Rights,* **2**, 223–41.

Pywell, S. (2001). Particular issues of public health: vaccination. In *Law and the Public Dimension of Health,* ed. R. Martin and L. Johnson, pp. 299–327. London: Cavendish.

R (Axon) v Secretary of State for Health [2006] EWHC 37.

R v Cambridge Health Authority, ex p. B [1995] 1 FLR 1055.

R. v Secretary of State for Social Services, ex parte Walker [1987] 3 BMLR 32.

R. v Secretary of State for Social Services, W. Midlands RHA and Birmingham AHA (Teaching), ex p. Hincks [1980] 1 BMLR 93.

Rachels, J. (1980). Active and passive euthanasia. In *Killing and Letting Die*, ed. B. Steinbock. Englewood Cliffs, NJ: Prentice-Hall.

Rachels, J. (1986). *The End of Life: Euthanasia and Morality*. Oxford: Oxford University Press.

Radcliffe Richards, J. (1998). The case for allowing kidney sales. *Lancet*, **352**, 143–67.

Rapp, R. (1998). Refusing prenatal diagnosis: the uneven meanings of bioscience in a multicultural world. In *Pragmatic Women and Body Politics*, ed. M. Lock and P. Kaufert, pp. 143–67. Cambridge: Cambridge University Press.

Rawls, J. (1971). *A Theory of Justice*. Oxford: Oxford University Press.

Raz, J. (1986). *The Morality of Freedom*. Oxford: Clarendon Press.

R (B) v *Ashworth Hospital Authority* [2005]. UKHL 20.

R (on the application of Burke) v *General Medical Council* [2005] 3 WLR 1132.

Re C [1994] 1 All ER 819 (FD).

Re C (A Child) (Immunisation: Parental Rights) [2003] EWCA Civ 1148.

Re E [1993] 1 FLR 386.

Re MB [1997] 2 FCR 541.

Re R [1991] 4 All ER 177.

Re R [1996] 2 FLR 99.

Re T [1992] 4 All ER 649.

Re W [1992] 4 All ER 627.

Re Y [1996] 2 FLR 787.

Re Y [1997] 2 WLR 556 (Connell J).

Re v *Bournewood Community and Mental Health NHS Trust, Ex parte L*, 2 WLR 764, opinions in the House of Lords delivered 25 June 1998.

Reich, W. (1998). Psychiatric diagnosis as an ethical problem. In *Psychiatric Ethics*, 3rd edn, ed. S. Bloch and P. Chodoff. Oxford: Oxford University Press.

Reiser, S. J., Dyck, A. J. and Curran, W. J. (ed.) (1977). Pope Pious XII. The prolongation of life. In *Ethics in Medicine – Historical Perspectives and Contemporary Concerns*, pp. 501–4. Cambridge, MA: MIT Press.

Robertson, D. W. (1996). Ethical theory, ethnography and differences between doctors and nurses in approaches to patient care. *Journal of Medical Ethics*, **22**, 292–9.

Robertson, J. (2003). The $1000 genome: ethical and legal issues in whole-genome sequencing of individuals. *American Journal of Bioethics*, **3**(3), W35–42.

Robertson, J. A. (1994). *Children of Choice: Freedom and the New Reproductive Technologies*. Princeton, NJ: Princeton University Press.

Robine, J-M. and Colvez, A. (1991). Quelle espérance pour la vie? *Futuribles*, **155**, 72–6.

Rodota, S. (1996). *Tecnolgie e Diritti*. Bologna, 11 Mulino.

Rodham, K., Hawton, K. and Evans, E. (2004) Reasons for deliberate self-harm: comparison of self-poisoners and self-cutters in a community sample of adolescents. *Journal of the American Academy of Child & Adolescent Psychiatry*, **43**(1), 80–7.

Rogers, W. (2002). Is there a tension between doctors' duty of care and evidence-based medicine? *Health Care Analysis*, **10**, 277–87.

Rose, H. (2001). Gendered genetics in Iceland. *New Genomics and Society*, **20**, 119–38.

Roth, L. H., Meisel, A. and Lidz, C. W. (1977). Tests of competence to consent to treatment, *American Journal of Psychiatry*, **134**(4), 279–84.

Rowland, R. (1992). *Living Laboratories: Women and Reproductive Technologies*. Bloomington, IN: University of Indiana Press.

Rowland, D. and Pollock, A. (2004). Editorial: Choice and responsiveness for older people in the 'patient centred' NHS. *British Medical Journal*, **328**, 4–5.

Royal College of Nursing (2008). *"Let's Talk about Restraint": Rights, Risks and Responsibility*. London: Royal College of Nursing

Royal College of Paediatrics and Child Health (1997). *A Framework for Practice in Relation to the Withholding and Withdrawing of Life-saving Treatment in Children*. Report of the Ethics Advisory Committee. London: Royal College of Paediatrics and Child Health edition.

Royal College of Paediatrics and Child Health (2004). *Withholding or Withdrawing Life-Saving Treatment in Children: A Framework for Practice*. London: Royal College of Paediatrics and Child Health.

Royal College of Physicians (1990). *Research Involving Patients*. London: Royal College of Physicians of London.

Royal Commission on New Reproductive Technologies (1993). *Proceed with Care: The Final Report of the Royal Commission on New Reproductive Technologies*, 2 vols. Ottawa, ON: Ministry of Supply and Services.

S v. *S, W* v. *Official Solicitor (or W)* (1972). AC 24, (1970). 3 All ER 107.

S v *S; W* v *Official Solicitor* [1970] 3 All ER 107.

Sacks, O. (1992). Tourette's syndrome and creativity. *British Medical Journal*, **305**, 1515–16.

Salles, A. L. F. (2004). Bioethics, difference and rights. In *Linking Visions: Feminist Bioethics, Human Rights and the Developing World*., ed. R. Tong, A. Donchin and S. Dodds, pp. 57–72. Lanham, MD: Rowman & Littlefield.

Sammet, K. (2007). Autonomy or protection from harm? Judgements of German course on care for the elderly in nursing homes. *Journal of Medical Ethics*, **33**, 534–7.

Sandel, M. (1982). *Liberalism and the Limits of Justice*. Cambridge: Cambridge University Press.

Savulescu, J. (2003). Is the sale of body parts wrong? *Journal of Medical Ethics*, **16**, 117–19.

Savulescu, J. (2007). In defence of procreative beneficence. *Journal of Medical Ethics*, **33**, 284–8.

Savulescu, J. and Dickenson, D. (1998). The time frames of preferences, dispositions, and the validity of advance directives for the mentally ill. *Philosophy, Psychiatry and Psychology*, **5**, 225–46.

Scarre, G. (ed.) (1989). *Children, Parents and Politics*. Cambridge: Cambridge University Press.

Schaefer, C. E., Briesmeister, J. M. and Fitton, M. E. (ed.) (1984). *Family Therapy Techniques for Problem Behaviours of Children and Teenagers*. San Francisco, CA: Jossey-Bass.

Scheper-Hughes, N. (2002). The global trade in human organs. In *The Anthropology of Globalization: A Reader*, ed. J. X. Inda and R. Rosaldo. Oxford: Blackwell.

Schmidt, U. and Frewer, A. (ed.) (2007). *History and Theory of Human Experimentation: The Declaration of Helsinki and Modern Medical Ethics*. Stuttgart: Franz Steiner.

Schuklenk, U. and Pacholczyk, A. (2009). Editorial: Dignity's woolly uplift. *Bioethics*, **24**, ii–iii.

Schwartz, S. (1991). Clinical decision-making. In *Handbook of Behaviour Therapy and Psychological Science: An Integrative Approach*, ed. P. R. Martin. New York, NY: Pergamon.

Scitovsky, A. A. (1984). The high cost of dying: what do the data show? *The Milbank Quarterly*, **62**, 591–608.

Scitovsky, A. A. (1988). Medical care in the last twelve months of life: the relation between age, functional status and medical expenditures. *The Milbank Quarterly*, **66**, 640–60.

Scitovsky, A. A. and Capron, A. M. (1986). Medical care at the end of life: the interaction of economics and ethics, *Annual Review of Public Health*, **7**, 59–78.

Scully, J. L., Porz, R. and Rehman-Sutter, C. (2007). 'You don't make genetic test decisions from one day to the next, – using time to preserve moral space. *Bioethics*, **21**(4), 208–17.

Scutt, J. A. (1990). Epilogue. In *The Baby Machine: Reproductive Technology and the Commercialisation of Motherhood*, ed. J. A. Scutt, pp. 208–17. London: Merlin.

Seedhouse, D. and Lisetta Lovett, L. (1992) *Practical Medical Ethics*. Chichester: John Wiley.

Senituli, L. (2004). They came for sandalwood, now the b . . . s are after our genes! Paper presented at the conference 'Research ethics, tikanga Maori/indigenous and protocols for working with communities'. Wellington, NZ, 10–12 June.

Sheldon, T. (2003). Being "tired of life" is not grounds for euthanasia. *British Medical Journal*, **326**, 71.

Sheldon, T. (2005). Dutch euthanasia law should apply to patients "suffering through living," report says. *British Medical Journal*, **330**, 61.

Sherwin, S. (1993). *No Longer Patient: Feminist Ethics and Healthcare*. Philadelphia, PA: Temple University Press.

Sherwin, S. (2002). Toward a feminist ethics of health care. In *Healthcare Ethics and Human Values*, ed. K. W. M. Fulford, D. L. Dickenson and T. H. Murray, pp. 5–28. Oxford: Blackwell.

Shotter, J. (1993). *Conversational Realities*. London: Sage.

Showalter, E. (1987). *The Female Malady: Women, Madness and English Culture 1830–1980*. London: Virago.

Sidaway v. Board of Governors of Bethlem Royal Hospital (1985) 1 All ER 643.

Sigurdsson, S. (2001). Yin-yang genetics, or the HSD deCODE controversy. *New Genetics and Society*, **20**, 103–17.

Sikan, A., Schubiner, H. and Simpson, P. M. (1997). Parent and adolescent perceived need for parental consent involving research with minors. *Archives of Pediatric and Adolescent Medicine*, **151**, 603–7.

Silva, M. L. P. (1997). Conceptual questions raised by the principles of current medical ethics: on the principle of autonomy. Paper presented at the Tenth European Biomedical Ethics Practitioner Education (EBEPE) Conference, Turku, Finland, June.

Singer, P. A. and Siegler, M. (1990). Euthanasia – a critique. *New England Journal of Medicine*, **322**, 1881.

Singer, P. (1993). *Practical Ethics*, 2nd edn. Cambridge: Cambridge University Press.

Singer, P. (ed.) (1991). *A Companion to Ethics*. Oxford: Blackwell.

Skloot. R. (2006). Taking the least of you: the tissue-industrial complex. *New York Times*, 16 April.

Skoe, E. E and Marcia, J. E. (1991). A measure of care based morality and its relation to ego identity. *Merrill Palmer Quarterly*, **37**, 289–304.

Sloan, J. M. and Ballen, K. (2008). SCT in Jehovah's Witnesses: the bloodless transplant. *Bone Marrow Transplantation*, **41**, 837–44.

Smail, D. (1994). Community psychology and politics. *Journal of Community and Applied Social Psychology*, **4**, 3–10.

Smajdor, A. (2007). Is there a right not to be a parent? *Bionews*, April, www.bionews.org.uk

Smart, A., Martin, P. and Parker, M. (2004). Tailored medicine – who is it designed to fit? The ethical aspects of stratified prescribing. *Bioethics*, **18**(4), 322–44.

Smith, M. L. and Glass, G. V. (1977). Meta-analyses of psychotherapy outcome studies. *American Psychologist*, **32**, 752–60.

Smith, M. L., Glass, G. V. and Miller, T. I. (1980). *The Benefits of Psychotherapy*. Baltimore, MD: Johns Hopkins University Press.

Smith, T. (1999). *Ethics in Medical Research: A Handbook of Good Practice*. Cambridge: Cambridge University Press.

Snowden, R. and Mitchell, G. D. (1983). *The Artificial Family: A Consideration of Artificial Insemination by Donor*. London: Unwin Paperbacks.

Sodergard, C.-G. (1996). Patients' rights in Finland. Paper presented at the Sixth European Biomedical Ethics Practitioner Education (EBEPE) Workshop, Naantali, Finland, September.

Spallone, P. (1989). *Beyond Conception: The New Politics of Reproduction*. Granby, MA: Bergin and Garvey Publishers.

Spar, D. (2006). *The Baby Business: How Money, Science and Politics Drive the Commerce of Conception*. Cambridge, MA: Harvard Business School Press,

Specter, M. (1999). Decoding Iceland. *New Yorker* 18 Jan, 40–51.

Spiker, D. G., Weiss, J. C., Griffin, S. J. *et al.* (1985). The pharmacological treatment of delusional depression. *American Journal of Psychiatry*, **142**, 243–6.

Stanko, E. (1990). *Everyday Violence*. London: Pandora.

Statman, D. (ed.) (1997). *Virtue Ethics*. Edinburgh: Edinburgh University Press.

Steinberg, D. L. (1997). *Bodies in Glass: Genetics, Eugenics, Embryo Ethics*. Manchester: University of Manchester Press.

Stichting Pati'ntenvertrouwenspersoon Geestelijke Gezondheidszorg (1994). *Verslag 1993* ('Report 1993'). Utrecht: SPGG.

Stirrat, G., Johnston, C., Gillon, R. and Boyd, K. (2010). Teaching and learning ethics: medical ethics and law for doctors of tomorrow – the 1998 consensus statement updated. *Journal of Medical Ethics*, **36**, 55–60.

Strathdee, R. (1993). *Children Who Run*. London: Centrepoint.

Sturgiss, S. N. and Davison, J. M. (1992). Effect of pregnancy on long-term function of renal allografts. *American Journal of Kidney Disease*, **19**, 167–72.

Sutton, A. (1997). Authority, autonomy, responsibility and authorisation with specific reference to adolescent mental health practice. *Journal of Medical Ethics*, **23**, 26–31.

SW Hertfordshire v. *KB* (1994). 2 FCR 1051 (FD).

Sykes, N. and Thorns, A. (2003). The use of opioids and sedatives at the end of life. *Lancet Oncology*, **4**, 312–18.

Szasz, T. (1974). *The Myth of Mental Illness*. New York, NY: Harper & Row.

Tan, J. O. A., Hope, T., Stewart, A. and Fitzpatrick, R. (2006). Competence to make treatment decisions in anorexia nervosa: thinking processes and values. *Philosophy, Psychology and Psychiatry*, **13**(4), 267–82.

Tauer, C. (1990). Essential considerations for public policy on assisted reproduction. In *Beyond Baby M: Ethical Considerations in New Reproductive Techniques*, ed. D. M. Bartels, R. Priester, D. E. Vawter and A. L Caplan, pp. 65–86. Clifton, NJ: Humana.

Taylor, C. (1989). *Sources of the Self*. Cambridge: Cambridge University Press.

Taylor, C. (1991). *The Ethics of Authenticity*. Cambridge: Cambridge University Press.

Taylor, M. (1996). A rebellious boy. Paper presented at the First European Biomedical Ethics Practitioner Education (EBEPE) Workshop, Rome, 25 May.

Ten Have, H. (2008). UNESCO's ethics education programme. *Journal of Medical Ethics*, **34**, 57–9.

Thomasma, D. C. (1996). When physicians choose to participate in the death of their patients: ethics and physician-assisted suicide. *Journal of Law, Medicine and Ethics*, **24**, 183–97.

Thompson, A. and Chadwick, R. (1999). *Genetic Information: Acquisition, Access and Control*. New York, NY: Kluwer.

Thompson, T., Barbour, R. and Schwartz, L. (2003). Adherence to advance directives in critical care decision-making: vignette study. *British Medical Journal*, **327**, 1011–14.

Thomson, J. J. (1971). A defence of abortion. *Philosophy and Public Affairs*, **1**, 47–68.

Thorslund, M., Bergmark, R. and Parker, M. G. (1997a). Allocation decisions concerning care and services for elderly people: the need for open discussion. Paper submitted to the Ninth European Biomedical Ethics Practitioner Education (EBEPE) Workshop, Maastricht, April.

Treece, S. J. and Savas, D. (1997). More questions than answers? *R* v. *Human Fertilisation and Embryology Authority ex parte Blood*. *Medical Law International*, **3**(1), 75–82.

Trew, A. (1998). Regulating life and death: the modification and commodification of nature. *University of Toledo Law Review*, **29**(3), 271–326.

Tronto, J. C. (1993). *Moral Boundaries. A Political Argument for an Ethic of Care*. New York, NY: Routledge

Turner, T. (1992). The indomitable Mr Pink. *Nursing Times*, **88**(24), 26–9.

UKCC (1988). *Ethical Guidelines for Nursing*. London: UKCC.

UK Department of Health (2003). Measles, mumps and rubella vaccine (MMR). Available at http://www.doh.gov.uk/mmr/index.html.

241

UK Department of Health and Welsh Office (1999). *Codes of Practice to the Mental Health Act 1983*. London: Department of Health.

UK Department of Health and Welsh Office (2008). *Codes of Practice to the Mental Health Act 1983*. London: Department of Health.

UK National Institute for Clinical Excellence (2004). *Self-harm. The Short-term Physical and Psychological Management and Secondary Prevention of Self-harm in Primary and Secondary Care*. London: NICE.

UNESCO (1997). *Universal Declaration on the Human Genome and Human Rights*. Geneva: UNESCO.

United Nations (1989). *Convention on the Rights of the Child*.

US National Institutes of Health and Centers for Disease Control and Prevention (1997). *The Conduct of Clinical Trials of Maternal–Infant Transmission of HIV Supported by the United States Department of Health and Human Services in Developing Countries*, July. Available at http://www.nih.gov/%20news/mathiv/mathiv.htm

Välimäki, M. and Helenius, H. (1996). The psychiatric patient's right to self-determination: a preliminary investigation from the professional nurse's point of view. *Journal of Psychiatric and Mental Health Nursing*, **3**, 361–72.

Välimäki, M., Leino-Kilpi, H. and Helenius, H. (1996). Self determination in clinical practice: the psychiatric patient's point of view. *Journal of Nursing Ethics*, **3**(4), 361–72.

Van Dienst, P. and Savulescu, J. (2002). For and against: no consent should be needed for using leftover body material for scientific purposes. *British Medical Journal*, **325**, 648–51.

Van den Eynden, B. and Van Bortel, P. (1997). Palliative care and ethics. Presented at the Seventh European Biomedical Ethics Practitioner Education (EBEPE) Workshop, Maastricht, 21–22 March.

Van der Maas, P. J. (1988). Ageing and public health. In *Health and Ageing*, ed. J. F. Schroots, J. E. Birren and A. Svanborg, pp. 95–115. New York, NY and Lisse: Swets.

Van der Maas, P. J., Delden, J. J. M. van, Pijnenborg, L. and Looman, C. W. N. (1991). Euthanasia and other medical decisions concerning the end of life. *Lancet*, **338**, 669–74.

Van der Maas, P. J., Van Der Wal, G., Bosma, J. M. *et al.* (1996). Euthanasia, physician-assisted suicide, and other medical practices involving the end of life in the Netherlands. *New England Journal of Medicine*, **335**(22), 1699–705.

Vanderpool H. Y. (ed.) (1996). *The Ethics of Research Involving Human Subjects: Facing the 21st Century*. Frederick, MD: University Publishing Group

Van der Wal, G. and Van der Maas, P. J. (1996a). *Euthanasie en andere medische beslissingen rond het levenseinde. De praktijk en de meldingsprocedure*. Den Haag: Sdu uitgevers

Van der Wal, G. and Van der Maas, P. J. (1996b). Evaluation of the notification procedure for physician-assisted death in the Netherlands. *New England Journal of Medicine*, **335**,(22), 1706–11.

Van der Wal, G. A. (1991). Geestelijk lijden. In *De dood in beheer. Morele dilemma's rondom het sterven*, ed. R. L. P. Berghmans, G. M. W. R. de Wert and C. van der Meer, pp. 112–37. Baarn: Ambo BV.

Varmus, H. and Satcher, D. (1997). Ethical complexities of conducting research in developing countries. *New England Journal of Medicine*, **337**(14), 1003–5.

Veatch, R. (1989). *Death, Dying and the Biological Revolution*. Revised edn. New Haven, CT: Yale University Press.

Verkerk, M. (1990). *De Mythe van de leeftijd. Ethische kwesties rondom het ouderenbeleid.*'s Gravenhage: Meinema.

Verkerk, M. (1998). Paper presented at the Fourth International Association of Bioethics Conference, Tokyo, November.

Vygotsky, L. S. (1978). *Mind in Society*. Harvard: Harvard University Press.

W. v. Egdell (1990). 1 All ER 835.

Wakefield, A. J., Murch, S. H., Anthony, A. *et al.* (1998). Ileal-lymphoid-nodular hyperplasia, non-specific colitis, and pervasive developmental disorder in children. *Lancet*, **351**, 637–41.

Waldby, C. and Mitchell, R. (2006).*Tissue Economies: Blood, Organs and Cell Lines in Late Capitalism*. Durham, NC: Duke University Press.

Walrond-Skinner, S. (1986). *Dictionary of Psychotherapy*. London: Routledge & Kegan Paul.

Warren, M. A. (1991). Abortion. In *Companion to Ethics*, ed. P. Singer. Oxford: Blackwell.

Warren, M. A. (2002). The moral status of the gene. In *A Companion to Genethics*, ed. J. Birley and J. Harris, pp. 147–57. Oxford: Basil Blackwell.

Washington DC: US Government Printing Office, (1949). *Trials of War Criminals Before the Nuremberg Military Tribunals Under Control Council Law No. 10*, Volume **2**, Nuremberg, October 1946 – April 1949 pp. 181–221.

Watchtower Bible and Tract Society of New York (1992). *Family Care and Medical Management for Jehovah's Witnesses*. Brooklyn NY: International Bible Students Association.

Weir, R. F. and Peters, C.(1997). Affirming the decisions adolescents make about life and death, *The Hastings Center Report*, **27**,(6) 29–45.

Whitty, P. and Devitt, P. (2005). Surreptitious prescribing in psychiatric practice. *Psychiatric Services* **56**, 481–3.

Widdershoven, G. (1996). Contribution to the Fourth Workshop of the European Biomedical Ethics Practitioner Education Project, Maastricht, September.

Wikler, D. (1987). Personal responsibility for illness. In *Health Care Ethics*, ed. D. Vanderveer and T. Regan, pp. 326–58. Philadelphia: Temple University Press.

Wilde, G. de and Bijl, R. (1993). *Afwenden van gevaar. Mogelijkheden om buiten het psychiatrisch ziekenhuis gevaar af te wenden*. [Aversion of dangerousness. Possibilities to avert dangerousness outside the mental hospital.] Utrecht: Nederlands centrum Geestelijke volksgezondheid.

Wilkie, T. (1993). *Perilous Knowledge*. London: Faber and Faber.

Wilkinson, S. (2003). *Bodies for Sale: Ethics and Exploitation in the Organ Trade*. London: Routledge.

Williams, B. (1973). A critique of utilitarianism. In *Utilitarianism: For and Against*, ed. J. J. C. Smart and B. Williams. Cambridge: Cambridge University Press.

Williams, B. (1985). *Ethics and the Limits of Philosophy*. London: Fontana.

Williams, G. (2005). Bioethics and large-scale biobanking: individualistic ethics and collective projects. *Genomics, Society and Policy*, **1**, 50–66.

Williams, J. R. (2004.) The promise and limits of international bioethics: lessons from the recent revision of the Declaration of Helsinki. *International Journal of Bioethics*, **15**: 31–42

Williams, J. R. (2006). The physician's role in the protection of human research subjects. *Science and Engineering Ethics*, **12**, 5–12.

Williams. J. R. (2008). The Declaration of Helsinki and public health. *Bulletin of the World Health Organization*, **86**, 650–1.

Winkler, E. (1995). Reflections on the state of the current debate over physician-assisted suicide and euthanasia. *Bioethics*, **9**, (3/4), 313–26.

Wittgenstein, L. (1974). *Philosophical Investigations*, 2nd edn. Oxford: Blackwell.

Wolf, R. (1996). Contribution to the Fourth Workshop of the European Biomedical Ethics Practitioner Education Project, Maastricht, September.

Wong, J. G. W. S., Poon, Y. and Hui, E. C. (2005) "I can put the medicine in his soup, Doctor!" *Journal of Medical Ethics*, **31**, 262–5.

World Medical Association (1964). *Declaration of Helsinki*. Amended 1975, 1983, 1989, 1996 and 2000.

World Medical Association. (2000). *The International Response to Helsinki VI – The WMA's Declaration of Helsinki on Ethical Principles for Medical Research Involving Human Subjects, as adopted by the 52nd WMA General Assembly*. Edinburgh: World Medical Association.

Yoshino, K. (2006). Fertility scandal at UC Irvine is far from over. *Los Angeles Times*, 22 January.

Zatz, J. (1996). I am definitely having it done. In *The Troubled Helix*, ed. Martin Richards and Theresa Martineau, pp. 27–31. Cambridge: Cambridge University Press, 1996.

Zaw, F. K. (2006). ECT and the youth: catatonia in context. *International Reviews of Neurobiology*, **72**, 207–31.

Zola, I. K. (1975). *De medische Macht*. Meppel: Boom.

Index